An Atlas of Foot Surgery

Volume I
Forefoot Surgery

O. A. Mercado, D.P.M.

Professor of Surgery
Illinois College of Podiatric Medicine, 1971–1984
Chief of Podiatric Surgery
Franklin Boulevard Community Hospital
Attending Podiatrist
St. Mary's of Nazareth Hospital Center
Diplomate, American Board of Podiatric Surgery

Foreword by:
Phillip R. Brachman, D.P.M.
Chancellor
Illinois College of Podiatric Medicine

Carolando Press, Inc.   *Oak Park, IL*

Copyright © 1979 by O.A. Mercado, D.P.M.

All rights reserved. No part of this publication may be reproduced or transmitted in any form or by any means, electronic or mechanical, including photocopy, recording, or any information storage and retrieval system without the written permission of the publisher.

Printed in the United States of America at the Illinois College of Podiatric Medicine.
Typesetting by TYPESOURCE, INC.
Graphic Designer: Robert Kramer

Third Printing 1986

Slides of all illustrations used in this book are available for teaching aids. Write the publisher for current price list:

                      Carolando Press
                      6545 W. North Ave.
                      Oak Park, Illinois 60302

Library of Congress Catalog Card Number: 86-71647

ISBN 0-940542-03-X

Other books by the author:
"An Atlas of Podiatric Anatomy"
"Hallux Abducto Valgus Surgery and Allied Deformities"
with Josh Gerbert and Tilden Sokoloff
"A Manual of Hospital Podiatry"
with Patrick A. DeMoon
**"Podiatric surgical dissection—
fundamental skills"**

Dedicated To:

Carol J. . . . . My best friend and wife
My Children . . . . Kent, Cindy, Marc and Matt

and

My late grandfather, Carmelo Mercado, a wonderful family man and hardworking farmer who would have never understood the content of this book; but, he would have known the hard work and love that went into it and he would have been . . . **Proud.**

Acknowledgement

No one ever writes a book alone for there are many individuals who help influence, steer and mold one's life. Here are but a few of the wonderful people who have helped along the way:

Phillip R. Brachman — My mentor who gave me a chance to teach.

Patrick A. DeMoon — Who opened his hospital to my work.

Earl G. Kaplan — Who chose to train me as a surgeon.

Lyle McCain — Who taught me anatomy.

Robert F. Triplett — Who taught me love for my profession.

FOREWORD

If I were to write a prescription for success in the field of Podiatric Medicine I would write for one part of inspiration, two parts of dedication, three parts of knowledge, four parts of perspiration, five parts of enthusiasm, plus a spark of genius. Mix them all together and label the solution "Dr. Orlando Mercado."

His energy, his ability to teach and inspire students, and his love for his profession continue to amaze me and many others with whom he comes in contact. The pages in this book are a living testimony of his great interest in expressing his ability to use the written word and line drawings to teach others.

The ideal simplicity of these pages are a most adequate illustration of the fact that Dr. Mercado's work has all the virtues of a labor of commitment and love.

Philip R. Brachman, D.P.M.
Chancellor
Illinois College of Podiatric Medicine

Contents

Chapter 1 — Anesthesia... 1
Chapter 2 — Nail Surgery... 15
Chapter 3 — Soft Tissue Surgery.. 35
Chapter 4 — Digital Surgery.. 45
Chapter 5 — Principles of Bone Surgery... 93
Chapter 6 — Metatarsal-Phalangeal Joint Surgery................................ 121
Chapter 7 — Hallux Valgus Surgery.. 185
            Bibliography.. 274
            Index... 288

CHAPTER 1—ANESTHESIA

History
Local Anesthesia
Modern Drugs
Preanesthetic Drugs
Toxic Reactions
Emergency Treatment
Clinical Application
Materials Used
Types of Blocks

1. Lesser Toe Block
2. Hallux Block
3. Tibial Nerve (posterior ankle) Block
4. Deep and Superficial Peroneal Nerve (anterior ankle) Block

Intravenous Regional (perfusion) Anesthesia

CHAPTER 1

ANESTHESIA

Pain is as old as man himself, and the search for its control has filled some of the finest pages of medical history. The road has not always been an easy one since the ancient dogma that "pain is the inescapable will of the Almighty" has blocked its way since the beginning of medicine. Nonetheless, courageous men in every century have experimented with the alleviation of pain.

The sixteenth century gave the world the greatest advances in human anatomy, the surgeons of this time experimented with such methods as applying digital pressure to the main branches of superficial nerves. This method which sounded to them anatomically correct, in reality, produced as much pain as it was supposed to relieve. In the sixteenth century, **Marco Aurelio Severino** described in his book "The Medical Use of Snow" some experiments in hypo thermia. This technique as we now know is successful, but it was too far advanced for the scientific knowledge of the day.

In 1842, in a small town of Georgia, **Crawford Williamson Long** performed the first operation under anesthesia using ether vapors. In spite of his monumental discovery Dr. Long never made an announcement of his great discovery. It remained for **Horace Wells,** and **William Thomas Green Morton,** two young dentists, to bring the analgesic qualities of nitrous oxide to the attention of medicine. The claim of these two to have been the first to use vapor or gases for the control of pain has given medicine one of its most controversial episodes to this day.

Local Anesthesia

Local anesthetics came into the limelight as surgeons became dissatisfied with general anesthetics during the latter part of the nineteenth century. The gases available for anesthesia and their method of application were hazardous and unreliable. Many researchers began looking for a drug which would create anesthesia. A young researchist in Vienna, who was later to become immortal for his work in psychoanalysis, **Sigmund Freud,** concluded that Cocaine could probably be used as an analgesic. He failed to experiment with it and consequently it was another German, **Koller,** who used Cocaine to anesthetize the cornea in 1884.

In the same year, the American Surgeon, **William Steward Halsted,** began a series of experiments with cocaine which proved that it could be used both for infiltration of the skin and direct nerve injection. He had no idea that cocaine was one of the most pernicious of all habit forming drugs and he carried on with his experiments, using himself as a guinea pig. Before long he was an addict. He spent a year in a mental hospital and left it, a changed man, to take over the Department of Surgery in the newly formed John Hopkins Medical School. He was no longer the rapid slash-happy surgeon, as was the fashion of the day, but careful and meticulous.

This overawareness to minute details is one of the symptoms of cocaine addiction and it was indeed his preoccupation for the minute and trivial details that made him the outstanding surgeon of the day and the father of **conservative surgery.**

Cocaine, continued to be used, but its high incidence of reaction, lack of a synthetic product and difficulty in sterilization led to research for a better anesthetic. In 1905, **Einhorn,** synthesized Procaine. Today, procaine is used as the standard for comparison with other anesthetics. Novocain (Winthrop-Stearns, Inc.) is the trade name for Procaine Hydrochloride.

Modern Drugs

There are many new drugs on the market today which have different characteristics and advantages. However, any local anesthetic with sufficient potency, low toxicity, rapid onset, adequate duration and non-irritating qualities should be satisfactory. It is of advantage for the practitioner to use an anesthetic with which he is familiar and has good results.

Vasoconstrictor Drugs

Vasoconstrictor drugs are incorporated in the anesthetic for a number of reasons. These are—1. Constriction of blood vessels, thereby slowing absorption and minimizing toxic reactions. 2. In local infiltration it will produce a bloodless field. 3. It prolongs the time of analgesia.

Adrenalin (epinephrine) is the most commonly used vasoconstrictor drug. Neo Synephrine (phenylphrine) and cobenfrin (cobarsil—a synthetic substitute for ephinephrine) are also used, but they are not readily available in the commercial local anesthetic preparations.

There seems to be a well ingrained belief that the use of epinephrine in local anesthetics used for digital blocks will cause permanent damage to blood vessels and hence cause gangrene. Where this began , it is hard to tell, but it is certainly lacking in clinical research. **Kaplan** and **Steinberg,** reporting their individual findings of **thousands of well documented cases,** emphatically disagree with this antiquated truism. The use of epinephrine in healthy patients with patent circulation is recommended whenever its actions are desirable.

Preanesthetic Drugs

These drugs are used to allay apprehension; sedation or hypnosis and elevation of the pain threshold. The drugs used are the following:
1. **Barbiturates**
2. **Non-Barbiturates**
3. **Belladonna Derivatives**
4. **Narcotics**

I. Barbituric Acid Derivatives

The barbiturates are classified as:
   a. Short Acting

   Example—1. Pentobarbital (Nembutal)
   2. Secobarbital (Seconal)

   b. Long Acting

   Example—1. Amytal
   2. Phenobarbital

Short acting barbiturates are most commonly used for **preanesthetic** medication, and reach their maximum effect in 1-1½ hours, and will last for 3-4 hours (orally). Intramuscularly they will have their maximum effect in ½ hour and last for 2-3 hours.

The usual dosage of seconal or nembutal is 50mg, (¾ grain) for sedation and 100mg. to 200 mg. (1½-3grs) for hypnosis.

The metabolization of the short and long acting barbiturates is different. The short acting conjugate principally in the liver. While the long acting are excreted mostly by the kidneys. This difference of metabolism may be of practical value in a patient with severe hepatic disease where the action of the short acting group may be exaggerated and prolonged. The long acting group would be used in this case since they are excreted by the kidney.

Barbiturates commonly cause agitation, excitement, and transient physchoses in the aged. Non-barbiturate sedatives (Valmid or Doriden 0.5-1.0gm) are used for these patients.

There is laboratory evidence that barbiturates have a tendency to decrease the toxic effects of local anesthetics. It should be noted, however, that the amounts used were closer to the anesthetic than to the sedative doses.

II. Non-Barbiturates

There are a number of excellent non-barbiturate sedatives available. Some that are ideal for patients over age fifty are Doriden, Valmid and Dalmane. The dosage for Doriden and Valmid is 0.5-1.0 gm and the dosage for Dalmane is 15-30 mg. Valium is also extremely useful as a premedication since it relieves anxiety and tension, and diminishes the recall of the procedure by the patient. Valium is best given IM 10 mg., one to two hours pre-op., or I.V. 2.5 mg.-10 mg. within five to ten minutes before Surgery. (Note: Intravenous injections of Valium should be given directly and slowly into the vein. Valium should not be mixed or diluted with other solutions or drugs.) Promethazine (phenergan) has gained popularity as a preanesthetic drug because of its anti-emetic effect; amnesic action; tendency to enhance the action of barbiturates; and potentiation of analgesics. Dosage: 12.5-25 mg. for children; 25-50 mg. for adults.

III. Belladonna Derivatives:

The most popular drugs of this group are Scopolamine and Atropine. These drugs are used in general anesthesia to reduce secretions within the respiratory tract. They also act on the central nervous system to produce a sedative and hypnotic effect.

Atropine is the most popular of the two. Its action is enhanced by the concomitant use of narcotics and barbiturates. The combination of Atropine and morphine produces the famous "twilight sleep" which is used so frequently in obstetrics.

Dosage: Scopolamine and atropine have identical dosage—0.2-0.6 mg hypodermically.

In patients over 60 years of age, scopolamine and barbiturates will often cause disorientation. Atropine and non-barbiturate sedatives may be substituted.

IV. Narcotics:

The alkaloids of opium and the synthetic opiate-like agents possess two very important actions:

1. A **sporific** action which tends to induce sleep.
2. An **analgesic** action which produces relief from pain.

The most commonly used drug for pre-anesthetic medication are morphine, demerol (meperidine) and nisentil (alphaprodine).

Dosages: Morphine 5mg (in older people) to 10 mg. in healthy males; Demerol .25-75 mg.; Nisentil 20-40 mg. It must be remembered that these drugs are primarily analgesics. They will allay apprehensions and quiet the patient; however, studies have proved that barbiturates and non-barbiturate sedatives produce better sedation and control apprehension more effectively than the narcotics.

Morphine or Demerol may be combined with barbiturates and scopolamine for profound hypnosis.

Nisentil may be combined with scopolamine but it should not be used concomitantly with barbiturates as respiratory depression may ensue.

The Rational Use of Preanesthetic Drugs

As we have seen there are many drugs that may be used alone or in combination to provide a certain pharmacologic action which may be desirable.

At Franklin Boulevard Community Hospital we use the following combinations with excellent results: For surgery at 8:00 a.m. (ages 15-65)

1. **Dalmane** 30 mg cap at hs. This is given to ensure the patient a good night's sleep, making the patient more cooperative and easy to work with the morning of surgery. We have tried other sedatives such as nembutal, placidyl, sodium seconal, etc., but have found Dalmane superior. (over 65 Placidyl 500 mg.).
2. **Inapsine** 5 mg IM at 6:30 AM. This sedative, anti-emetic agent is given 1½ hours before surgery. Following trials of various other drugs, we found this drug to be more satisfactory for the patient's need before surgery.
3. **Meperidine** 75 mg IM at 7:15 AM. This narcotic is given 45 minutes before surgery for analgesic purposes, and will raise the patient's pain threshold 60 to 65%.
4. **Atropine** 0.4 mg IM at 7:15 AM. This drug is given 45 minutes before surgery to reduce secretions within the respiratory tract.

For office surgery, the **belladonna drugs** should not be used as these will sedate the patient too deeply and too long to allow them to leave the office immediately after the surgery. A barbiturate (or synthetic barbiturate) orally or IM will give the desired sedation.

Although preanesthetic medications, if used intelligently, will allay the fears and apprehension of the patient, they **MUST NEVER** replace the proper rapport between patient and doctor.

We do not have to over medicate the patients or render them amnesic to allay their fears. A few comforting, assuring, and explanatory words will never be replaced by any amount of drugs. The patient who is well oriented, and confident will have a rapid and unremarkable recovery.

Toxic Reactions

With any local anesthetic untowards reactions may occur, however, these reactions are often exaggerated and are not quite as common nor as serious as it is commonly thought.

Basically, there are two causes for the reactions to the local anesthetics.

I. **Allergy** to the drug employed. Symptoms suggestive of true Anaphylaxis are *rare*! The symptoms consist of:
Histamine release
Bronchio spasm
Circulatory collapse
Failure in the blood to coagulate

The reaction may take place after only a few drops of the anesthetic have been given.

The treatment is **symptomatic;**
1. **Apply tourniquet above injection site.**
2. **Start I.V.**
3. **Epinephrine (vasopressor)**
4. **Supportive Therapy**

A good history will save a lot of trouble and embarrassment later. **Always** find out if the patient is allergic to any drug. Find out particularly if they have ever had any local anesthetics. Most of them will have been injected by a dentist at one time or another.

A lot of the so-called allergic patients to local anesthetics have merely been mis-diagnosed. What was a simple psychogenic reaction may have been diagnosed as an Anaphylactoid reaction. Even if they had a reaction to the drug it may have been because of an overdosage or more frequently, because of intravascular injection. These patients will do well if care is taken in the injection and a weaker solution is used. If they, however, are truly allergic to one local anesthetic, then another anesthetic with a different chemical formula may be used.

II. **High Blood Levels** of the drug injected. This occurs because of rapid absorption of intravascular injection of the drug. The highest incidence of reaction occurs in vascular regions such as the head, face, and neck.

The symptoms will appear with a varying degree of rapidity and intensity, depending on the rate of absorption. Most reactions will occur five to fifteen minutes following injection. If a reaction has not developed within thirty minutes, it is very unlikely to develop at all.

ANESTHESIA

Emergency Treatment

The success of the treatment will depend upon the correct diagnosis of the symptoms and the quick action taken to correct or ameliorate them.

I. **SYNCOPE (Fainting)**

The most common reaction. This is a psychogenic reaction and it is not necessarily a reaction to the drug.

Symptoms:

Patient will feel faint
Pallor
Rapid and/or weak pulse

Treatment:

A. Make the patient comfortable (in supine position with feet elevated)
B. Apply cold wet towel to face
C. Spirits of Ammonia
D. Comfort the patient

Do NOT leave the patient, be prepared to treat a more severe reaction.

II. **RESPIRATORY DEPRESSION**

Symptoms:

Sudden cessation of breathing
Cyanosis
Pulse is present

Treatment:

A. Open Airway
B. Oxygen
C. Metrazol 100mg. 3-5 cc I.M. or I.V.
D. Artificial respiration

III. **CONVULSIONS**

Restlessness, talkativeness, and muscle twitching may precede the onset of convulsions.

Treatment:

A. Intravenous injection of short acting barbiturate 5% Sodium Amytal until convulsions cease
B. Oxygen

IV. **CIRCULATORY COLLAPSE**

Symptoms:

Absence of blood pressure and pulse
Unconsciousness, gasping type of breathing

Treatment:

A. .5cc of 1:1000 Epinephrine subcut or I.M. repeat in two minutes if no response
B. Oxygen
C. External Cardiac Massage

Clinical Application

To the patient the most important thing is the assurance that the surgery will be painless. Many patients refuse or are hesitant of undergoing any procedure under local anesthesia because of a fear that they will feel something. Part of this difficulty resides in the ineffectual approach to the patient and lack of skill in the use of local anesthetics.

Enough cannot be said about the importance of a knowledgeable use of local anesthesia. It cannot be emphasized too strongly that blind poking and infiltration with a needle and anesthetic in the tissues will result in incomplete analgesia and may lead to deleterious effects. There is no substitute for a direct approach based on a secure knowledge of anatomy.

A common practice is to anesthetize the area after the patient has been scrubbed and draped. The surgeon, gowned and gloved asks: "DOES THIS FEEL SHARP OR DULL? DOES THIS HURT?"

Not only does this routine take up unnecessary time, but certainly, it arises the apprehension of the patient.

The anesthetic should be given before the preparation of the patient. By the time that the patient is scrubbed and draped, the anesthetic has had more than sufficient time to work, and consequently, the surgeon can begin without the unnecessary ritual of "DOES THIS FEEL SHARP OR DULL? DOES THIS HURT?"

Materials Used

In addition to the standard emergency drugs and equipment, the following is all that is required for achieving anesthesia to the foot:

1. 3 c.c. disposable syringe (with luer lock)
2. Disposable 1¼" needle (25-27 gauge)
3. Anesthetic solution of choice

Types of Blocks

The types of blocks most suitable for foot surgery are:

1. **Lesser toe block**
2. **Hallux block**
3. **Tibial nerve (posterior ankle) block**
4. **Deep and superficial peroneal nerve (anterior ankle) block.**

In addition to the above blocks, there is also intravenous regional (perfusion) anesthesia which can be extremely useful in foot surgery.

1. Lesser Toe Block

The skin on the dorsum at the base of the toe is pinched with the thumb and forefinger (Fig. 1-1A). The needle is quickly inserted and a wheal is raised. The needle is slowly pushed plantarly, injecting the anesthetic as it descends, on the lateral aspect of the toe. Note, it is not necessary to aspirate during digital blocks as the lumen (caliber) of the vessels is smaller than the 25-27 gauge needle used.

A **wheal** is then raised with ¼ to ½ c.c. of the anesthetic (Fig. 1-1B). The needle is withdrawn, but not all the way. The needle is then aimed towards the medial aspect of the toe and it is pushed slowly plantarly, depositing the anesthetic as it descends to the medial-plantar aspect of the toe. A wheal is raised with one-half c.c. of the anesthetic. (Fig. 1-1C). The needle is withdrawn all the way, the block is complete. On the fifth toe, since it is usually rotated, it is necessary to deposit an additional ¼ to ½ c.c. on the plantar aspect (Fig. 1-1D) to insure a complete block.

ANESTHESIA

Lesser Toe Block

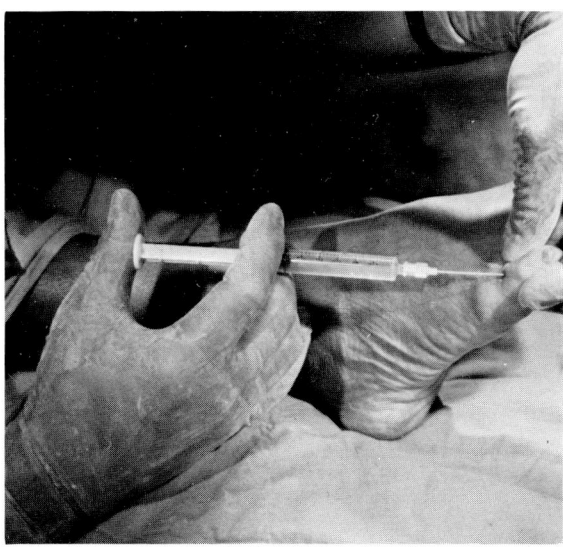

Fig. 1-1A. Lesser toe block. The skin on the dorsum of the toe is pinched and the needle is quickly inserted.

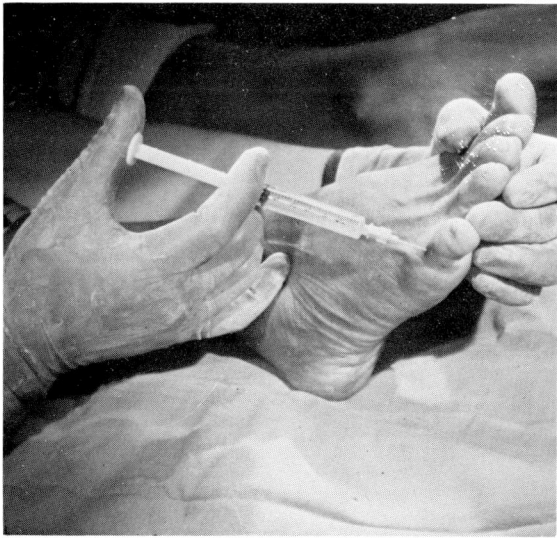

Fig. 1-1B. Injecting slowly a wheal is raised (using ¼ to ½ c.c. of the anesthetic solution) on the Lateral-plantar aspect of the toe.

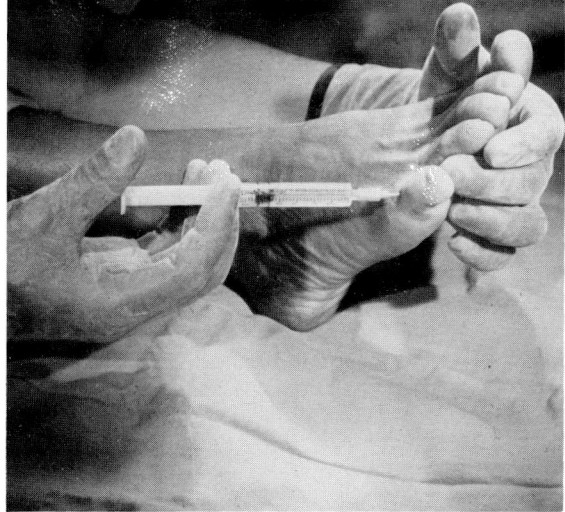

Fig. 1-1C. Another wheal is raised (using ¼ to ½ c.c. of the anesthetic solution) on the Medial-plantar aspect of the toe.

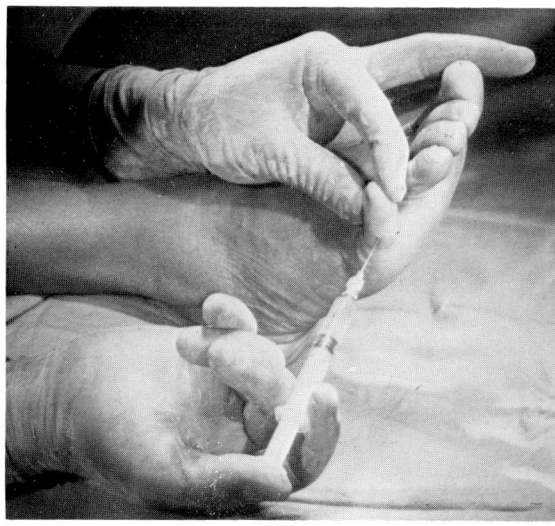

Fig. 1-1D. Since the fifth toe is usually rotated it is necessary to deposit an additional ¼ c.c. on the plantar aspect to insure a complete block.

2. Hallux block

The great toe is held as illustrated in Figure 1-2A. The needle is quickly inserted at the base of the toe just medial to the tendon of extensor hallucis longus and a wheal is raised. The needle is slowly pushed plantarly. One-half c.c. of the anesthetic is used to raise a wheal on the medial-plantar aspect of the Hallux. The needle is withdrawn all the way and reinserted at the base of the hallux just lateral to the tendon of extensor hallucis longus.

A wheal is raised and the needle is slowly pushed to the lateral-plantar aspect of the toe where one-half c.c. of the anesthetic is used to raise a wheal. The needle is completely withdrawn, the block is complete. Using lidocaine, hydrochloride 1% with epinephrine, digital blocks will last 4-6 hours.

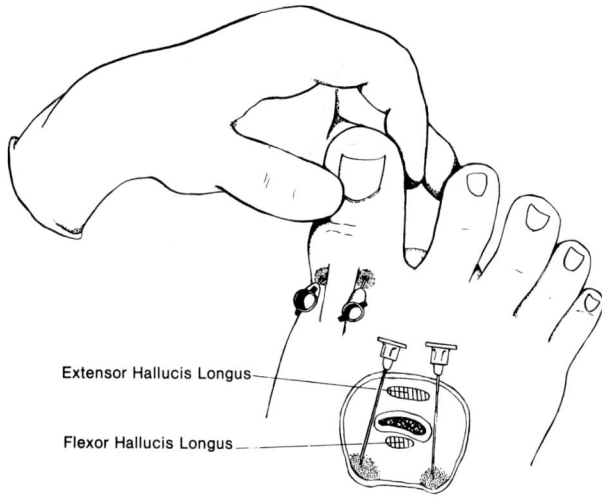

Fig. 1-2A. Hallux Block

3. Tibial Nerve (Posterior Ankle) Block

The Tibial Nerve gives the supply to the bottom of the foot. It gives off three branches, **the calcaneal branch; the medial plantar** and **lateral plantar branches.** The anatomy books describe this ramification of the Tibial Nerve as taking place between the first and second layer of the plantar muscles. In reality, as surgical dissection and surgery to release entrapped Tibial Nerves have shown us, this bifurcation occurs much higher up, usually at the level of the medial malleolous.

A cross section of the ankle (Fig. 1-2B) reveals the following: From anterior to posterior there are three tendons; **the tibialis posterior; the flexor digitorum longus** and **flexor hallucis longus.** The posterior tibial artery has two veins to either side. The tibial nerve is approximately **twice** as big as the artery and it lies somewhat posterior to it. The artery, the two veins and the tibial nerve comprise the **neurovascular bundle.** The Tendo Achilles is seen at the most posterior aspect of the cross section.

From medial to lateral we first have **the skin; the laciniate ligament** which forms the retinaculum around the Flexor Tendons; and the **neurovascular bundle.** Please note that the Tibial Nerve lies somewhat deeper and behind the posterior tibial artery.

ANESTHESIA

Tibial Nerve (Posterior Ankle) Block

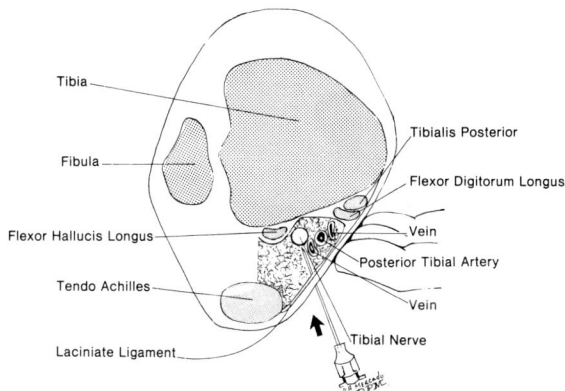

Fig. 1-2B. Cross Section of left ankle

Technique

The location of the Neurovascular bundle is ascertained by palpating for the pulse of the posterior tibial artery (fig. 1-3A). A wheal is then raised on the skin immediately over the Neurovascular bundle (fig. 1-3B).

Once the wheal is raised, the needle is advanced slowly into the subcutaneous tissues in search of the Tibial Nerve (fig. 1-3C and D). When the Tibial Nerve is hit the patient will get **paresthesia,** an involuntary jerk reflex with a shooting electric shock-like sensation running to the toes.

We then aspirate, to make certain that we are not in the artery, and inject 1 c.c. of the anesthetic solution. Within minutes, the plantar of the foot will be totally anesthetized.

The **important points** to remember in the Tibial Nerve Block is to: 1. ascertain the location of the neurovascular bundle. 2. to make certain that you elicit paresthesia before injecting the anesthetic. 3. inject high enough (at the level of the malleolous) in order to get the Tibial Nerve before it bifurcates.

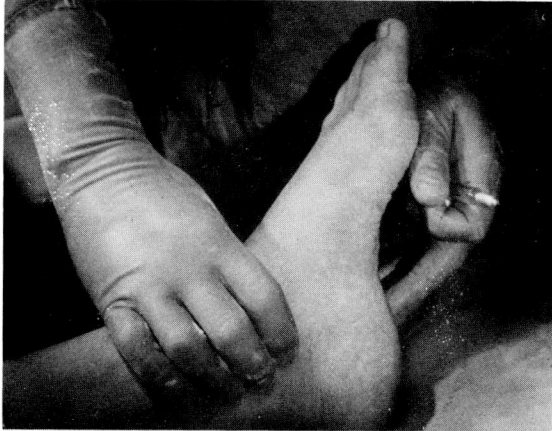

Fig. 1-3A. Palpating for the pulse of the posterior tibial artery.

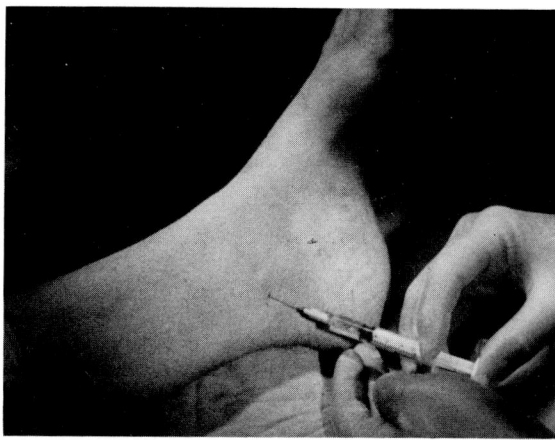

Fig. 1-3B. A wheal is raised under the skin immediately over the Neurovascular bundle.

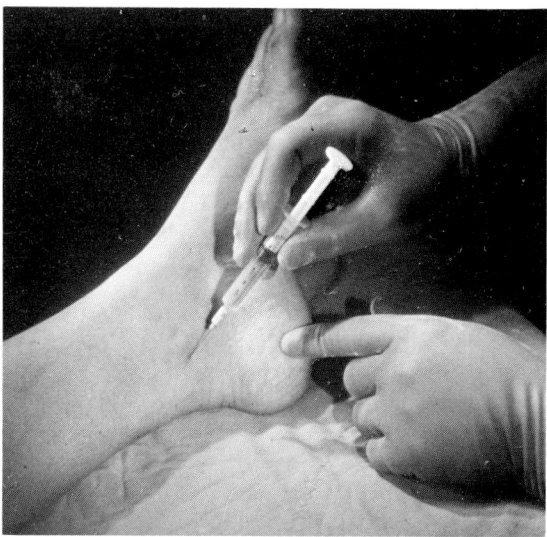 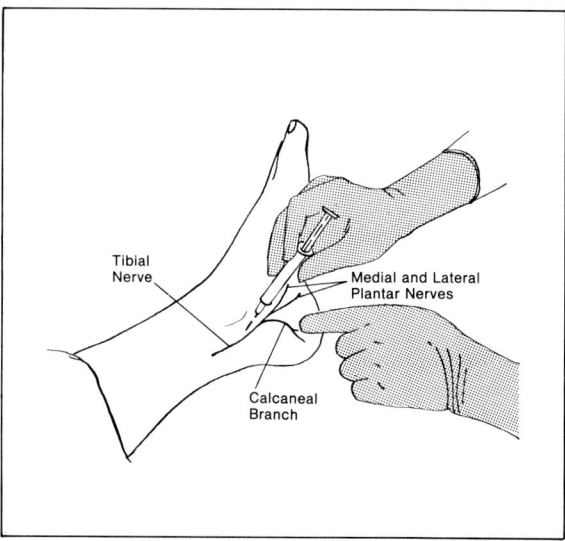

Fig. 1-3C. Once the wheal is raised, the needle is advanced slowly in search of the tibial nerve. When the nerve is hit, the patient will get paresthesia. One c.c. of the anesthetic is injected after aspiration.

Fig. 1-3D. If paresthesia is **not** obtained, we then deposit two additional c.c.'s of the anesthetic solution at different levels.

4. Deep and Superficial Peroneal Nerve (Anterior Ankle) Block

The nerve supply to the dorsum of the foot comes by way of the deep and superficial peroneal nerves; the saphenous nerve; and the sural nerve.

Technique

The Deep Peroneal Nerve runs in close proximity to the anterior tibial artery as part of the neurovascular bundle on the anterior aspect of the ankle. The location of this neurovascular bundle can be ascertained by palpating for the anterior tibial artery at the level of the malleoli (Fig. 1-4A).

A wheal is raised immediately over the neurovascular bundle. The needle is slowly advanced, keeping the needle at a 45° angle to the skin, all the way to its hub (see fig. 1-4B). After aspirating, 1 c.c. of the anesthetic solution is slowly infiltrated into the area. The needle is withdrawn, the block is complete. Unlike the Tibial Nerve Block, no paresthesia is elicited. Also, the block will take a little longer to take effect than the Tibial Block.

Incidentally, the deep peroneal nerve can also be blocked (for forefoot surgery) by infiltrating one c.c. of the anesthetic solution in between the first and second metatarsal bases.

The Superficial Peroneal Nerve divides into two cutaneous branches, the **medial dorsal cutaneus nerve** and the **intermediate dorsal cutanous nerve.** These nerves along with the saphenous (on the lateral aspect) lie immediately under the skin along with the superficial veins. They can easily be blocked by infiltrating a continuous wheal immediately under the skin medially (fig. 1-4C) and laterally (fig. 1-4D) making sure to descend to the plantar skin on the lateral aspect, to insure blocking of the Sural Nerve.

ANESTHESIA

Deep and Superficial Peroneal Nerve (Anterior Ankle) Block

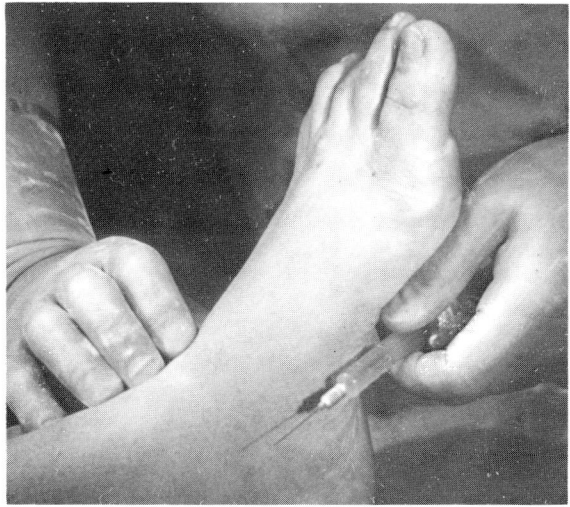

Fig. 1-4A. Palpating for the pulse of the anterior tibial artery.

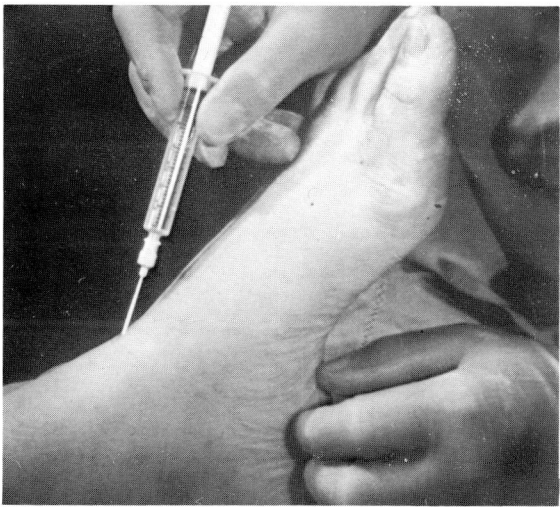

Fig. 1-4B. After a wheal is raised, the needle is slowly advanced all the way to its hub (note angle of needle to skin is 45°) and 1 c.c. of the anesthetic solution is injected after aspirating. This will block the deep peroneal nerve.

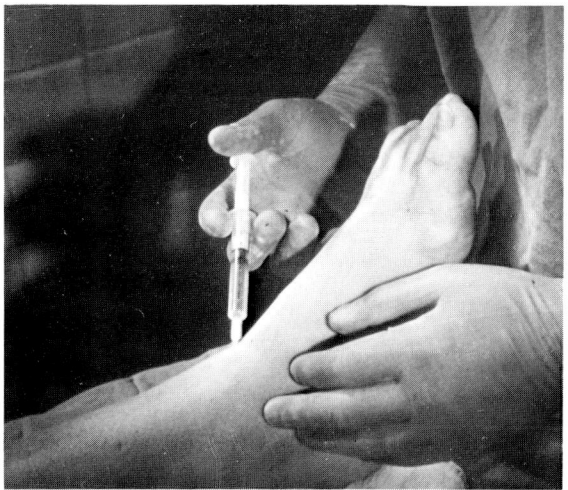

Fig. 1-4C. The superficial nerves lie immediately under the skin. They can be blocked by raising a continuous wheal immediately under the skin. Here we are aiming our needle medialwards to block the medial dorsal cutaneous and saphenous nerves.

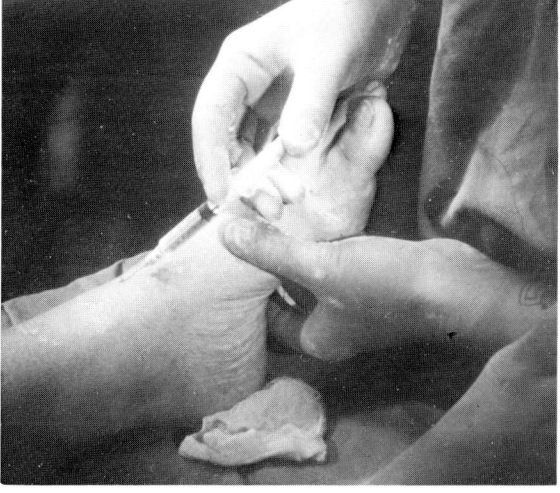

Fig. 1-4D. Our needle is directed lateralwards depositing a continuous wheal under the skin. If surgery is to be done around the fifth metatarsal head area make sure to carry the wheal far enough laterally to ascertain blocking of the sural nerve.

Perfusion Anesthesia

Perfusion anesthesia is not new to medicine. It dates back to 1908, but not too much was done with this technique until the 1930's when surgeons began using it for upper extremity work. Its use on the lower extremities has been tried intermittently since then.

Essentially, perfusion anesthesia is nothing more than **intravenous regional anesthesia.** A double compartment cuff is placed on the patient's mid-leg, a PRN catheter is introduced into any available superficial vein. The leg is then drained for 3 minutes, then the upper compartment cuff is inflated to 400 mm/Hg pressure. 1% Lidocaine HCL/2 mg's per pound of body weight is drawn on a 50 c.c. syringe (usually about 15-20 c.c.). Saline solution is then used to fill up the 50 c.c. syringe. This is then injected slowly into the veins. Blanching will occur and the anesthesia will be effective almost immediately.

If the patient complains of pain around the upper cuff area, then (after 10 minutes) the lower cuff will be inflated with 400 mm/Hg and the upper cuff deflated. Since the area underneath the lower cuff has been anesthetized, the patient should experience no discomfort. The patient is then simply preped in the usual manner and surgery can begin.

The anesthetic solution perfuses rapidly into the tissues and remains in the tissues until the tourniquet is released. The anesthetic will then be gradually reabsorbed into the veins and returned to the general circulation where it is eventually detoxified in the liver.

Precautions

We have successfully used perfusion anesthesia on hundreds of patients with consistently good results and few complications. However, it is important to remember the following points:

1. Do not use this technique in patients with Thrombophlebitis or any type of circulatory impairment.
2. Tourniquet failure could result in an escape of a large quantity of the anesthetic into the general circulation. Negative reactions will result, the most common being convulsions. For this reason, it is important to have an I.V. started, so that a port for emergency drugs can be available at all times.
3. This technique should only be performed by someone who is trained thoroughly in all techniques of resuscitation, including intubation.

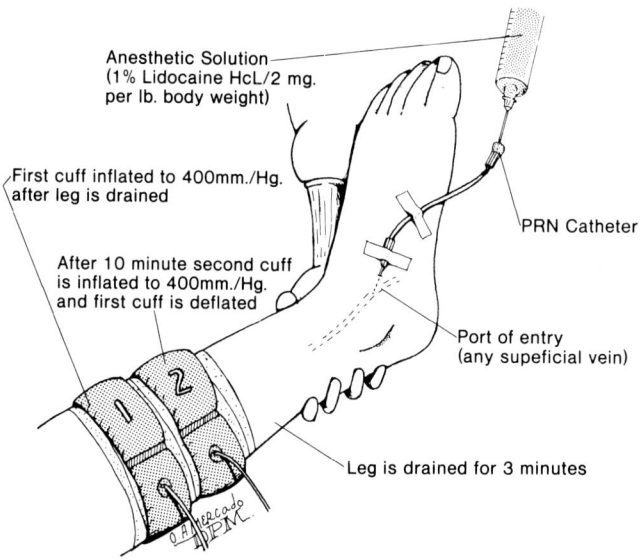

Fig. 1-5. Perfusion anesthesia

CHAPTER 2 — NAIL SURGERY

The Nail Matrix
Surgical Techniques
    1. Frost Technique
    2. Winograd Technique
    3. Kaplan Technique
    4. Mini-Kaplan Technique
    5. Terminal Syme
    6. Osteotripsy Technique
    7. Sub-Ungual Exostosis

CHAPTER 2

THE ANATOMICAL LANDMARK OF THE NAIL MATRIX

No adequate study of nail surgery can begin without first understanding the importance of the **nail matrix** and its anatomical location. The success or failure of any nail surgery operation depends on the complete removal of the portion of offending nail matrix.

Through clinical experience we have learned that unless the periosteum is removed at the site of the matrix, recurrence of horny-like portions of nail are unavoidable. In order to ascertain the anatomical landmark of the nail matrix and its intimacy with the phalanx and periosteum, a study was done to correlate our clinical findings with roentgenographic studies and cadaveric dissection.

Roentgenographic Studies

Urokon (Sodium Acetrizoate), a radiopaque substance commonly used in radiology for intravascular radiography, was injected under the eponychium deep to the base of the nail and the phalanx (Fig. 2-1A).

Lateral and oblique x-rays were then exposed. The lateral view revealed the nail plate descending to the bone. In some cases where too much Urokon was deposited, some of the solution overlapped into the mesa area at the phalanx and clearly outlined the insertion of the dorsal tendon (Fig. 2-1B).

NAIL SURGERY

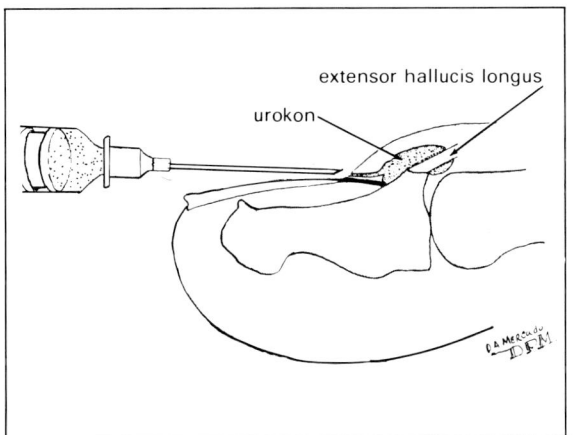

Fig. 2-1A. Urokon (Sodium Acetrizoate) a radiopaque substance is injected under the eponychium.

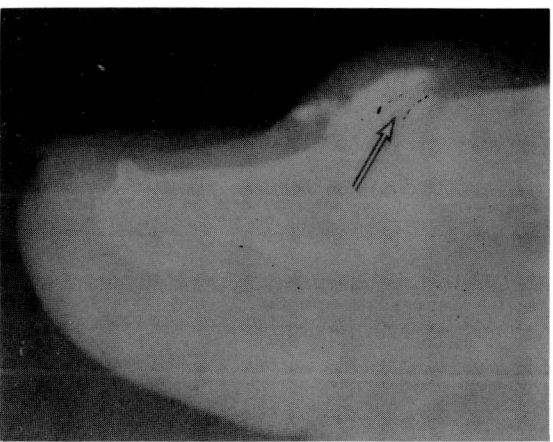

Fig. 2-1B. Lateral x-ray view reveals the nail plate descending to the bone. Some of the radiopaque solution overlapped into the **mesa** area of the phalanx and clearly outlines the insertion of the dorsal tendon (arrow).

Cadaveric Dissection

A sagittal section of the left great toe was obtained from a well preserved cadaver (Fig. 2-1C and D).

This longitudinal section upon careful examination revealed that:

1. There is a definite attachment, or rather **intimacy** between the nail matrix, the phalanx, and the periosteum. This area of intimacy seems to fall at the base of the phalanx, specifically at the point where the phalanx slopes superiorly and proximally.

2. The summit of the phalangeal slope flattens out into a **mesa**, and runs proximally a few millimeters and becomes continuous with the articulating surface of the phalanx. On the mesa there is a groove running from medial to lateral which serves for the attachment of the extensor hallucis longus tendon (Fig. 2-1E).

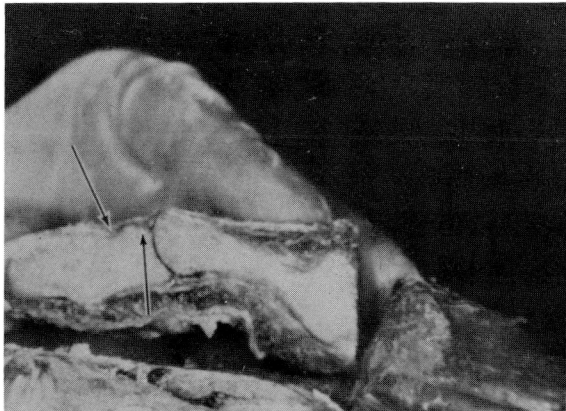

Fig. 2-1C. Longitudinal cadaver section. Top arrow shows anatomical landmark of nail; bottom arrow points to the insertion of extensor hallucis longus into the mesa.

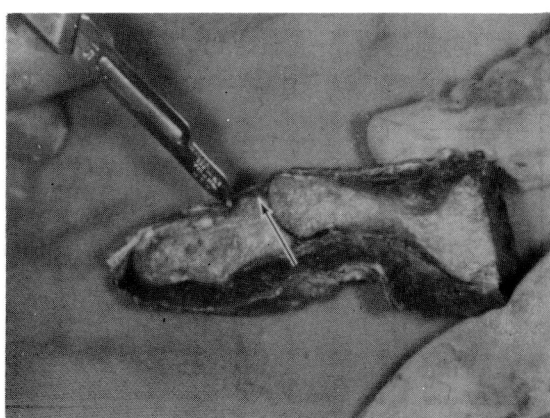

Fig. 2-1D. Note how nail descends **down** to the periosteum. Arrow points to the mesa, where the **dorsal** tendon attaches.

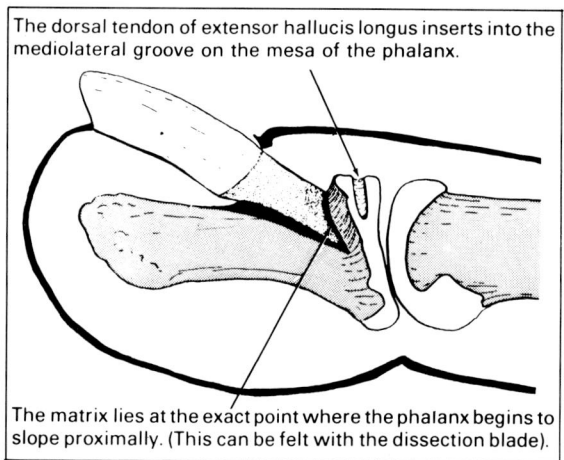

Fig. 2-1E.

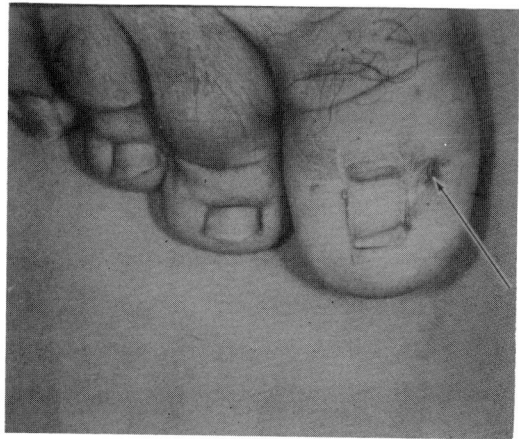

Fig. 2-1F. Recurrence of spicule (arrow) after nail surgery — the result of faulty dissection and failure to remove the nail matrix.

Conclusion

An anatomical landmark for the attachment of the nail matrix along with some observations as to the dorsal anatomy of the distal phalanx was described. This landmark will prove to be of great clinical (specifically surgical) value if the Surgeon remembers that:

1. The matrix lies at the exact point where the phalanx begins to slope proximally. (This can be felt with the dissection blade).
2. The matrix extends farther medially and laterally than it is commonly imagined.

The guesswork in partial and complete nail matrix resections will then be eliminated and the number of recurrences due to faulty dissection greatly reduced (Fig. 2-1F).

Surgical Techniques for Nail Surgery

Regardless of the etiology, nail surgery aims at the following:

1. **Partial** eradication of the nail matrix.
2. **Complete** eradication of the nail matrix.

The Techniques of Choice are:

1. **Frost Technique**
2. **Winograd Technique** } For partial eradication of the Nail Matrix
3. **Kaplan Technique**
4. **Mini-Kaplan Technique** } For Complete eradication of the Nail Matrix
5. **Terminal Syme**

NAIL SURGERY

Frost Technique

The Frost Technique takes its name from its originator, **Dr. Lawrence Frost.** Dr. Frost has given us a technique that will give excellent exposure to the nail matrix area and, when performed correctly, yields gratifying results.

Indications

The Frost Technique is used for the correction of an ingrown toe nail when the underlying problem is an **incurvated nail** with little or no proud flesh (hypertrophic nail lip).

Technique

A cut is started on the nail plate with a bone forceps (Fig. 2-2A). A No. 10 blade is placed on the groove made by the bone forceps and an incision is made **deep** to the bone, extending 1 cm past—proximal to—the eponychium.

A second incision is then made at 90° to the proximal end of the first incision, extending plantarwards for approximately 1.5 cm. A No. 15 blade is placed on the nail plate and worked under the nail groove from distal to proximal, with great care, thus forming an "L-shaped" eponychial flap (Fig. 2-2C). This flap is carefully retracted with a thumb and finger forceps or skin hooks. Remember, the flap is very **fragile** and any undue rough handling can lead to ischemia.

After the flap is retracted, two pie-wedge incisions are made—deep to the bone—to resect the offending nail plate, nail bed, and nail matrix (Fig. 2-2D).

The periosteum of the phalanx is rasped to expose the bone. This is important in order to eradicate the offending portion of the nail matrix and prevent recurrence. Remember that there is a close intimacy between the nail matrix and the periosteum. The removal of the periosteum will **insure** the removal of the nail matrix. Also, rasping of the phalanx should include the plantar margin of the bone, since the matrix does extend plantarwards (Fig. 2-2E and 2-1G).

The L-shaped flap is then repositioned to its original site and sutured with the material of choice (usually 5-0 nylon). Healing is uneventful.

Frost Technique

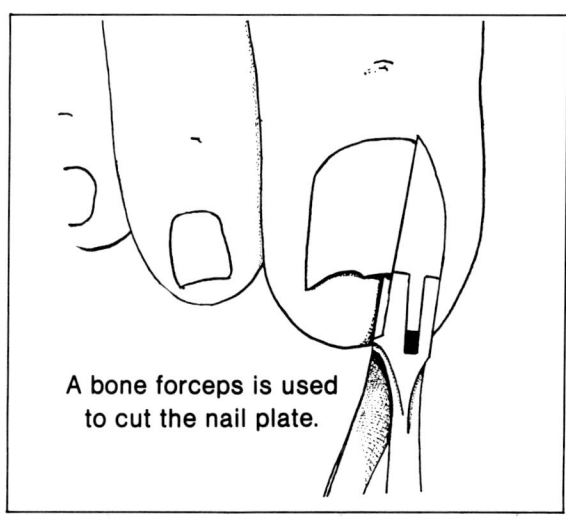

A bone forceps is used to cut the nail plate.

Fig. 2-2A

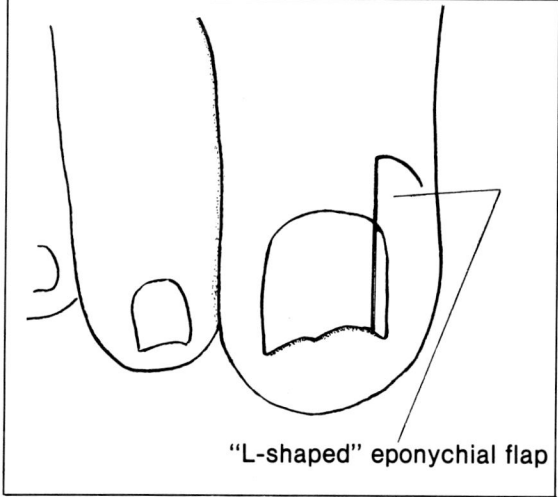

"L-shaped" eponychial flap

Fig. 2-2B

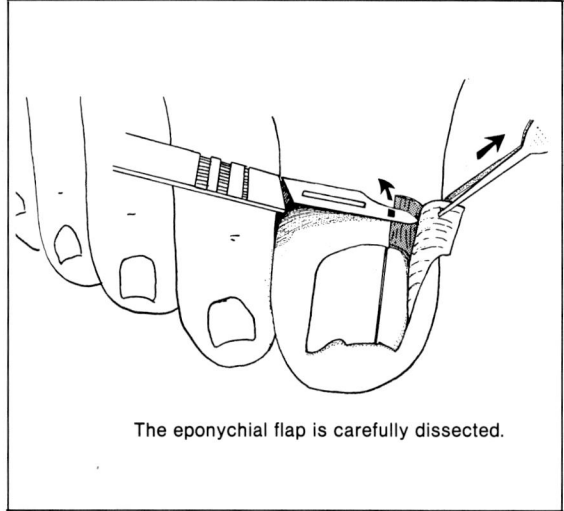

Fig. 2-2C

The eponychial flap is carefully dissected.

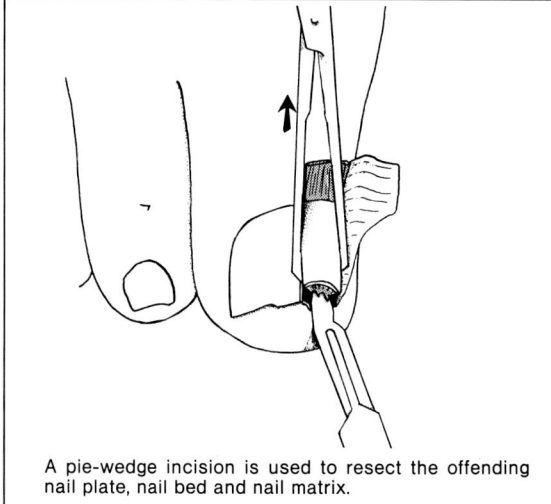

Fig. 2-2D

A pie-wedge incision is used to resect the offending nail plate, nail bed and nail matrix.

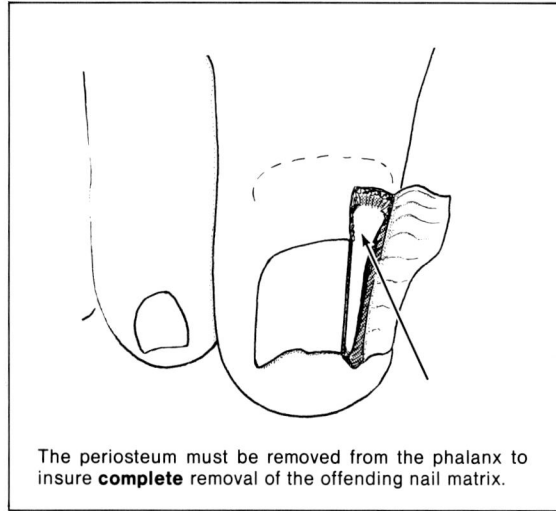

Fig. 2-2E

The periosteum must be removed from the phalanx to insure **complete** removal of the offending nail matrix.

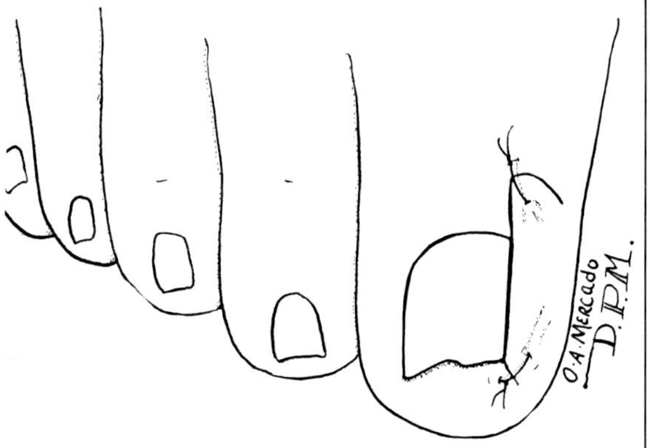

Fig. 2-2F

Precautions

1. The Frost Technique has the advantage that the flap allows **maximum exposure** to the nail matrix area. However, care must be exercised so as not to carry the flap incision too far plantarly as this could cause localized ischemia.
2. As with **any nail surgery,** it is important to clear up any infections pre-operatively.

Winograd Technique

The Winograd Technique is probably the most common operation used for the relief of an ingrown toenail. When performed properly, it will yield consistently good results.

Indications

This technique is used where the underlying problem is an incurvated nail with **proud flesh.** It is the best technique available for the reduction of the hyperthropic nail lip (Fig. 2-3A).

Technique

A cut is started on the nail plate with a bone forceps or an English nail splitter. A No. 10 blade is placed on the groove made by the bone forceps and an incision is made deep to the bone to one centimeter past, proximal to, the eponychium.

A second semi-elliptical incision is made, joining the two ends of the first incision. Here it is important to use a sawing (up and down) motion when cutting through the **hypertrophic tissues.** The hypertrophic nail lip has varying thickness and density and the sawing motion of the blade will insure an even cut and prevent accidental slipping and cutting of good tissues. The two incisions are then deepened with a No. 15 blade to the bone and the hypertrophic nail lip and offending nail plate are resected (Fig. 2-3B).

The fibrotic tissue around the phalanx is removed and the periosteum of the phalanx is rasped to expose the bone. This will eradicate the offending portion of nail matrix and will prevent recurrence of the incurvated nail plate (Fig. 2-3C).

The excessive nail lip is then remodeled so as to create a more normal looking nail groove. The best method of doing this remodeling is to hold the nail lip against the nail plate by applying pressure with the fingertips and cutting the hypertrophic nail lip with a No. 10 blade (Fig. 2-3D). While this maneuver might seem difficult at first, it allows for the complete removal of the hypertrophic nail lip leaving behind a normal looking toe that will heal with little induration and with excellent cosmetic results.

Two sutures of 5-0 Nylon are used to approximate the wound. One proximal to the eponychium and one distal at the tip of the toe (fig. 2-3E). Steri-strips are then used to approximate the newly-formed nail lip to the nail margin (Fig. 2-3F). Healing is usually uneventful.

Precautions

The Winograd technique is used where there is a lot of proud flesh accompanying the incurvated nail problem. Some important points to keep in mind in this technique are the following:

1. Make the first (longitudinal) incision long enough. This will make closure easier.
2. The second (semi-elliptical) incision should not be made too wide as this will make closure harder.
3. **Take as much of the indurated nail lip as possible during the nail lip remodeling portion of the operation (Fig. 2-3D).**

Conclusion

I have been performing Winograd techniques for almost two decades and I would be hard pressed to find one which didn't turn out well. I say this to emphasize the great and lasting results that can be obtained when a technique is performed meticulously and with respect for the tissues.

I find often that the students have a tendency early in their training to lean towards the chemo-surgical corrections for ingrown toenails. While there is nothing wrong with these techniques; they do not give the consistently **good** results and cosmesis that can be obtained with a well executed Winograd. Also, a Winograd technique will afford the student a chance to deal with bone, soft tissues and plastic remodeling of indurated tissues which will help the students improve their surgical skills.

Winograd Technique

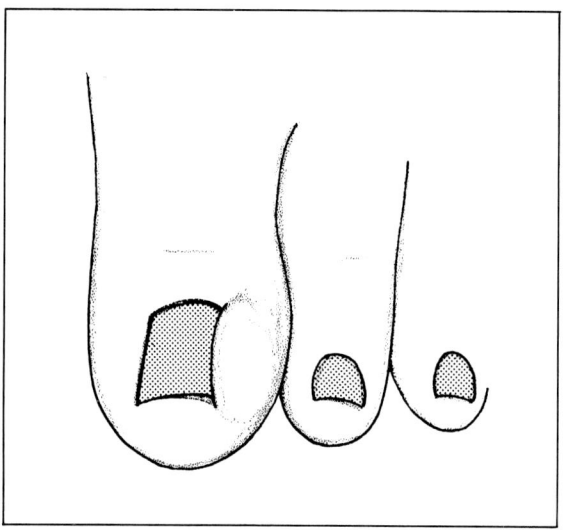

Fig. 2-3A

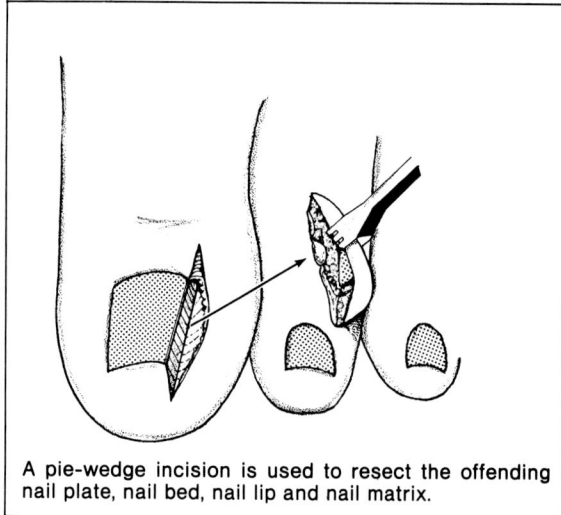

A pie-wedge incision is used to resect the offending nail plate, nail bed, nail lip and nail matrix.

Fig. 2-3B

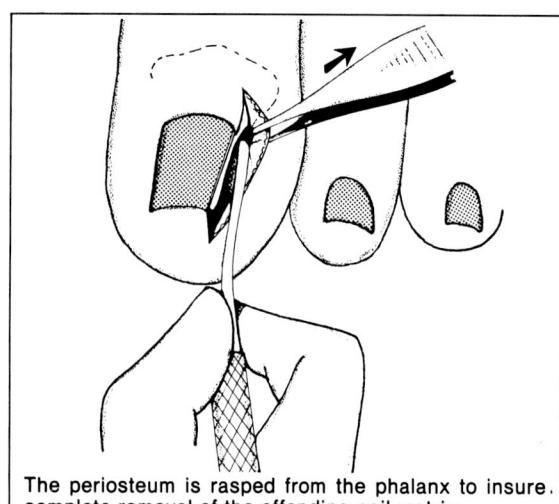

The periosteum is rasped from the phalanx to insure complete removal of the offending nail matrix.

Fig. 2-3C

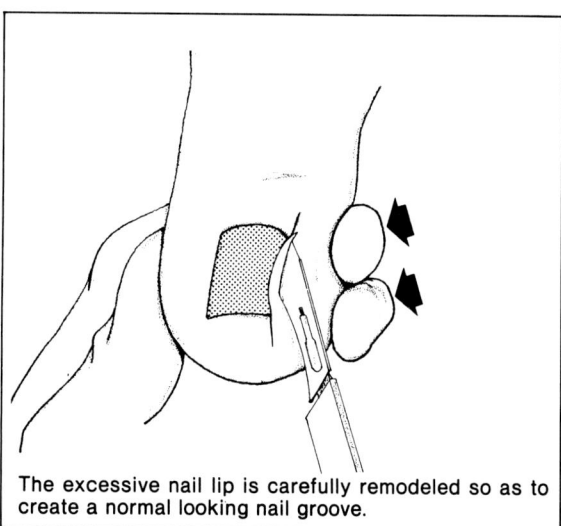

The excessive nail lip is carefully remodeled so as to create a normal looking nail groove.

Fig. 2-3D

NAIL SURGERY

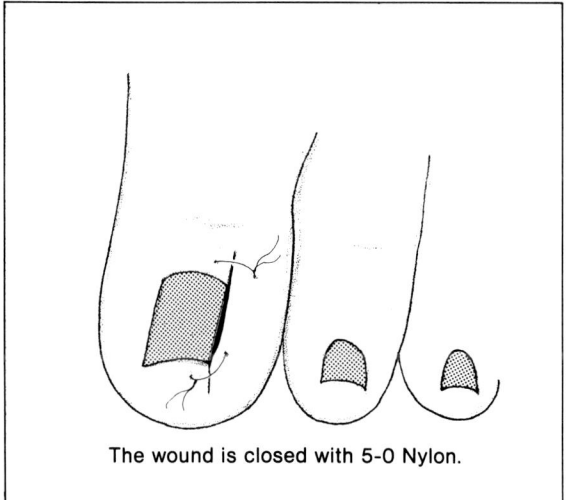

Fig. 2-3E

The wound is closed with 5-0 Nylon.

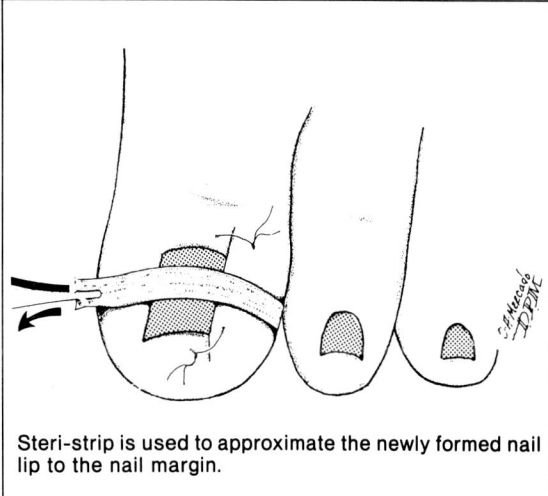

Fig. 2-3F

Steri-strip is used to approximate the newly formed nail lip to the nail margin.

Kaplan Technique

One of the best methods for **complete** excision of the hypertrophic (onychomycotic) nail is the operation devised by **Dr. Earl Kaplan.** His technique gives excellent cosmetic results and may be used successfully on the **hallux** or **second toe;** it does not work as well for the lesser three toes.

The technique is not used as often as it should because many surgeons feel that it is too radical and that it takes too long to heal. In reality, the technique is simple, safe and the healing time is about the same as for a partial phalangectomy.

Indications

The technique is used when the offending nail, nail bed and nail matrix require excision in-toto. It may be performed on patients with patent circulation and used on the first and second toes.

Technique

The offending nail plate is resected (Fig. 2-4A). Two incisions are made to either side of the nail grooves, extending 1.5 cm. past the eponychium (Fig. 2-4B). The **eponychial flap** thus made, is carefully underscored and retracted (Fig. 2-4C).

Two incisions are then made just outside the nail grooves. These incisions are carried distally and joined by a third incision in front of the toe. Care is taken to make this incision even with the dorsal aspect of the phalanx. The incisions are then underscored and a **nail bed flap** is made. This flap is carefully underscored even with the dorsum of the phalanx and resected in-toto all the way back to the attachment of the nail matrix (Fig. 2-4D).

Two wedge sections of tissue are taken from either side of the base of the phalanx to ascertain the complete resection of the matrix (Fig. 2-4E). At this time, if a sub-ungual exostosis is present, it is easily removed. The eponychium is then carefully resected, with straight scissors, from the eponychial flap. The flap is sutured with 5-0 Nylon. Care is taken to angulate the sutures so that the flap sits back without overlapping.

Gel-foam can then be used, if desired, to cover the exposed phalanx. Two more sutures of 4-0 Dexon are placed from one margin of the incision to the other (Fig. 2-4F). These sutures are important as they will reduce the size of the wound and thus cut down considerably the healing time.

In a week the exposed bone is covered completely with granulation tissue and the superficial portion of the suture is easily removed. The deeper portion stays in the wound and is dissolved by the granulation tissues.

Kaplan Technique

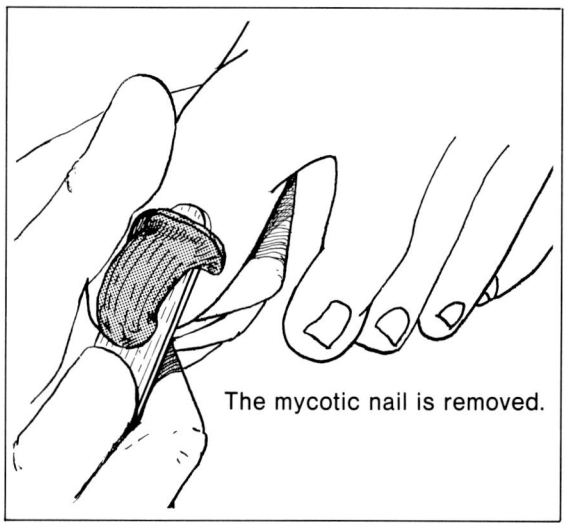

The mycotic nail is removed.

Fig. 2-4A

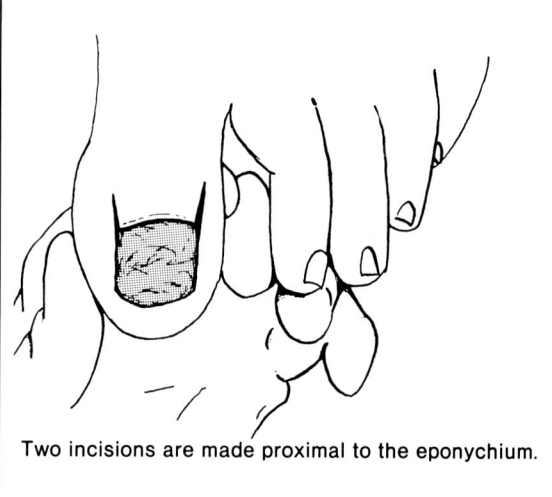

Two incisions are made proximal to the eponychium.

Fig. 2-4B

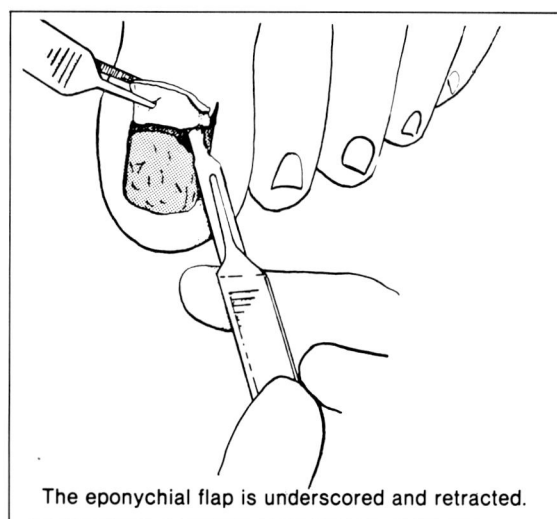

The eponychial flap is underscored and retracted.

Fig. 2-4C

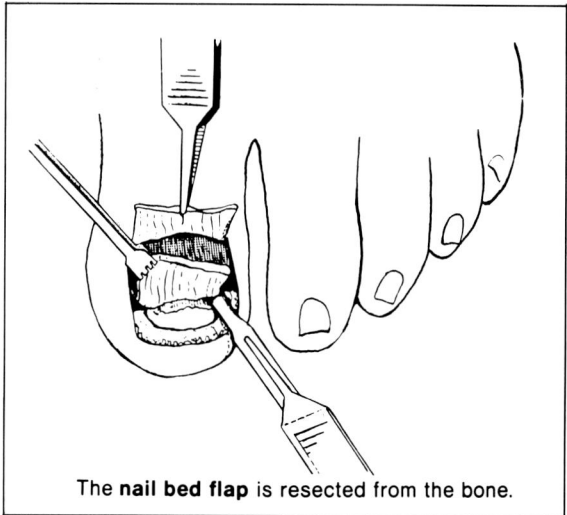

The **nail bed flap** is resected from the bone.

Fig. 2-4D

NAIL SURGERY

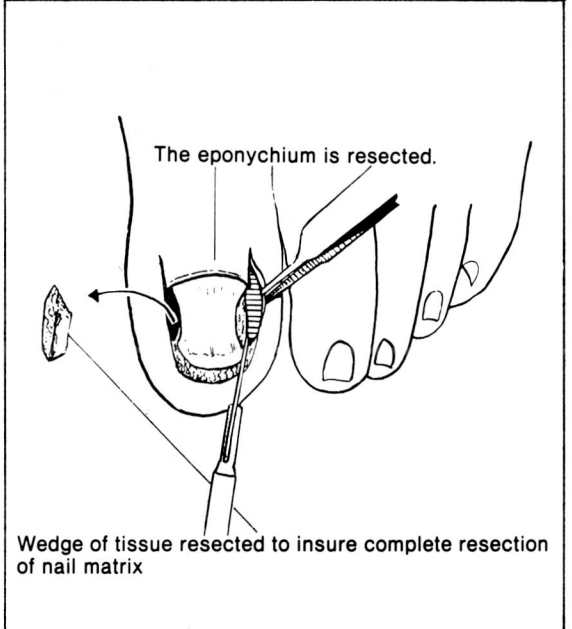

Fig. 2-4E

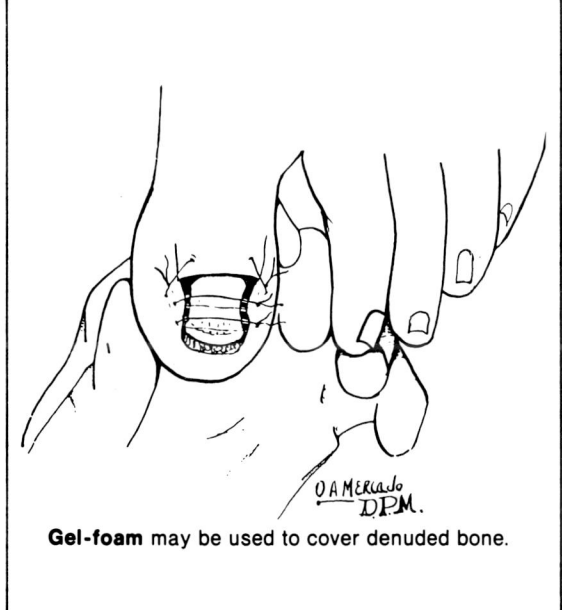

Fig. 2-4F

Dressing the Wound

It is important to use vaseline gauze (or adaptic dressing, etc.) to cover the wound immediately post-op. A snug dressing is then applied.

The bandage which will be completely soaked with dry blood, is removed in one week after soaking with bactine. The sutures are also removed at this time. An antibiotic ointment is then used and the wound is dressed with vaseline gauze and kling bandages.

The post-operative period is essentially unremarkable with the patient wearing a Band-Aid or light dressing after three weeks and complete healing taking place in five to six weeks.

Precautions

The technique yields consistently good results with excellent cosmetic appearance.

These are the important points to keep in mind:
1. Patient must have good **patent** circulation.
2. The dorsum of the phalanx must be completely denuded.
3. Suture the wound as shown in Fig. 2-4F.
4. Perform technique only on the first and second toes.

Mini-Kaplan Technique

The Mini-Kaplan Technique is our modification of Earl Kaplan's operation for the complete resection of a nail plate.

Indications

As with the Kaplan Technique, the Mini-Kaplan is used when complete excision of the nail matrix is desired. It can be used on **all toes,** and it is particularly useful in a geriatric patient with onychomycosis.

Technique

The mycotic nail (Fig. 2-5A) is underscored at its proximal end by inserting a small periosteal elevator under the eponychium and freeing all around the nail's base (Fig. 2-5B).

We like to remove the nail plate from proximal to distal in the following manner. First, a small curved hemostat is introduced under the proximal end of the nail plate (Fig. 2-5C). Next, the tips of the hemostat are spread open and closed a number of times to help loosen the nail plate. Then the nail plate is removed from proximal to distal (Fig. 2-5D). We find that by removing a mycotic nail plate in this fashion, as opposed to removing the plate by inserting an instrument under the anterior aspect of the nail, the nail bed is left smooth and clean (Fig. 2-5E).

Two incisions are made to either side of the nail groove to create an **eponychial flap** (Fig. 2-5E). The eponychial flap is gently retracted and a transversed incision is made across the proximal end of the nail bed deep to the bone (Fig. 2-5F).

The proximal end of the nail bed is then resected to the bone, exposing the dorsum of the distal phalanx, more specifically, the area of the phalanx where the **nail matrix** attaches. The bone is rasped to insure complete resection of the nail matrix. A small piece of Gel-foam is then used to cover the denuded bone (Fig. 2-5G).

The eponychium is then resected from the flap. The flap is returned to its original position and sutured with 5-0 Nylon as illustrated in Fig. 2-5H. Healing is usually uneventful.

Precautions

The Mini-Kaplan technique is easy to perform and yields consistently good results when performed as described here.

However, the surgeon will do well to keep the following points in mind:

1. **Do not** use the Mini-Kaplan on a hallux where the nail plate is greatly deformed; a regular Kaplan technique should be performed in these cases.
2. On a greatly deformed fifth toenail, a **Terminal Syme** will be the technique of choice.
3. Make sure that the periosteum is removed from the exposed phalanx (dorsally, medially and laterally) to insure complete removal of the nail matrix.

NAIL SURGERY

Mini-Kaplan Technique

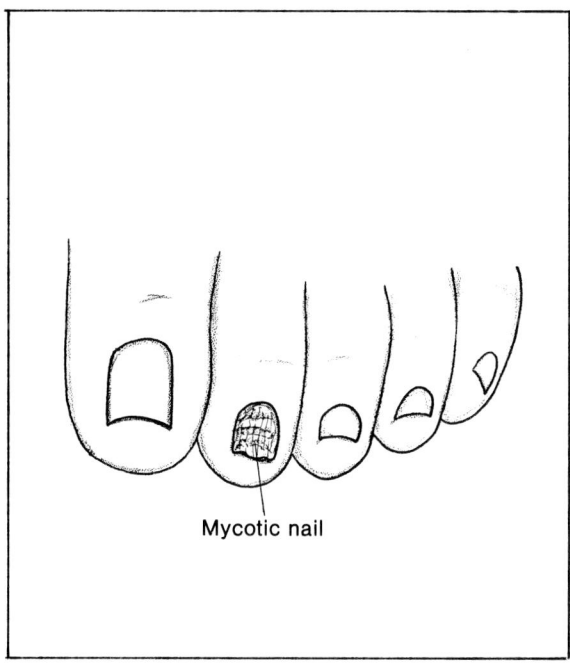

Fig. 2-5A — Mycotic nail

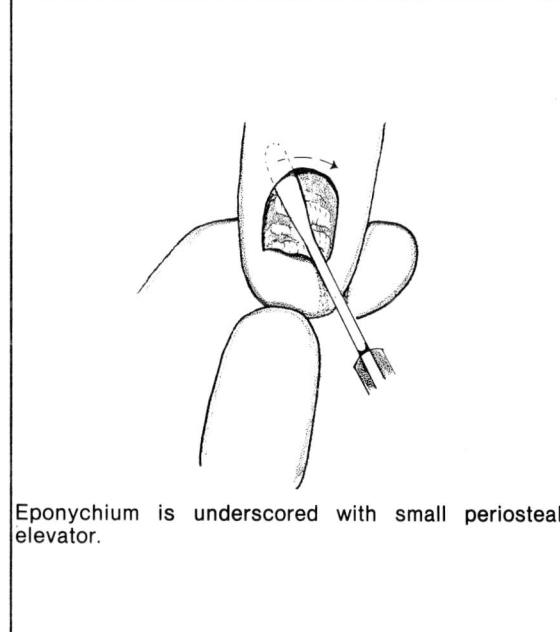

Fig. 2-5B — Eponychium is underscored with small periosteal elevator.

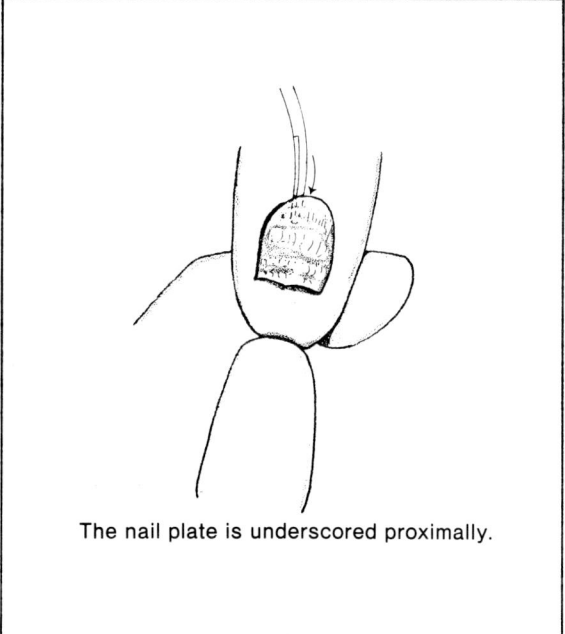

Fig. 2-5C — The nail plate is underscored proximally.

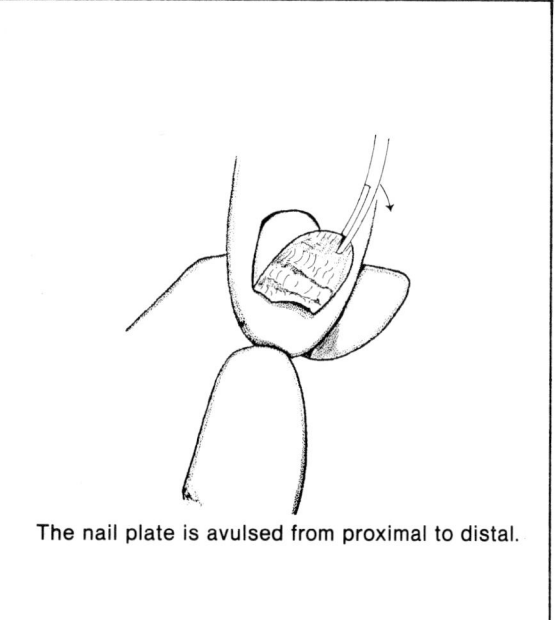

Fig. 2-5D — The nail plate is avulsed from proximal to distal.

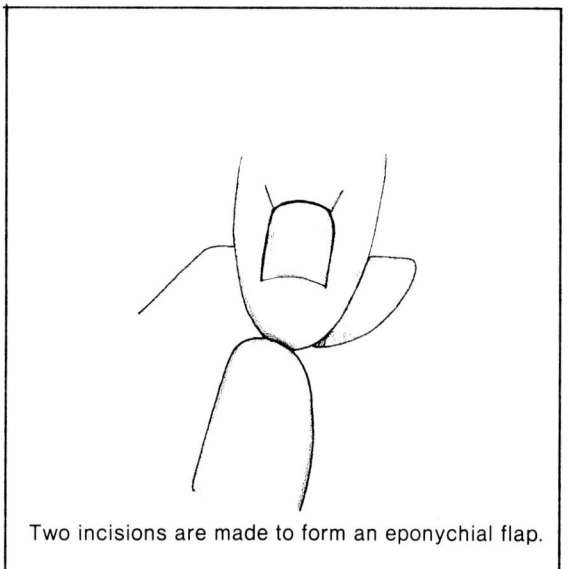

Two incisions are made to form an eponychial flap.

Fig. 2-5E

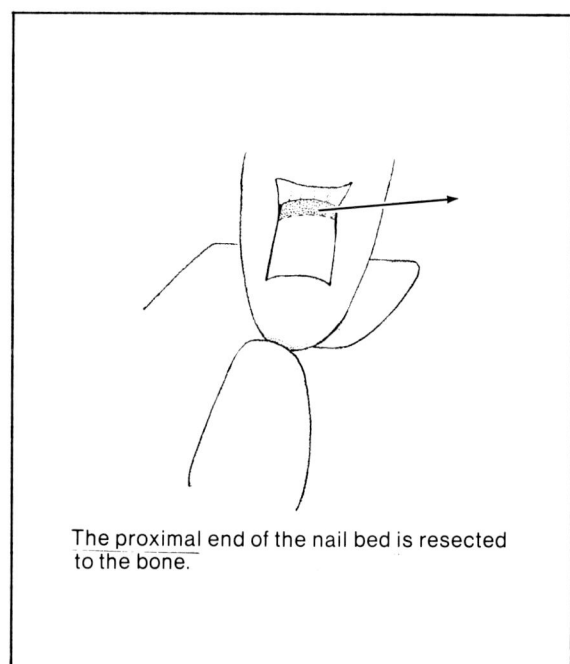

The proximal end of the nail bed is resected to the bone.

Fig. 2-5F

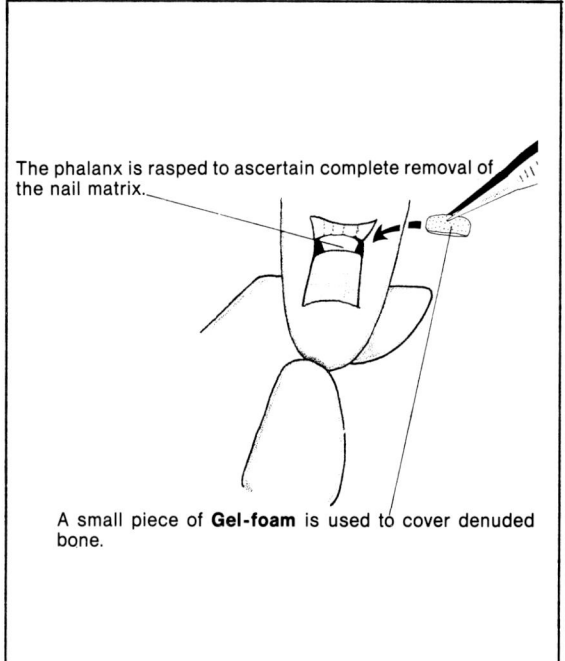

The phalanx is rasped to ascertain complete removal of the nail matrix.

A small piece of **Gel-foam** is used to cover denuded bone.

Fig. 2-5G

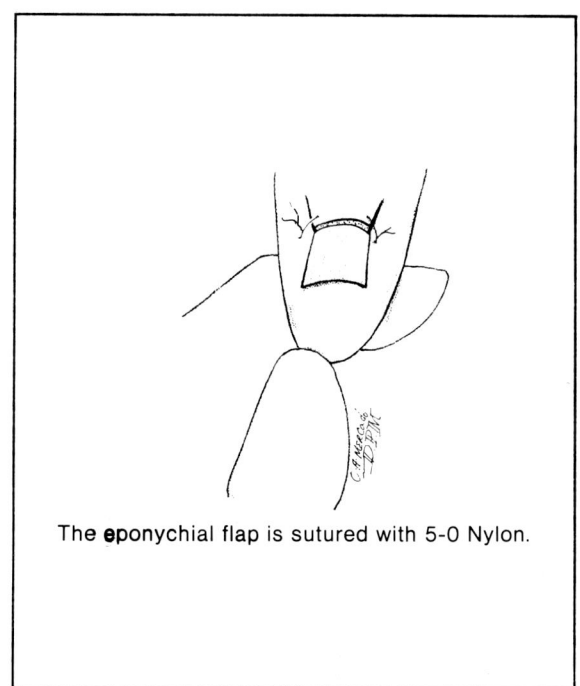

The eponychial flap is sutured with 5-0 Nylon.

Fig. 2-5H

Terminal Syme

The Terminal Syme, or **partial amputation** technique is used to eradicate the complete nail matrix. However, since it does deform the toe, **it should only be used on the lesser three toes.**

Indications

The technique is used when the offending nail, nail bed and nail matrix require excision in-toto.

It may be performed on patients with patent circulation and used on the lesser three toes **only.** It works particularly well on the fifth toe where the shortening of the toe is minimal.

Technique

A transversed incision is made just behind the eponychium. Two lineal incisions are made from the medial and lateral margins of the first incision running distally on either side of the nail grooves to the tip of the toe.

Another incision is made at the tip of the toe connecting the two lineal incisions (Fig. 2-6A). The nail plate and surrounding tissues are resected in-toto (Fig. 2-6B).

The distal phalanx of the toe is then exposed and underscored. Approximately **one-third** of the distal phalanx is then resected (Fig. 2-6C and D). The tip of the toe is then pushed dorsally and proximally and held in place with a horizontal mattress suture (2-6E); this will shorten the toe somewhat, as can be seen when figures 2-6D and E are compared. The excessive tissue found at either side of the wound resemble **dog-ears.** These dog-ears are resected with a No. 15 blade and sutured with simple sutures of 5-0 Nylon (2-6F).

Precautions

The Terminal Syme Technique is used to eradicate the complete nail matrix. This technique should be used only on the **lesser three toes.** The technique itself is quite simple, however some points should be kept in mind.

1. **Do not** resect more than one-third of the distal phalanx; the more bone resected, the more will the disfiguration of the toe be noticed.
2. When closing the wound, use a horizontal mattress suture in the center and one or two simple sutures to either side after the excess skin (dog-ears) have been excised.
3. Since the technique will shorten the toe, the patient should be warned beforehand. However, when performed on the lesser three toes, the amount of shortening that occurs is so slight that the cosmetic results are excellent.

Terminal Syme

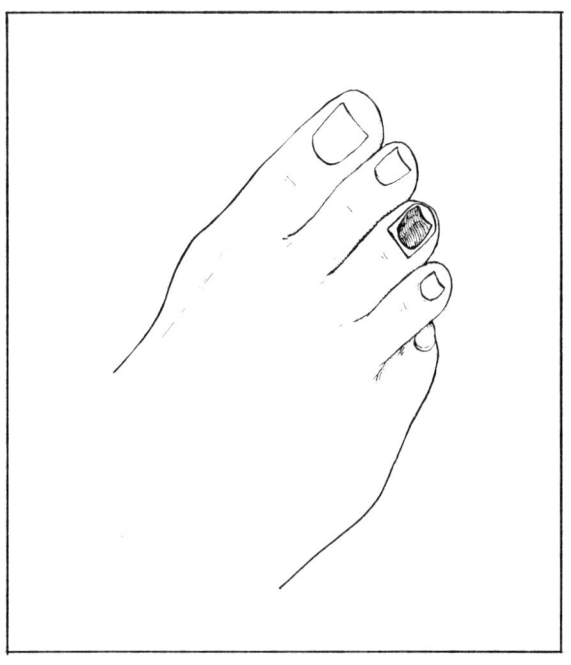

Fig. 2-6A

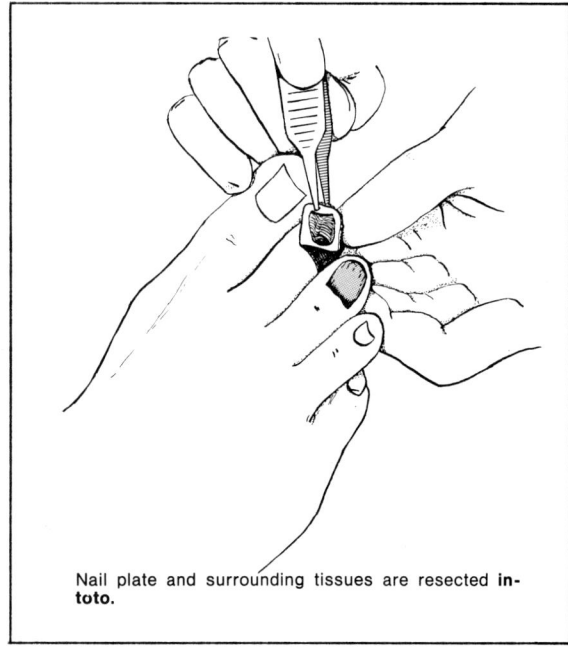

Nail plate and surrounding tissues are resected **in-toto.**

Fig. 2-6B

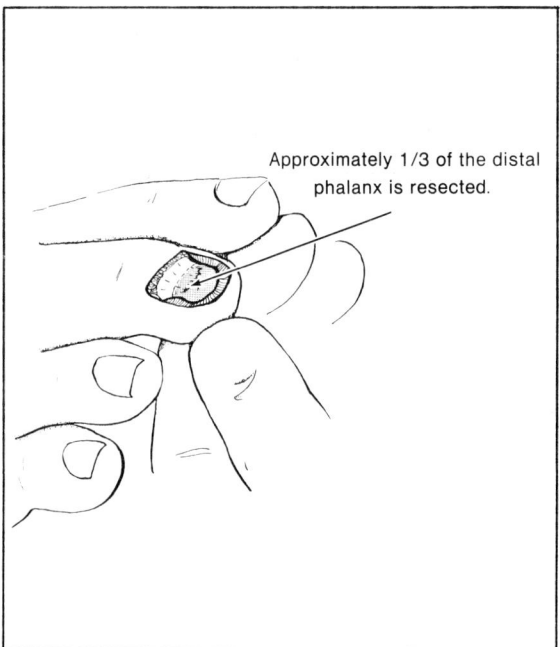

Approximately 1/3 of the distal phalanx is resected.

Fig. 2-6C

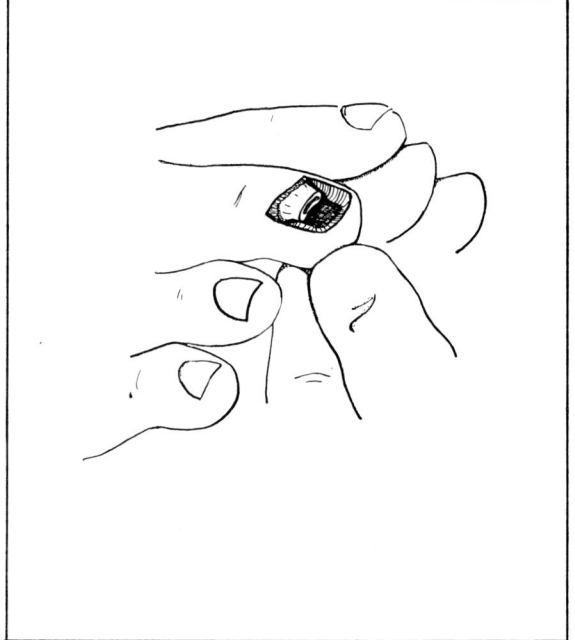

Fig. 2-6D

NAIL SURGERY

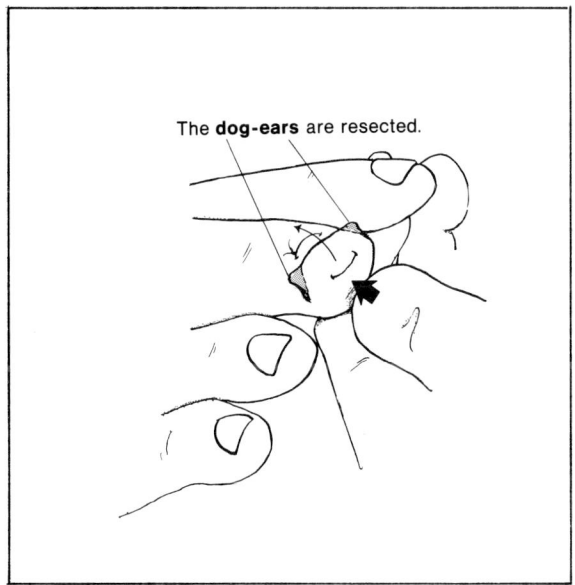

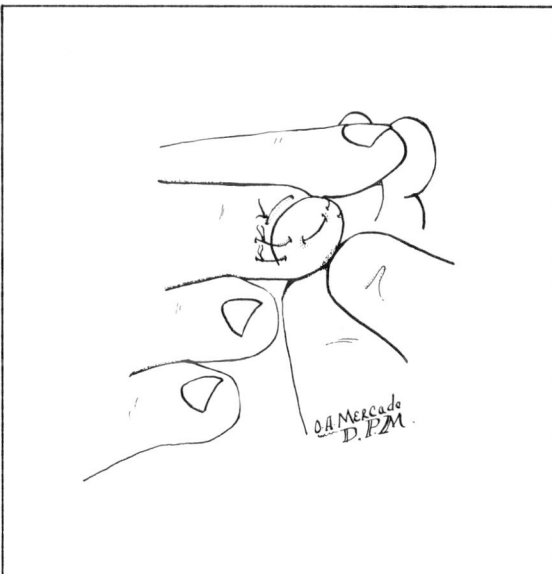

Fig. 2-6E *Fig. 2-6F*

Osteotripsy Technique

The Osteotripsy, or bone rasping techniques have been in vogue for a number of years. They are simple to perform and when done properly will yield good results.

Indications

The Osteotripsy Technique may be used for partial or complete eradication of the nail matrix. It should be used where the underlying problem is an incurvated nail with little or no proud flesh or for a mycotic nail.

The Osteotripsy Techniques work particularly well on the geriatric patients.

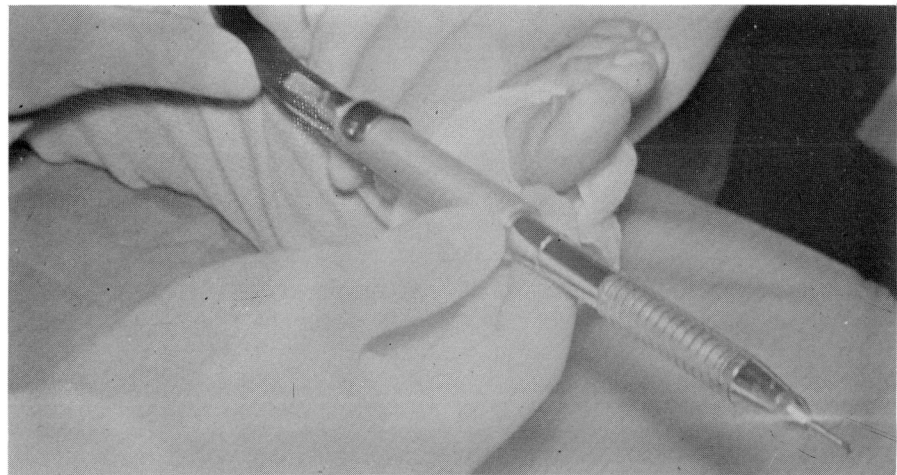

Fig. 2-7A. Typical power drill used for osteotripsy technique.

Partial Eradication of the Nail Matrix

A nick is started on the nail plate with a nail-splitter and the offending portion of nail is removed. **The eponychium is not cut.**

The fibrotic tissue is resected from around the phalanx with tissue nippers. With a hand rasp or power equipment, the periosteum is removed from the bone.

The wound is then flushed with one c.c. of Xylocaine (1% with epinephrine) or the anesthetic solution of choice and one c.c. of Prednisolone Acetate Suspension (25 mg.) and packed with Gel-foam. Vaseline gauze is applied and the wound is dressed in the usual manner.

The post-operative period is unremarkable with the patient wearing a Band-Aid or light dressing by the second post-op visit.

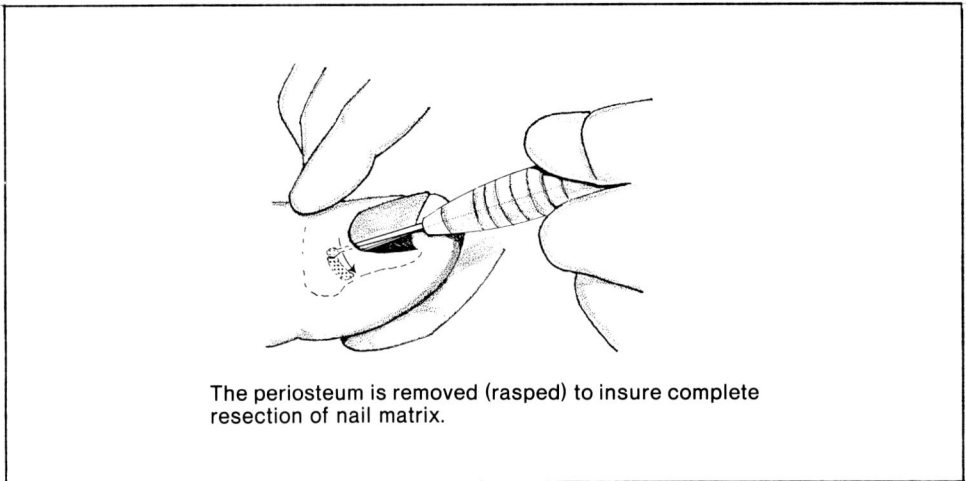

The periosteum is removed (rasped) to insure complete resection of nail matrix.

Fig. 2-7B

Complete Eradication of the Nail Matrix

The nail plate is avulsed. A No. 15 blade is slipped under the eponychium and the wound is underscored, thus forming an eponychial envelope. A hand rasp or power equipment is then used to remove the periosteum from the bone. A mixture of one c.c. Xylocaine and Prednisolone Acetate Suspension, is used to flush the wound. Gel-foam is used to pack the wound. The toe is then dressed in the usual manner.

Precautions

Perhaps the greatest inherent problem with the Osteotripsy techniques is that they are so simple to perform that there is a tendency towards misuse.

We must keep in mind that:
1. Osteotripsy techniques will work best on simple nail incurvations, where there is no proud flesh.
2. There is a greater percentage of failures with Osteotripsy than with open techniques.
3. As with any surgery, routine laboratory tests and strict aseptic conditions are mandatory.

NAIL SURGERY

Sub-Ungual Exostosis

A common finding in nail problems is that of an enlargement on the dorsal tip of the distal phalanx. This osteal enlargement usually progresses until it becomes a **sub-ungual exostosis** (Fig. 2-8A). Often the exostosis will grow so large that it will actually deform the nail plate (Fig. 2-8C).

Technique

If the nail plate is mycotic, then a Kaplan technique is performed. The sub-ungual exostosis is easily removed since the Kaplan technique calls for the resection of all the tissues from the dorsum of the phalanx.

If, however, the nail plate is normal, then the following technique is performed; a fish-mouth incision is made on the anterior aspect of the toe, making sure to place the incision inside one of the many **papillary ridges** found in this area. This will insure good apposition of the tissues and an almost invisible scar (Fig. 2-8D).

The sub-ungual exostosis is carefully dissected, taking care to preserve the nail plate above it. The exposed sub-ungual exostosis is then resected using small rongeur bone forceps (Fig. 2-8E).

The bone is rasped smooth. The wound is carefully closed with simple sutures of 5-0 Nylon (Fig. 2-8F) and dressed in the usual manner. Healing is usually uneventful.

Precautions

The resection of a sub-ungual exostosis is a simple matter. However, the surgeon should keep the following points in mind to insure consistently good results.

1. Place the fish-mouth incision inside a papillary ridge to insure almost scar free healing.
2. Be gentle when retracting the dorsal portion of the wound. Use skin hooks, as these will not damage the fragile nail plate.

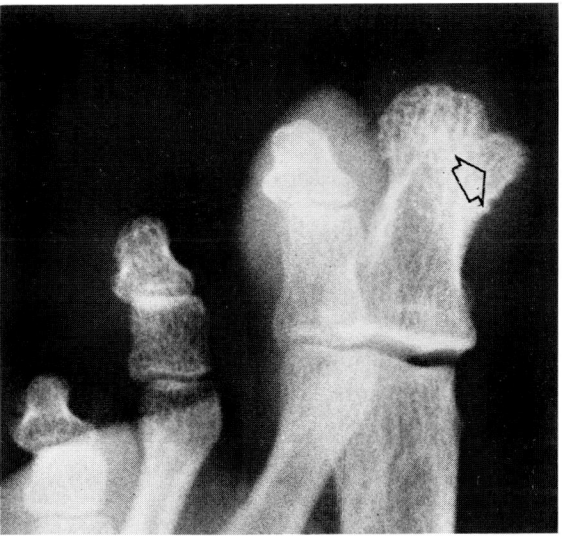

Fig. 2-8A. Note large sub-ungual exostosis on hallux (arrow).

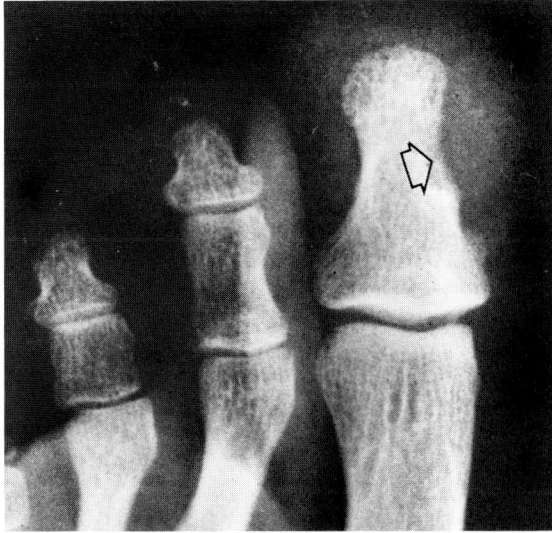

Fig. 2-8B. Post-operative view. Sub-ungual exostosis has been resected (arrow).

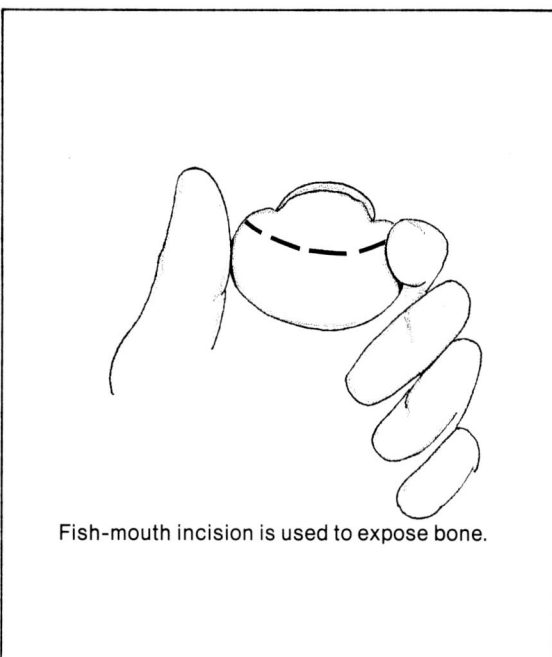

Fish-mouth incision is used to expose bone.

Fig. 2-8C

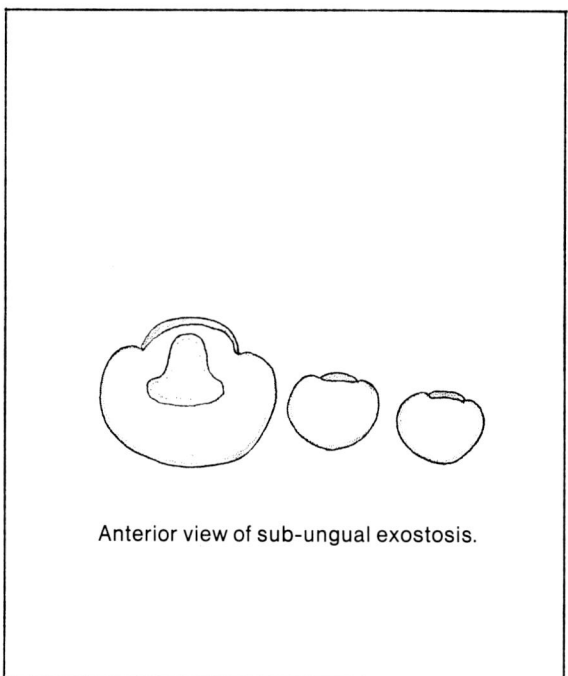

Anterior view of sub-ungual exostosis.

Fig. 2-8D

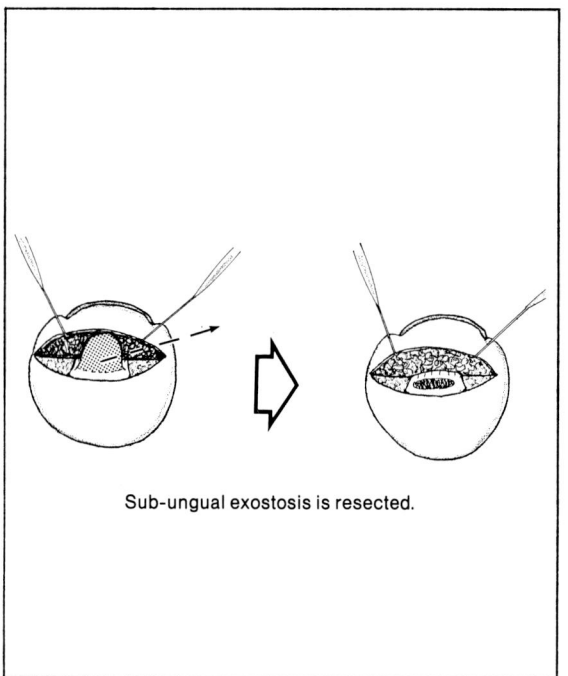

Sub-ungual exostosis is resected.

Fig. 2-8E

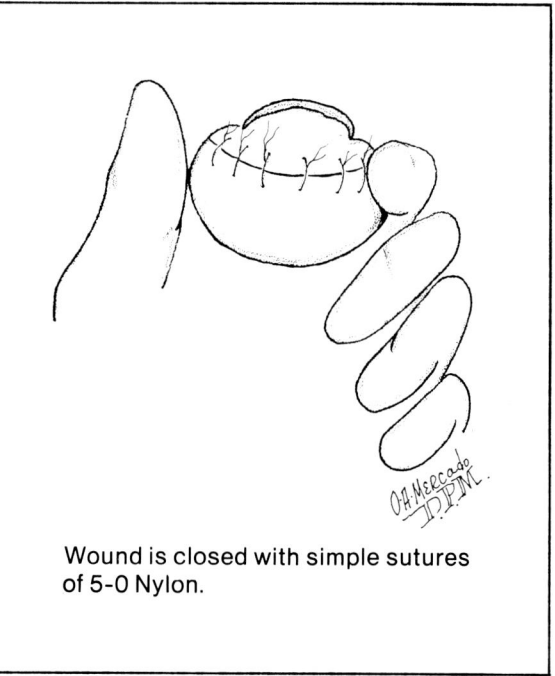

Wound is closed with simple sutures of 5-0 Nylon.

Fig. 2-8F

CHAPTER 3—SOFT TISSUE SURGERY

Verruca Plantaris
Excision Technique
The Cleavage Lines
The Papillary Lines
The Needling Technique
Neuroma

CHAPTER 3

Soft Tissue Surgery

Perhaps the most common lesion found on the foot is Verruca Plantaris. This small, but often excruciatingly painful, entity has been the subject of scores of articles dealing with its eradication. From simple salicylic acid plasters to ultra sound therapy to even amputation of the involved part have been recommended.

For the most part, Verruca Plantaris is essentially a **surgical problem.** Surgical correction is simple and the results are good enough to justify it being the treatment of choice. There are two simple methods used for the surgical correction of Verruca Plantaris, these are:
1. **The Excision Technique**
2. **The Needling Technique**

Excision Technique

This technique is simply the resection of the verruca by the use of two semi-elliptical incisions.

The pitfall of this procedure is that often the surgeon sadly neglects his surgical training which stresses the importance of the cleavage lines and the papillary lines (ridges) in the production of a sound and inconspicuous scar.

SOFT TISSUE SURGERY

The Cleavage Lines

The cleavage lines (Fig. 3-1A and B), sometimes known as **Langer's lines,** were described in the early 1800's. They are simply the lineal direction in which the skin splits when a rounded, sharp pointed instrument is thrust through it. Nowhere in the surface of the body does a stab with a sharp cylindrical instrument leave a rounded hole in the skin. The skin will always split in a lineal direction and the line of the slit will run in a definite direction in any region of the body.

Papillary Lines

The plantar surface of the foot and toes shows, like the palmar surface of the hand and fingers, the furrows and ridges of the horny layer of the epidermis that make the well-known patterns that constitute the basis for the system of fingerprint identification (Fig. 3-1C).

The apical digital pads of the toes are marked by papillary patterns of the looped and spiral type seen in the fingers, but the pattern is generally simpler.

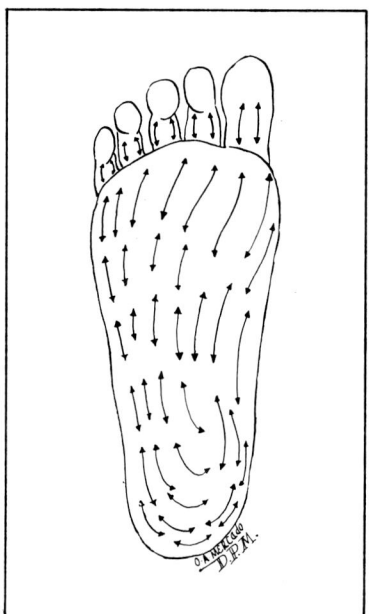
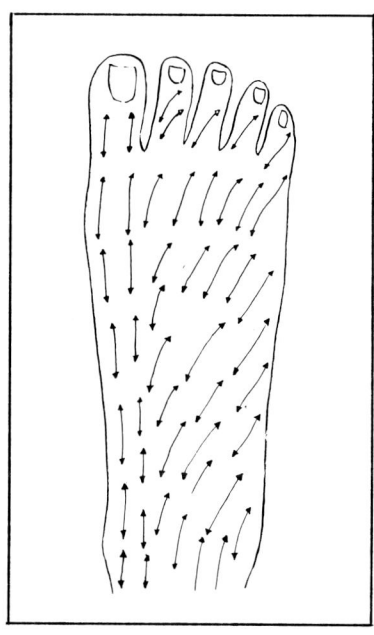
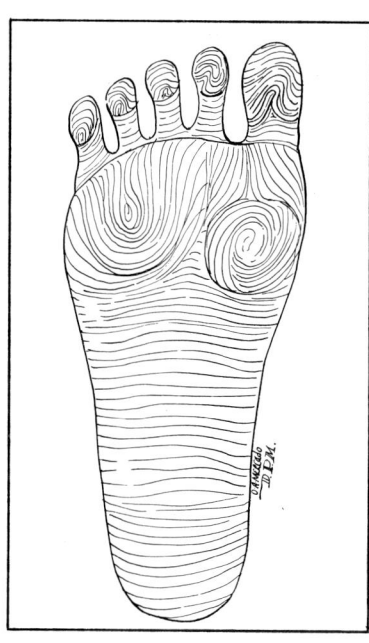

Fig. 3-1A. The cleavage lines on the plantar aspect of the foot.

Fig. 3-1B. The cleavage lines on the dorsal aspect of the foot.

Fig. 3-1C. The papillary lines on the sole of the foot.

Technique

A typical site for a verruca plantaris is shown in figure 3-2A. Here we see a large verruca plantaris with two smaller satellite lesions.

Our surgery aims at the resection of the larger verruca, taking care to place our incisions to coincide with the papillary lines. The verruca is excised in-toto. The skin is then underscored (Fig. 3-2B) and the satellite verruca is needled. The wound is then closed using a continuous lock suture with the material of choice (Fig. 3-2C).

Plantar incisions will **heal** as well as any other incision if the surgeon remembers the importance of using the cleavage and papillary lines in choosing the direction of his incision.

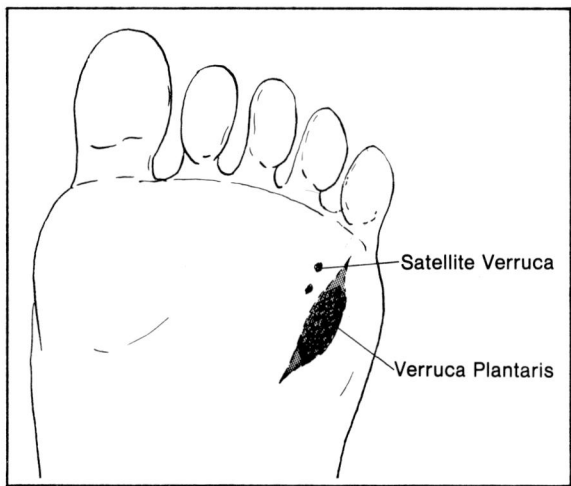

Fig. 3-2A. Verruca plantaris with two satellite verrucae.

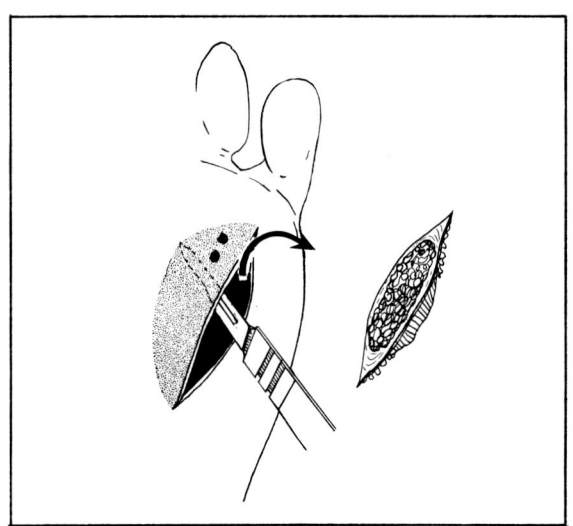

Fig. 3-2B. The large verruca is resected. The small satellites are needled.

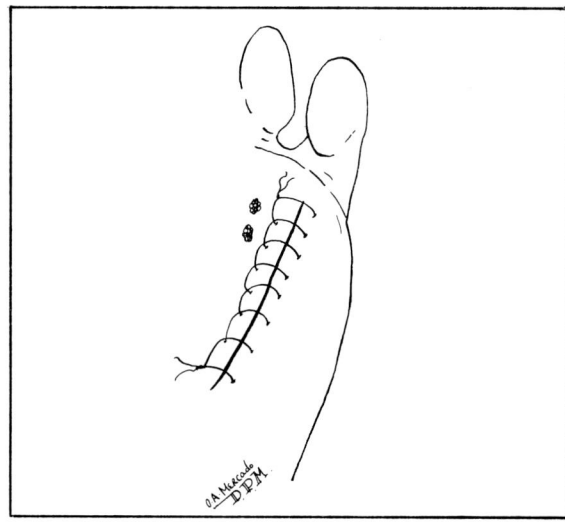

Fig. 3-2C. The wound is closed with a continuous lock suture.

SOFT TISSUE SURGERY

The Needling Technique

The Needling Treatment was described by **Dr. Gordon W. Falknor,** and essentially it is nothing more than the destruction of the verruca by rapid needling (puncturing), up-and-down, until the encapsulated warty tissues are no longer identifiable.

The technique is simple and efficacious, however it will only work on **single** and **satellite verrucae**. It **will not** work on the mosaic type. Sometimes it is necessary to use adjunct acid therapy to insure total destruction (i.e. verzone, monochloracetic acid, etc.)

Technique

The surgical area can be anesthetized with a field block (Fig. 3-3A) or by utilizing a tibial nerve block (Chapter I). The foot and ankle are scrubbed and draped in the usual manner.

A large bore needle (22 gauge) is held between the thumb, forefinger and middle finger (Fig. 3-3B). The needle is inserted in-and-out in rapid succession until the verruca and capsular tissues are no longer identifiable (Fig. 3-3C). The wound is dressed in the usual manner, healing is uneventful.

Five days post-op. the area will look very much like a dryed-up hematoma. The upper layers of the lesion are then reduced in three to four visits until the skin is normal.

Sometimes if some verrucanous tissue remains, it can be treated with acid therapy.

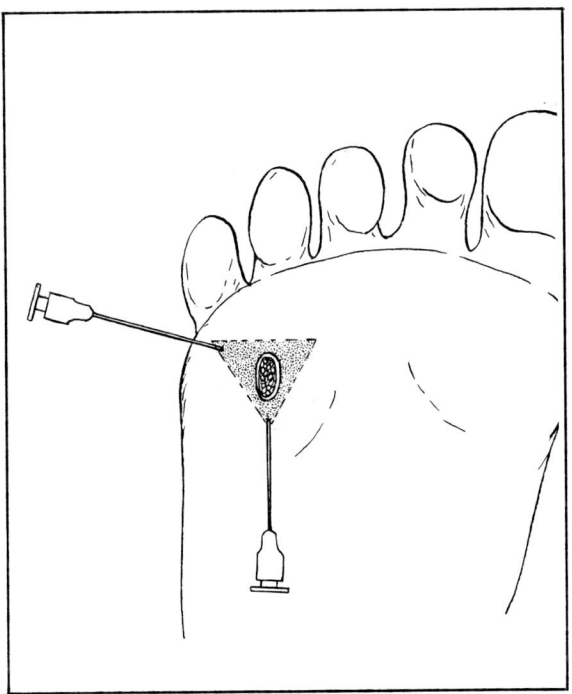

Fig. 3-3A. The area can be anesthetized with a field block, as shown, or with a tibial nerve block (Chapter 1).

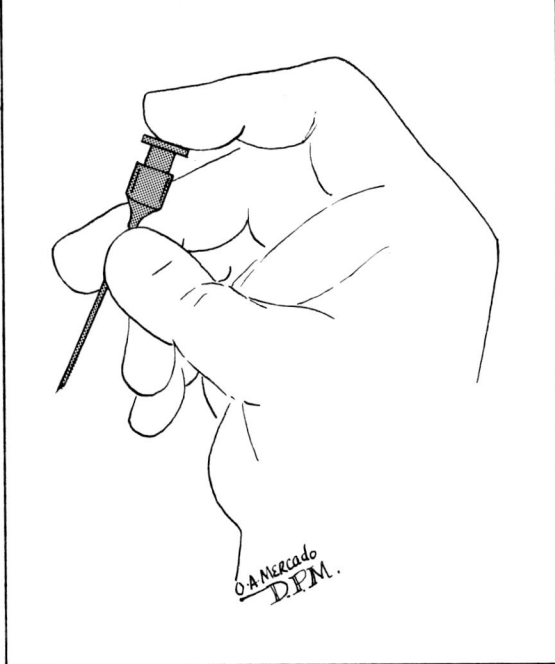

Fig. 3-3B. Proper way of holding needle for needling technique.

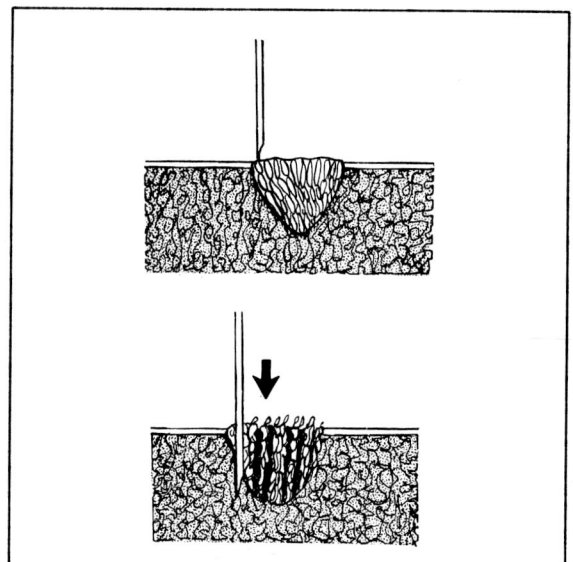
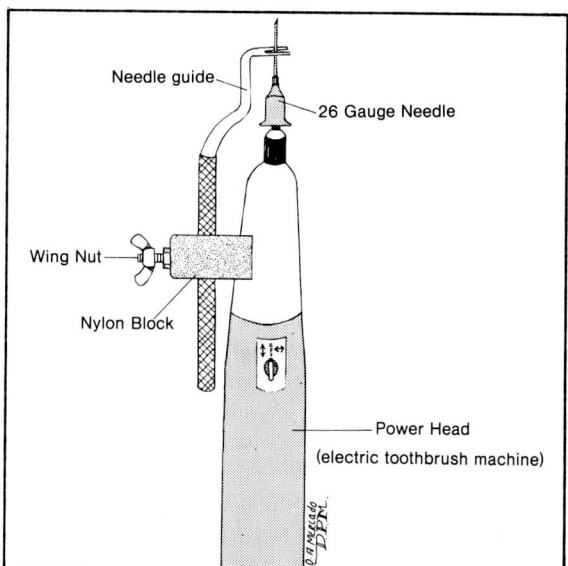

Fig. 3-3C. The verrucanous tissue is destroyed by rapid needling (puncturing) up-and-down, until the encapsulated warty tissue are no longer identifiable.

Fig. 3-3D. The Chrencik reciprocal dermal puncturing (needling) instrument affords the surgeon a rapid method of needling.

The Chrencik Reciprocating Dermal Puncturing (Needling) Instrument

Dr. E. W. Chrencik, of Hopkins, Minnesota, has devised an ingenious instrument which he fashioned utilizing the power head of an electric toothbrush. He attaches a pre-cut nylon block to the power unit and threads through the block, a needle guide made from a flat nail splitter instrument.

A slot is cut on the nail splitter to allow for the passage of the needle and to adjust the desired depth of penetration. The needle guide is held in place by a wing nut.

When the motor is turned on, the needle will penetrate in-and-out of the wart at a rate of **1,100 times a minute!** (Fig. 3-3D)

The Chrencik instrument affords the surgeon a rapid and accurate method of needling a verruca.

Precautions

The Needling Technique is an excellent method of eradicating a verruca plantaris, however the surgeon should remember that:

1. This technique is used only on single and satellite verrucae.
2. It **will not** work on the mosaic type verruca.
3. Sometimes it is necessary to use adjunct acid therapy to insure total destruction.

The Mosaic Verruca

A Mosaic Verruca is nothing more than a coalition of numerous small verrucae into an irregular, moisac-like pattern which often becomes recalcitrant.

The treatment of choice is conservative acid therapy (i.e. monochloracetic acid, salicylic acid, etc.). This mode of treatment, albeit slow, will usually resolve the problem or at least **reduce** the verruca in size to the point where surgical excision is feasible.

Neuroma

A Neuroma can occur in almost any nerve of the foot but the most prevalent site is the 3rd intermentatarsal space.

Numerous writers in the past have expounded on the etiology of the neuroma and almost all of them (with the notable exception of **Kelikian**) blame it on an impingement by the metatarsal heads of the **3rd common digital branch** of the **medial plantar nerve** on its **communication** with the **common digital branch** of the **lateral plantar nerve.**

The impingement of this nerve by the 3rd and 4th metatarsal heads would be an anatomical impossibility as the heads are connected plantarly by the strong fibrous transverse metatarsal ligament and the nerve lies below it (Fig. 3-4A).

That there is an impingement however, can be readily demonstrated by the surgeon compressing the forefoot with his hands. This will elicit an acute shooting pain in the patient's foot.

The probable etiology of a neuroma **is not** an impingement by the metatarsal heads, but, probably by the bases of the proximal phalanges (Fig. 3-4B).

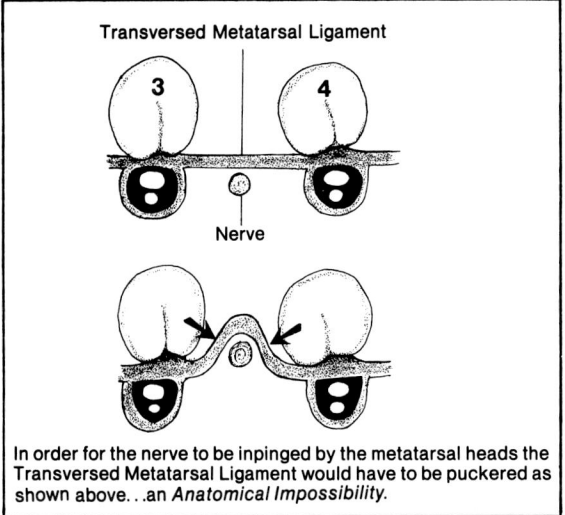

Fig. 3-4A

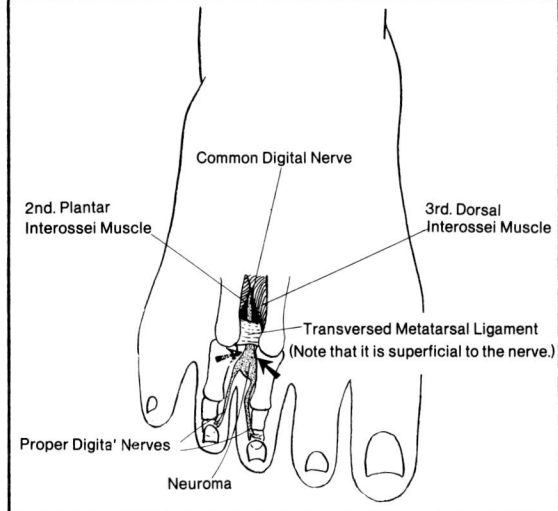

Fig. 3-4B. Arrow shows impingement of nerve by the proximal phalangeal bases.

Technique

An incision is made in the intermetatarsal area extending from the junction of the proximal and middle one-third of the metatarsal shaft to just into the interdigital space (Fig. 3-4C). The incision is deepened and retracted. The surgeon then spreads the 3rd and 4th toes and using his index finger pushes up just anterior to the metatarsal heads (Fig. 3-4D).

The fatty tissue is retracted and the vessels are preserved by gentle retraction. A glistening, grayish, indurated mass will then be easily identified. The mass is then carefully dissected. Usually the indurated common digital nerve can be traced running proximally, plantarly, and descending under the transversed metatarsal ligament.

A curved hemostat is placed underneath the ligament and spread apart. The ligament is then cut for better exposure and the common digital nerve is excised (Fig. 3-4E).

The resected mass will have an indurated central mass, a tail made-up of the indurated common digital nerve and two tendril-like arms made up of the proper digital nerves (Fig. 3-4F).

The wound must be closed carefully, layer by layer to avoid any dead spaces which may lead to a hematoma formation. The skin is closed with a continuous lock suture of 5-0 Nylon. The lock suture is used to the beginning of the interdigital space. The part of the incision in the interdigital space is closed with two simple sutures of 5-0 Nylon (Fig. 3-4G).

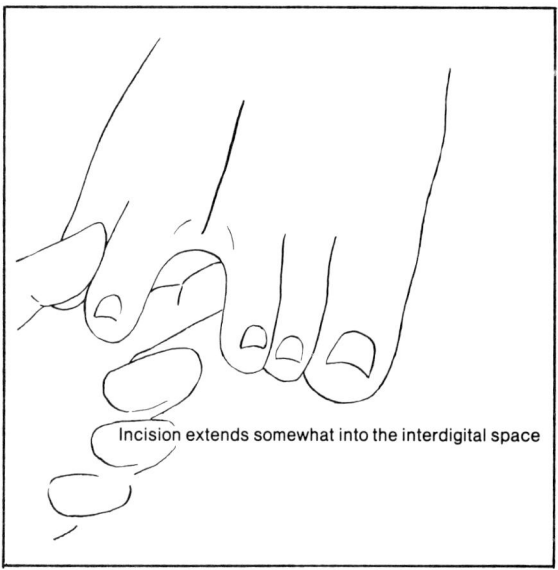

Fig. 3-4C

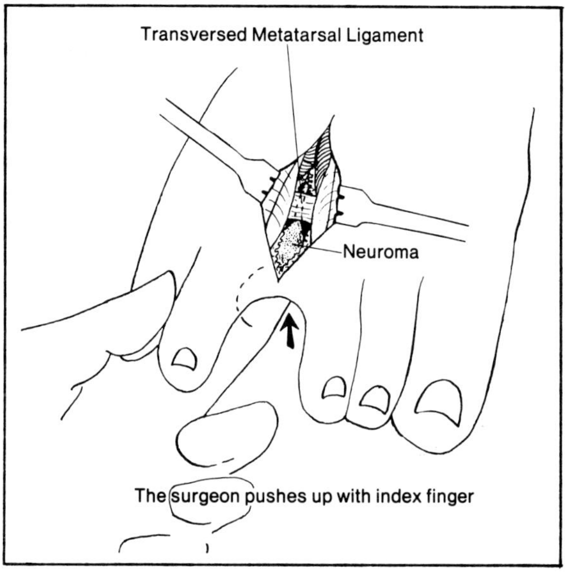

Fig. 3-4D

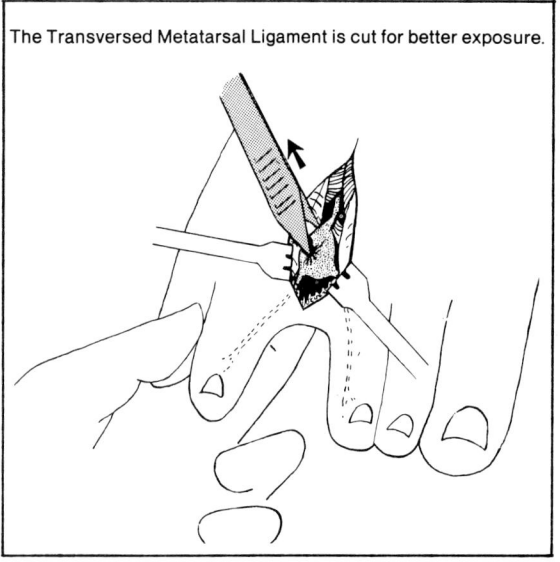

Fig. 3-4E

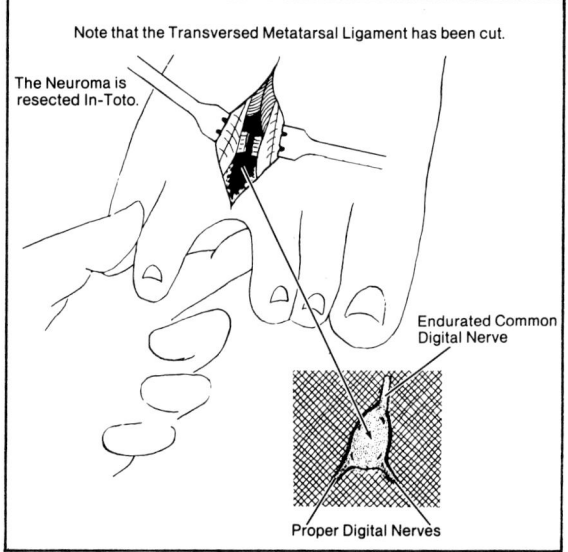

Fig. 3-4F

SOFT TISSUE SURGERY

The continuous Lock suture is used to the beginning of the interdigital space. Two simple sutures are used to close the remaining space.

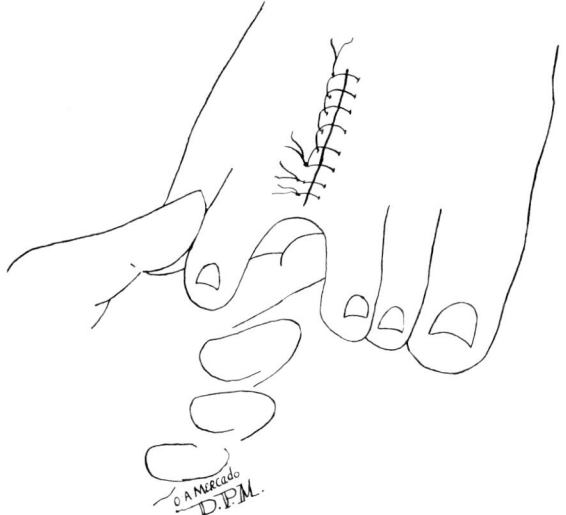

Fig. 3-4G

Precautions

The surgeon should keep the following points in mind when performing neuroma surgery:

1. The neuroma actually lies anterior to the metatarsal heads, hence the incision should be made somewhat into the interdigital space. However, avoid extending the incision **too far** into the interdigital space.
2. Good surgical dissection and hemostasis are essential in order to preserve vessels and afford adequate visualization of the neuroma.
3. One last point—do not be afraid to suggest to the patient an **exploratory operation** in this area if you have good suspicion of a neuroma.

CHAPTER 4—DIGITAL SURGERY

Pressure Deformities
1. Fifth Toe Heloma Durum
2. Hammer Toe
3. Contracted Toe
4. Mallet Toe
5. Heloma Molle
6. Distal Heloma Durum
7. Pinch Callus
8. Interphalangeal Joint Callus
9. Deviated Toe

Congenital Deformities
1. Overlapping Fifth Toe
2. Syndactylism
3. Polydactylism

CHAPTER 4

Digital Surgery

Digital Surgery can be divided into procedures for the correction of **Pressure Deformities** and **Congenital Deformities.**

The Pressure Deformities are the most common and are associated with shoe pressure which usually result in the formation of digital corns. The **Pressure Deformities** include:
1. Fifth Toe Heloma Durum
2. Hammer Toe
3. Contracted Toe
4. Mallet Toe
5. Heloma Molle
6. Distal Heloma Durum
7. Pinch Callus
8. Plantar Interphalangeal Joint Callus
9. Deviated Toe

The **Congenital Deformities** include:
1. Overlapping Fifth Toe
2. Syndactylism
3. Polydactylism

Fifth Toe Heloma Durum

The fifth toe is usually rotated (see Fig. 4-1A) by the shoe and consequently the formation of the hyperkeratotic lesion occurs on the **lateral** aspect of the toe.

Our aim in fifth toe heloma durum surgery is to remove the hypertrophic bone and realign the toe. The hypertrophic bone usually occurs on the lateral-dorsal aspect of the proximal phalangeal head and the dorsal-lateral aspect of the base of the middle phalanx (Fig. 4-1B).

The technique used for the correction of a fifth toe heloma durum is a Partial Phalangectomy (Ostectomy) of the offending bone. This technique is also referred to as an Arthroplasty.

DIGITAL SURGERY

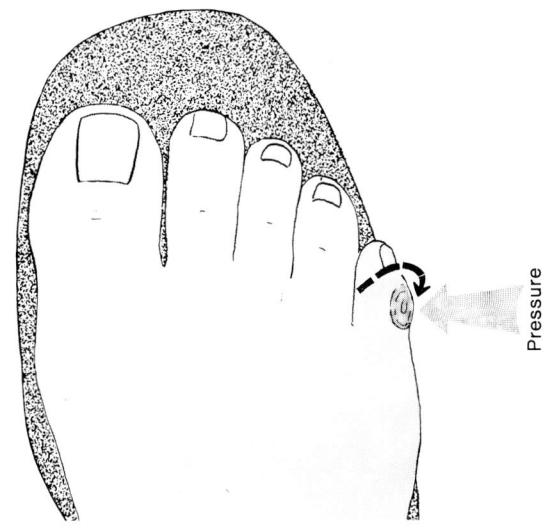

Fig. 4-IA. The fifth toe is usually rotated by the shoe and consequently the formation of the keratotic tissue occurs on the lateral aspect of the toe.

Technique

A lineal skin incision, bisecting the toe in half, is made on the dorsal aspect. A second semi-elliptical incision (Fig. 4-1C) is made joining the ends of the first incision. Care is taken so as not to make this incision too wide as this will create difficulty in closure. One reason for the combination of a straight and semi-elliptical incision is that since most of the lesion is on the lateral aspect of the toe, we want to remove as much of the keratotic tissue as possible. Another important reason is to remove the excessive skin that is created by the resection of the proximal phalangeal head. In essence, when an Arthroplasty is performed, the toe is shortened by the amount of bone that is removed. If the excessive skin is not removed, then there will be a greater likelihood of a **fat toe** forming.

The wedge of skin formed by the two skin incisions is resected and the skin is carefully underscored to either side of the proximal interphalangeal joint. Remember to use clean sharp dissection and avoid cutting or button-holing the skin.

The wound is retracted and the tendon is exposed. A transversed incision is made on the tendon at the widest point of the joint, actually the head of the proximal phalanx (Fig. 4-1D). The tendon is carefully retracted proximally and the collateral ligaments are cut with a collar and crown scissors or a No. 15 blade (Fig. 4-1E).

The head of the proximal phalanx is delivered dorsally for better exposure and cut with a bone forceps just proximal to the articular cartilage (Fig. 4-1F). It is **not** necessary to resect a great deal of bone, just resecting the articular head will give enough movement for the toe to be properly aligned. Also, it is important to cut the bone on an even plane so as to avoid angulation of the shaft.

The bone is then rasped smooth and the toe is pulled distally and plantiflexed. The lateral aspect of the middle phalangeal base is underscored and the hypertrophic bone is resected and rasped smooth. It is important to remove this area of bone as failure to do so may result in recurrence of the hyperkeratotic tissue (Fig. 4-1G).

The toe is then held in proper alignment and the tendon is sutured with two simple sutures of 3-0 Dexon (Fig. 4-1H). The suturing of the tendon is an important step in the procedure as it will:

1. **Derotate** the toe.
2. Prevent a **flail toe.**
3. After the toe is healed, the tendon will become a **viable** part of the digital extensor mechanism.

The wound is then carefully closed with a continuous lock suture, using the material of choice (Fig. 4-1I).

Precautions

Fifth toe Heloma Durum surgery is one of the most common procedures performed in the foot. As such it is extremely important that **good** results be predictable and consistent. The most frequent **pitfalls** encountered are:

1. A **fat toe,** sometimes called a **sausage toe,** is usually the result of too much bone being removed from the proximal phalanx. This creates a dead space in the interphalangeal joint space resulting in an excessive amount of skin left over. The dead space fills up with fibrotic tissue and the excessive skin hypertrophies, leading to the formation of a fat toe. A fat toe can be prevented by taking a wedge of skin with the initial incisions (thus removing the excessive skin which will be left over when the bone is removed); and by resecting very little bone from the proximal phalanx. Remember that the basic problem causing the heloma durum is the position of the toe. All that we have to do is to remove enough bone to allow for the **repositioning** of the toe.

    Incidentally, I have heard a number of speakers advocate that, "...on black patients, the head and part of the proximal phalangeal shaft should be resected to prevent recurrence of the corn". This is an **erroneous statement.** In my own experience, and those of close colleagues, we have performed the Partial Phalangectomy as advocated here (removing very little bone) on **all races** with the same **good** results.

2. **Recurrence** of the corn is usually the result of **failure** to remove the hypertrophic bone on the **lateral aspect** of the middle phalangeal base. The removal of just a small amount of bone from this area (Fig. 4-1G) will prevent recurrence of the corn.

3. A **flail,** or flaccid toe is caused by failure to suture the tendon. It can also be caused by too much bone being removed. Remember that the **suturing** of the tendon is essential in order to retain the tendon as a viable part of the extensor mechanism.

DIGITAL SURGERY

Partial Phalangectomy

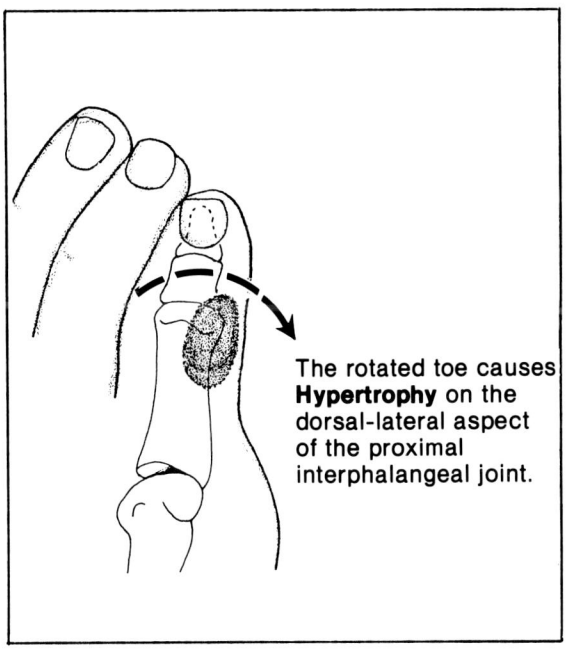

The rotated toe causes **Hypertrophy** on the dorsal-lateral aspect of the proximal interphalangeal joint.

Fig. 4-IB

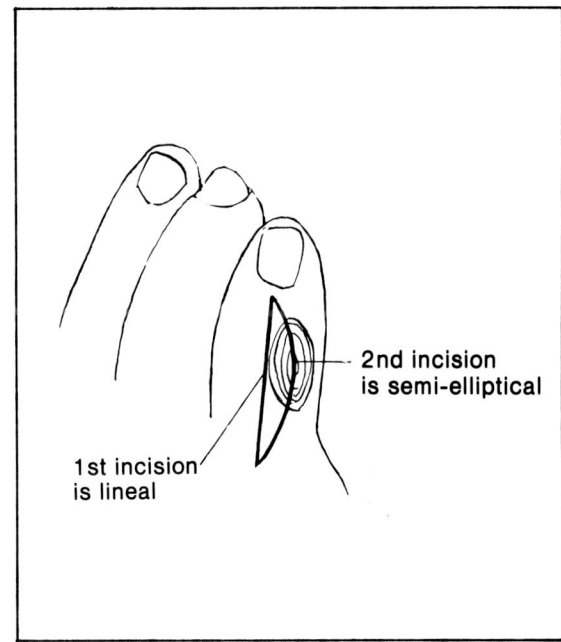

1st incision is lineal

2nd incision is semi-elliptical

Fig. 4-IC

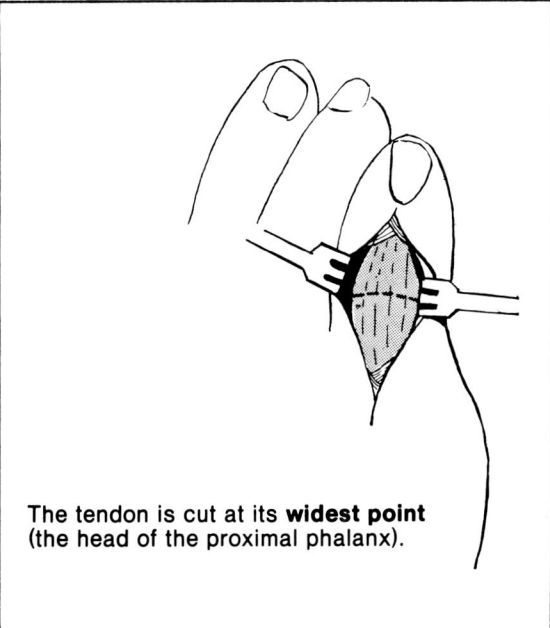

The tendon is cut at its **widest point** (the head of the proximal phalanx).

Fig. 4-ID

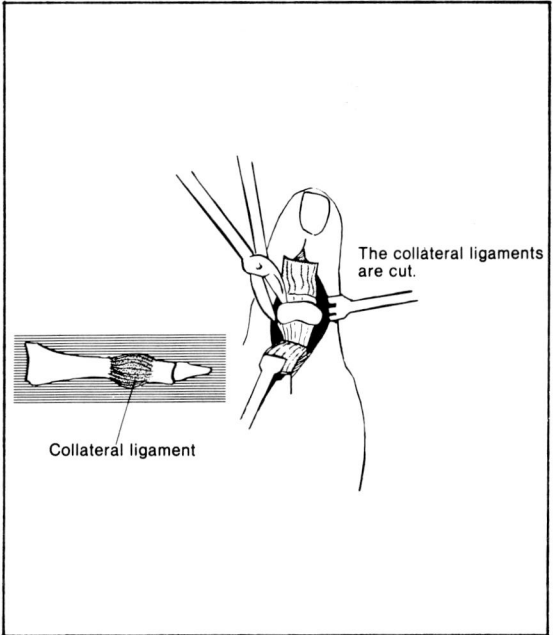

The collateral ligaments are cut.

Collateral ligament

Fig. 4-IE

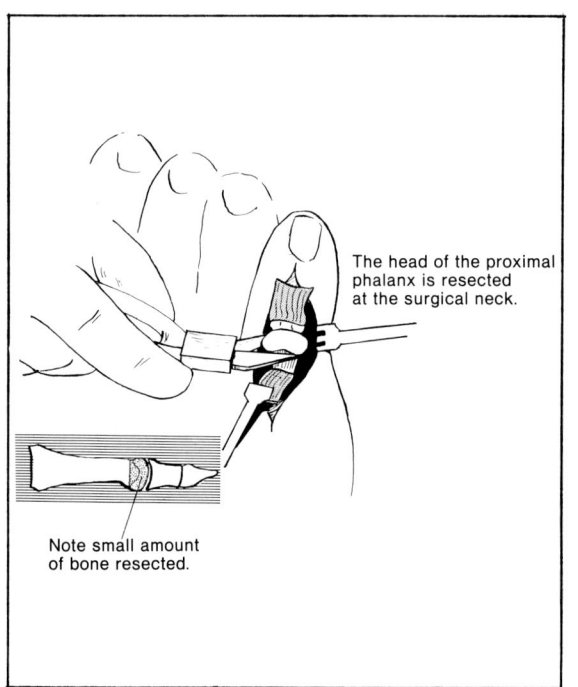

Fig. 4-1F

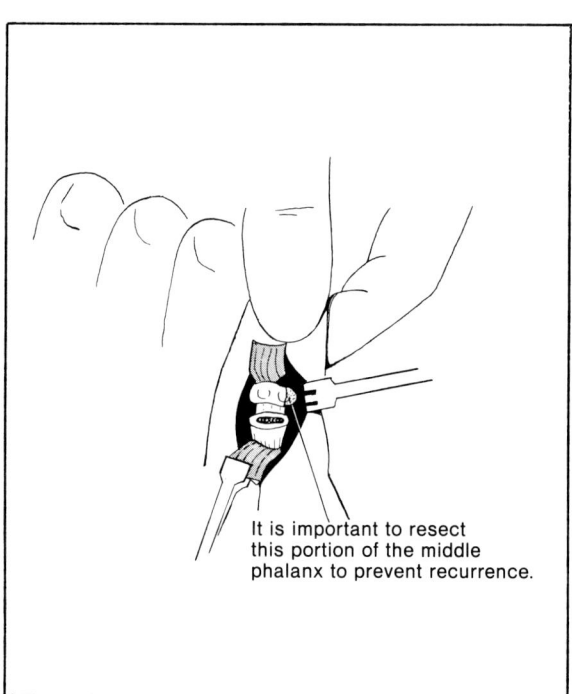

Fig. 4-1G

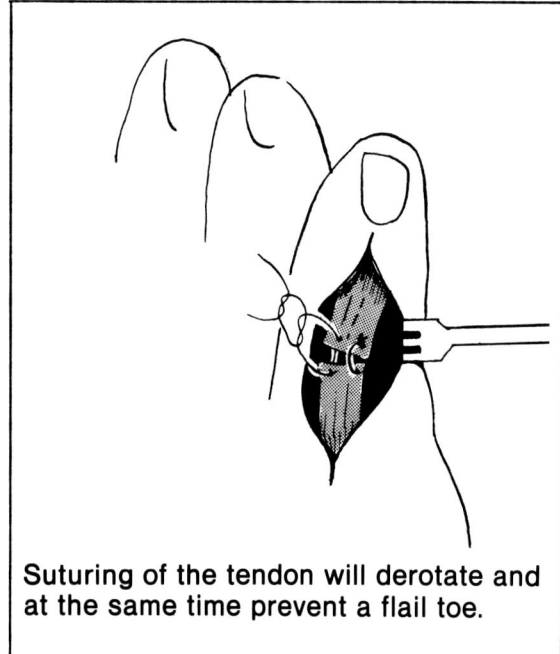

Fig. 4-1H

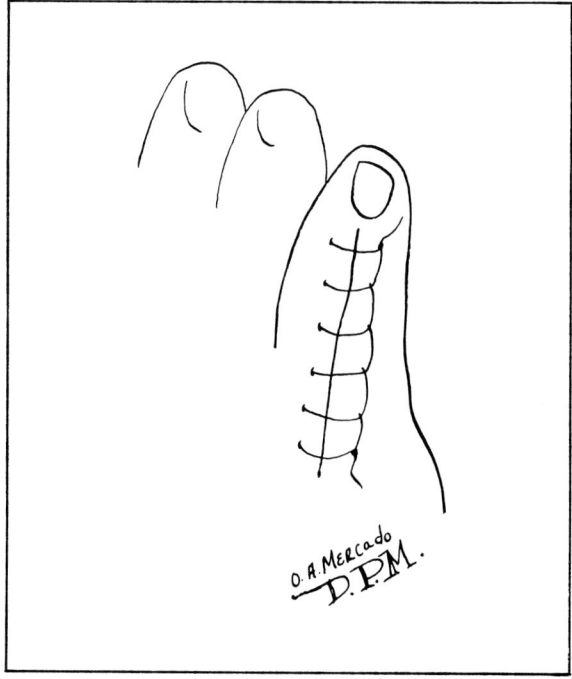

Fig. 4-1I

DIGITAL SURGERY

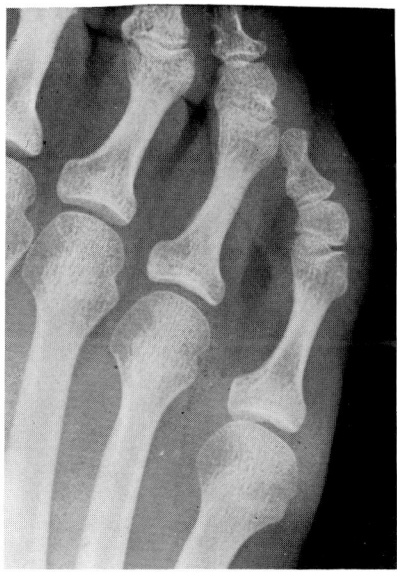

Fig. 4-IJ. Pre-operative x-rays. Patient has painful heloma durum on fourth and fifth toes. Note rotation of fifth toe.

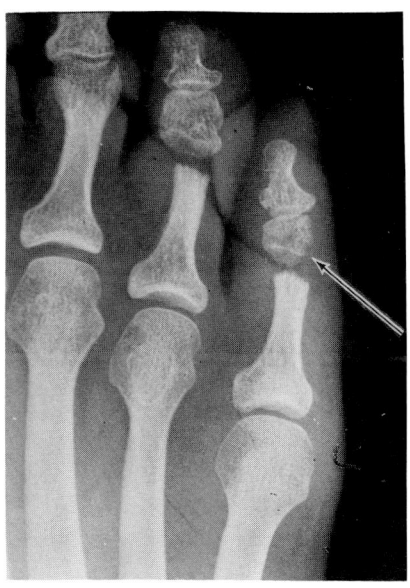

Fig. 4-IK. Post-operative view. Resection of fourth and fifth proximal phalangeal heads is seen. Arrow points to resection of the lateral dorsal aspect of the middle phalanx.

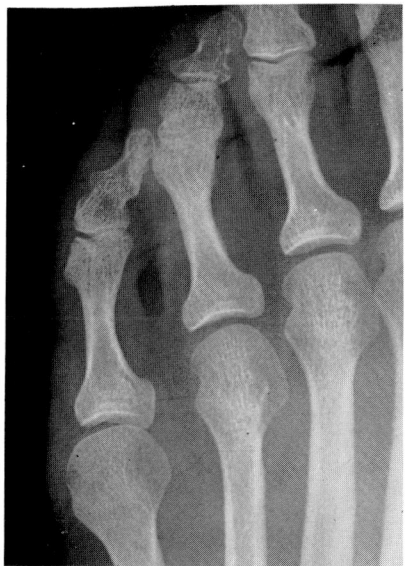

Fig. 4-IL. Pre-operative view. Patient has painful heloma durum on fourth and fifth toes.

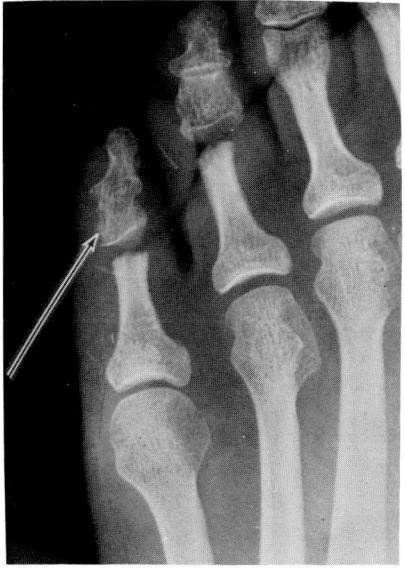

Fig. 4-IM. Post-operative view. Resection of fourth and fifth proximal phalangeal heads and ostectomy lateral-dorsal aspect middle phalanx (arrow). Note also that the toes have been realigned into a normal position.

Hammer Toe

A Hammer Toe will usually occur on the 2nd, 3rd, and 4th toes. It is caused by the buckling of the proximal phalanx on the metatarsal head and a plantar dislocation of the two most distal phalanges. The shoes rub on the dorsum of these toes and a hyperkeratotic lesion is formed. As time passes, the toe is permanently fused in its **deformed** state and surgery is required to correct the problem.

Our surgery aims at the resection of the proximal phalangeal head (Partial Phalangectomy) to release the buckling effect and allow the toe to lay in a straight, more normal position.

Technique

Since most of the hyperkeratotic lesion is on the dorsal aspect of the toe, our approach is by two semi-elliptical incisions. (See Fig. 4-2A).

It is important not to make these skin incisions too wide as this would create difficulty in closure. The reason for the two semi-elliptical incisions is to take up the excess skin which will be left over after the bone is removed.

The incisions are deepened and the wound is underscored staying close to the interphalangeal joint. We stick close to the joint when underscoring because most of the blood vessels and nerves are in the fatty layer beneath the skin and they must be **preserved** (Fig. 4-2B).

The wound is retracted and the tendon is exposed. The Extensor Digitorum Longus tendon at this level expands into an aponeurosis which blends in with the capsular ligament. Very seldom do we see the classical dorsal tendon which bifurcates into three slips, one going to the middle phalanx and the other two slips inserting into the distal phalanx.

The Tendo-aponeurosis is cut at its widest point with a transversed incision (Fig. 4-2C). The tendon is then carefully underscored and retracted proximally and distally so as to expose the joint. The only tissues holding the joint now are the collateral ligaments. These ligaments are cut and the proximal phalangeal head is exposed (Fig. 4-2D). The head is cut just proximal to the articular facet. It **is not** necessary to resect a great deal of bone to obtain the desired correction (Fig. 4-2E).

The bone is rasped smooth, the toe is held in the corrected position and the tendon is sutured with two simple sutures of 3-0 Dexon (Fig. 4-2F). The wound is closed with a continuous lock suture using the material of choice (Fig. 4-2G, H).

Precautions

Hammer Toe surgery will yield **consistently good results** if the Surgeon remembers to do the following:

1. Remove only the amount of bone which is needed to correct the deformity.
2. Suture the tendon to maintain the corrected alignment of the toe and insure extensor mechanism viability.

Hammer Toe Operation

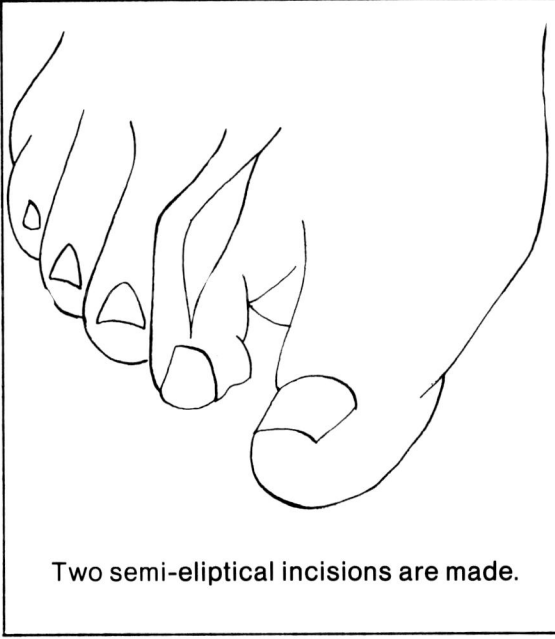

Two semi-eliptical incisions are made.

Fig. 4-2A

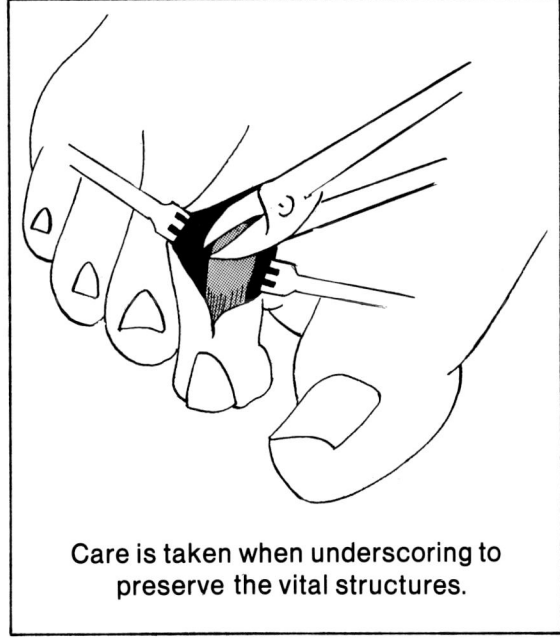

Care is taken when underscoring to preserve the vital structures.

Fig. 4-2B

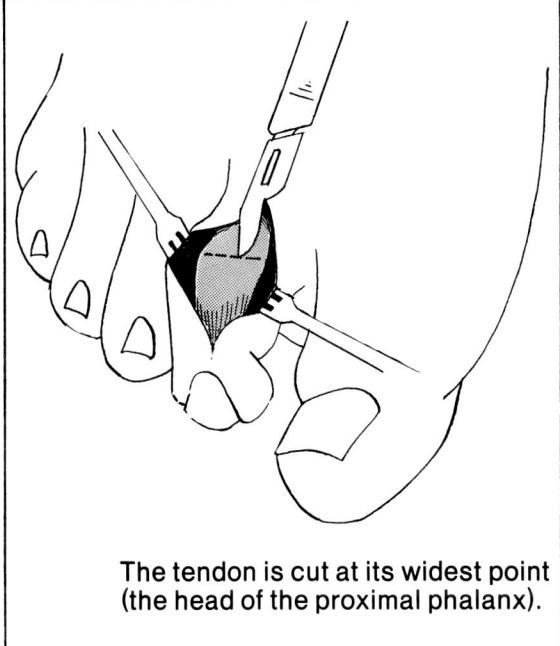

The tendon is cut at its widest point (the head of the proximal phalanx).

Fig. 4-2C

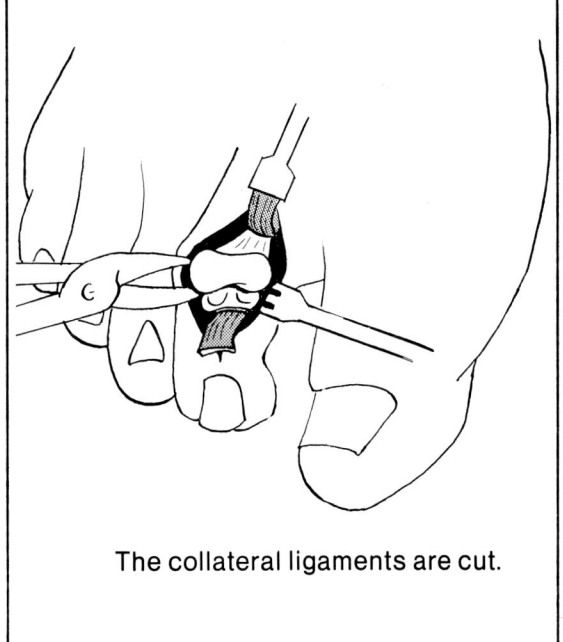

The collateral ligaments are cut.

Fig. 4-2D

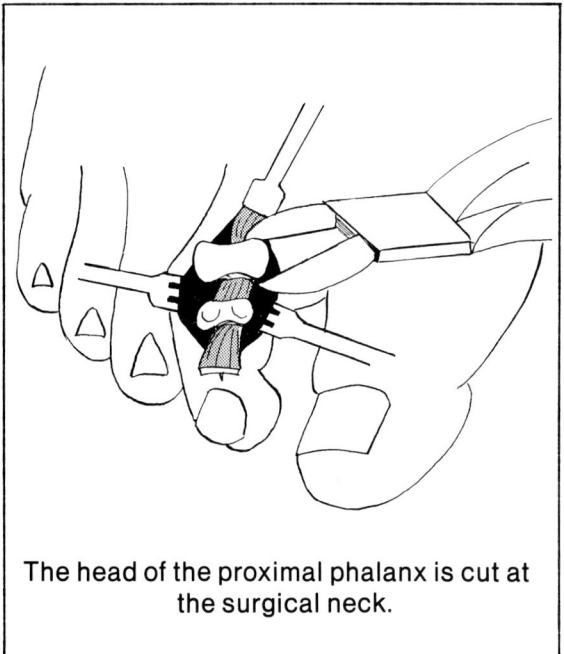

The head of the proximal phalanx is cut at the surgical neck.

Fig. 4-2E

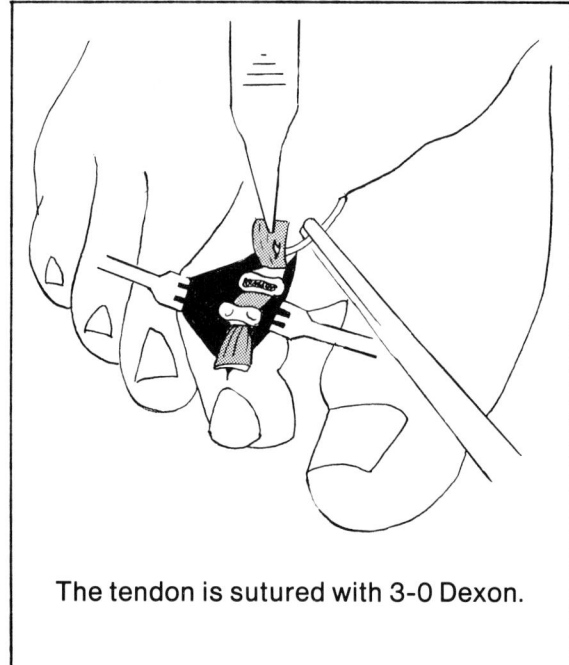

The tendon is sutured with 3-0 Dexon.

Fig. 4-2F

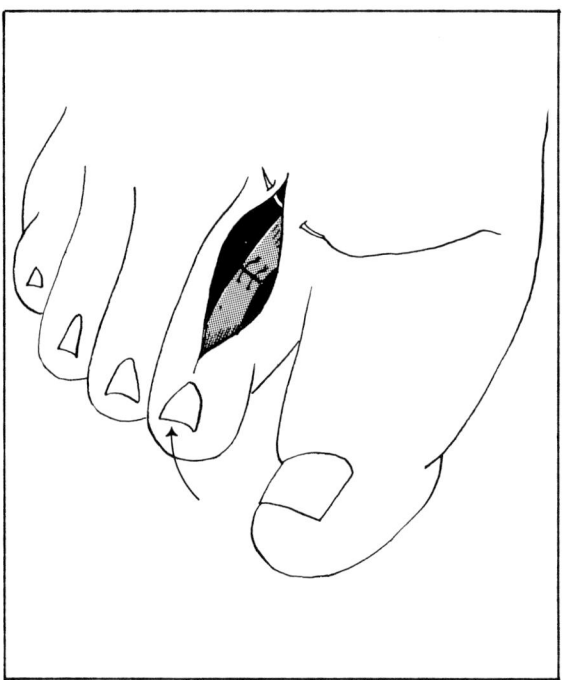

Fig. 4-2G

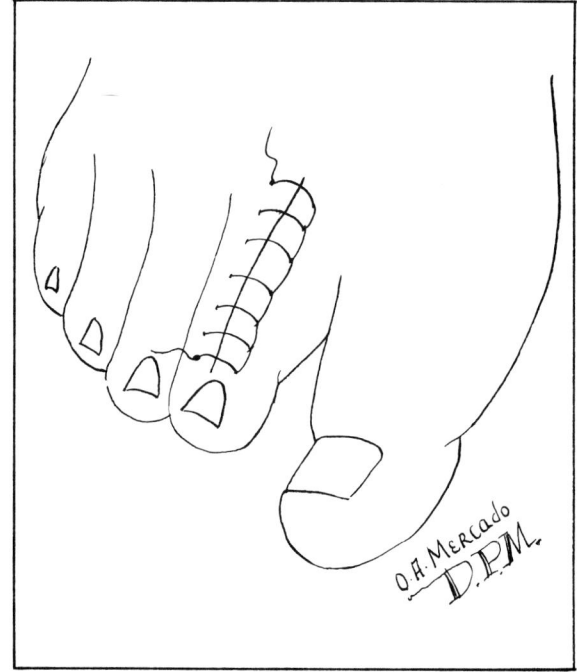

Fig. 4-2H

DIGITAL SURGERY

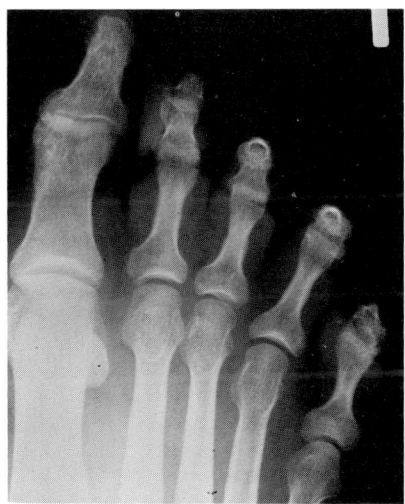

Fig. 4-2I. Pre-operative x-rays. Hammer toes 2, 3, 4 and 5. Note 3rd and 4th distal phalanges are not visible.

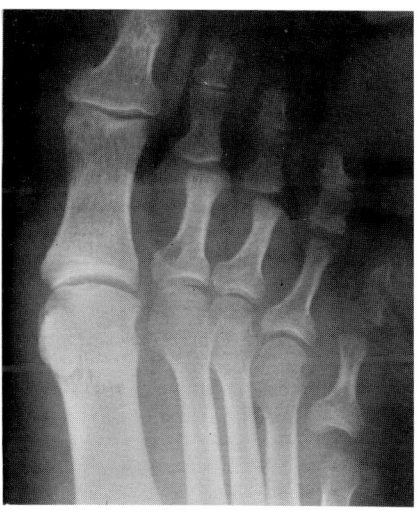

Fig. 4-2J. Post-operative x-rays. Note proper alignment of toes — all phalanges are now visible.

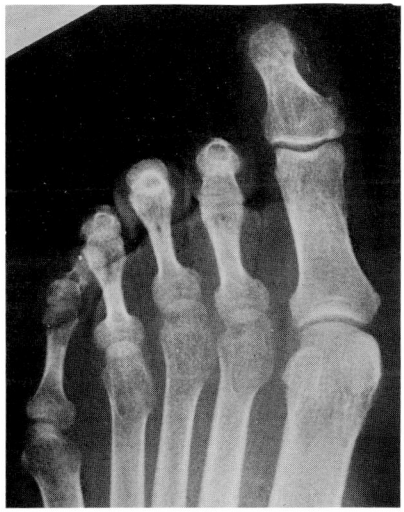

Fig. 4-2K. Pre-operative x-rays reveal hammer toes 2, 3 and 4. Note marked planti-flexion of distal phalanges.

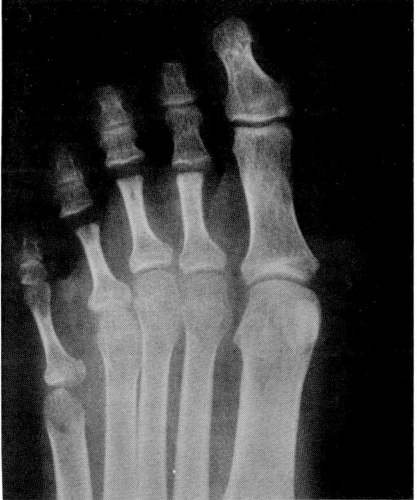

Fig. 4-2L. Post-operative x-rays reveal normal alignment of phalanges.

Contracted Toe

A contracted toe is nothing more than a **flexible hammer toe.** The proximal phalanx is buckled against the head of the metatarsal and the two most distal phalanges are planti-flexed due to the strong pull of the Flexor Digitorum Longus. A contracted toe is found usually on the second, third, and fourth toes, and as a rule occurs on younger individuals.

Our surgery aims at the correction of the problem by the resection of the proximal phalangeal head, to create a joint space and the release of the strong Flexor Digitorum Longus pull by a tenotomy and dorsal relocation (transfer).

Anatomy

On a lateral view, we can see two extensor tendons (Extensor Digitorum Longus and Brevis) and two flexor tendons (Flexor Digitorum Longus and Brevis).

On the **dorsal aspect** the Extensor Digitorum Longus is the most superficial tendon. The Extensor Digitorum Brevis is plantar and lateral to the longus and blends in with it to form a single tendon.

On the **plantar aspect,** the Flexor Digitorum Brevis is the most superficial tendon and, since it has to insert into the base of the middle phalanx, it bifurcates to allow for the passage of Flexor Digitorum Longus and rejoins again to form an aponeurotic insertion (Fig. 4-3A) into the base of the middle phalanx.

In a **contracted toe,** the pull of the flexor is such that it causes a buckling effect on the proximal interphalangeal joint. The proximal phalanx dorsiflexes, thus pulling on the plantar capsule of the metatarsal phalangeal joint and causing an anterior displacement of the fat pad (Fig. 4-3A).

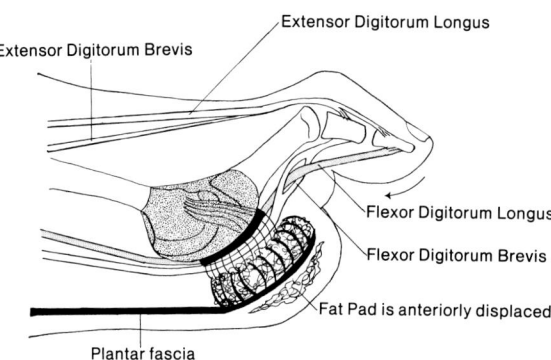

Fig. 4-3A

Technique

Our approach is the same as for a hammer toe. After the head of the proximal phalanx is resected, the shaft is underscored and retracted dorsally as far as it can go to expose the tendon of Flexor Digitorum Brevis which lies immediately under the phalanx.

A lineal incision is then made on the tendon (Fig. 4-3B). The incision is retracted and with a curved hemostat the Flexor Digitorum Longus tendon is delivered dorsally through the incision (Fig. 4-3C). The tendon of Flexor Digitorum Longus is pulled vigorously and cut as far distally as possible. The tendon is then split into two slips (Fig. 4-3D).

The slips are pulled around the shaft of the proximal phalanx and sutured in place (Fig. 4-3E) with 3-0 Dexon. The dorsal tendon is also sutured with 3-0 Dexon. The skin is closed using a continuous lock suture with the material of choice.

The transfer of the Flexor tendon will planti-flex the proximal phalanx and in time the contracted plantar metatarsal phalangeal joint capsule and displaced fat pad, will return to their normal position (Fig. 4-3F).

DIGITAL SURGERY

Flexor Tendon Transfer Operation

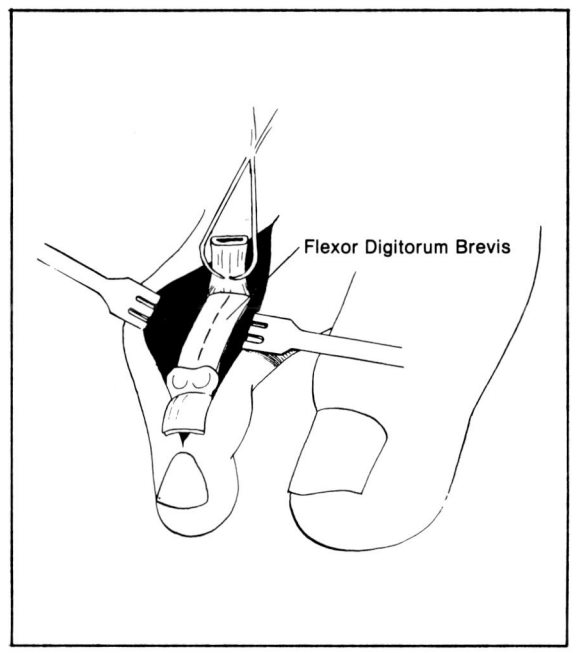

Fig. 4-3B

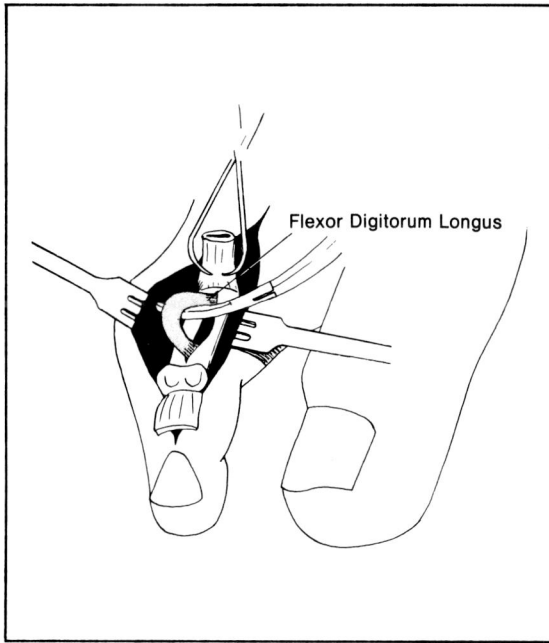

Fig. 4-3C

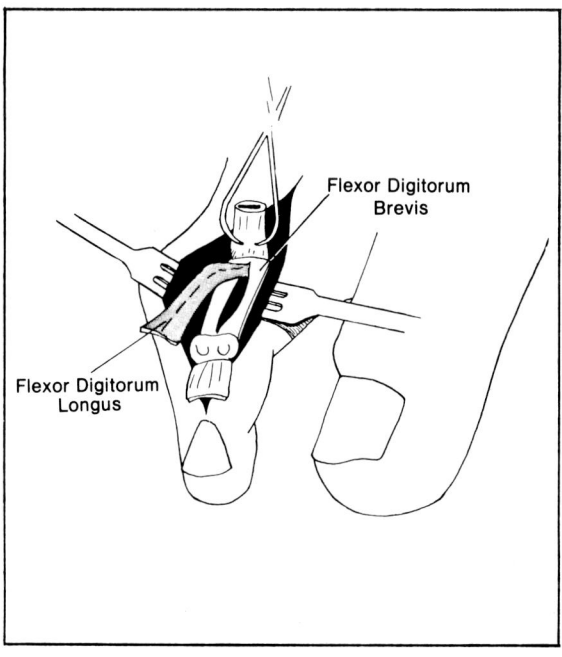

Fig. 4-3D

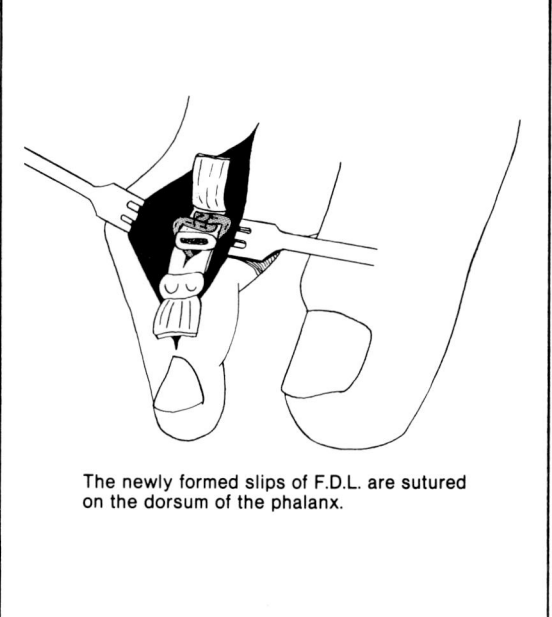

The newly formed slips of F.D.L. are sutured on the dorsum of the phalanx.

Fig. 4-3E

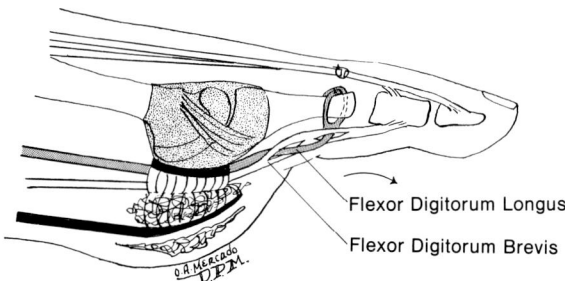

Fig. 4-3F

Precautions

The flexor transfer operation is one of those operations which make a great deal of sense from an anatomical standpoint but, with the exception of a few cases, will not live up to its expectation.

This is not to say that the operation is useless, but rather, that its application is **very limited.** In order to obtain the best results with this operation the surgeon should keep these points in mind:
1. This procedure will work best on **younger** individuals where the tissues are still pliable enough to allow them to return to their normal position.
2. This procedure will work best on the second digit since the anatomical structures are larger and hence easier to work with.
3. It is important to cut the flexor tendon as far distally as possible. The longer the tendon is, the easier it will be to relocate (transfer) the slips to the dorsum of the phalanx.
4. While this procedure, if it works well, will alleviate a mild plantar callus under the metatarsal phalangeal joint. It is **not** intended to be used primarily for the correction of an intractable plantar keratosis.

Mallet Toe

A mallet toe is formed by a marked planti-flexion deformity of the distal phalanx on the middle phalangeal head.

This acute planti-flexion often leads to the formation of hyperkeratotic lesion on the dorsal aspect of the distal interphalangeal joint and frequently on the plantar aspect of the tip of the toe (Fig. 4-4A).

Our surgery for the mallet toe deformity aims at the resection of the middle phalangeal head, to create a joint space, and the realignment of the distal tip of the toe.

DIGITAL SURGERY

Technique

Two semi-elliptical incisions are made surrounding the dorsal hyperkeratotic lesion on the distal interphalangeal joint. It is important **not** to carry these incisions too far plantarly on the medial or lateral side of the toe as this could interfere with the fragile vascular supply (Fig. 4-4A).

The incisions are deepened and the wedge of skin formed is resected. The wound is carefully underscored to expose the tendon over the joint. A transversed incision is made on the tendon immediately over the middle phalangeal head (Fig. 4-4B).

The tendon is carefully retracted and the collateral ligaments are cut. The head is exposed and retracted out of the wound as much as possible. The head of the phalanx is then resected and the bone is rasped smooth (Fig. 4-4D).

The toe is realigned into its proper position and the tendon is sutured with two simple sutures of 3-0 Dexon (Fig. 4-4E). The wound is closed with a continuous lock suture and the foot is dressed in the usual manner (Fig. 4-4E).

Precautions

Mallet toe surgery will yield consistently good results and may be performed on any patient with patent circulation and no medical contraindications. The most important precautions are:

1. Take care not to carry the skin incisions too far plantarly on the medial or lateral side. The circulation to the distal tip of the toe is **very fragile** and any interruption will have deleterious effects.
2. Because of the semi-elliptical incisions, the exposure to the phalangeal head will be somewhat cramped. The Surgeon must fight off the temptation to overexpose the area, as this could lead to an **ischemic digit.**

Mallet Toe Operation

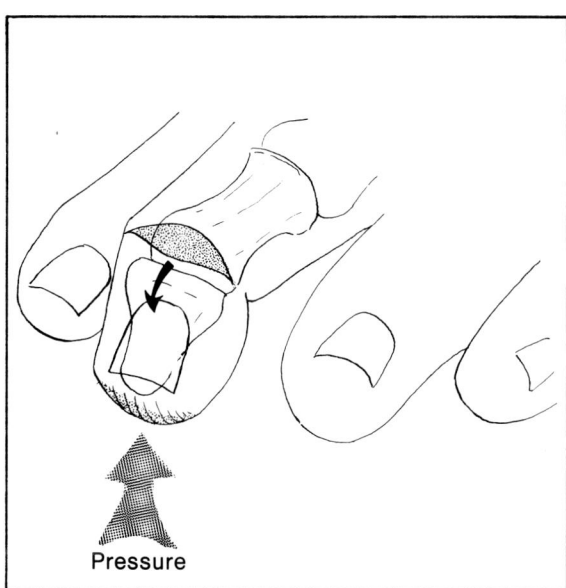

Fig. 4-4A

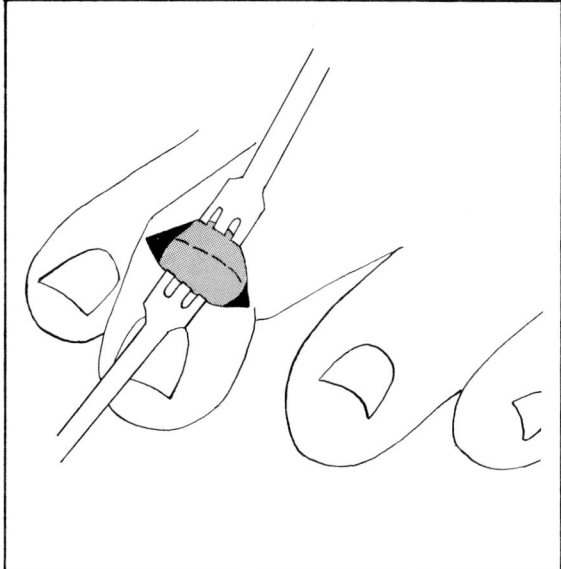

Fig. 4-4B

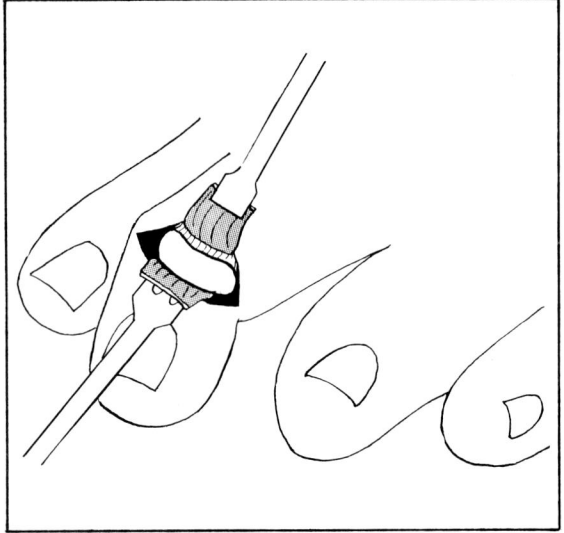

Fig. 4-4D

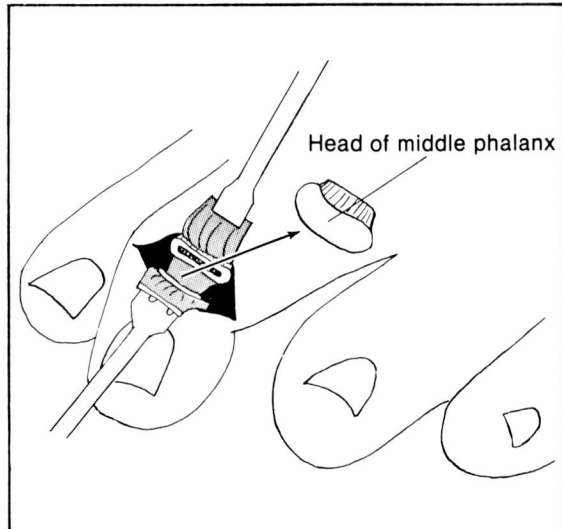

Head of middle phalanx

Fig. 4-4C

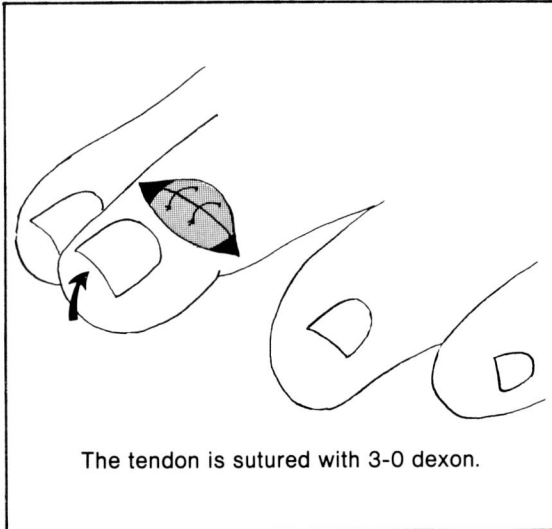

The tendon is sutured with 3-0 dexon.

Fig. 4-4E

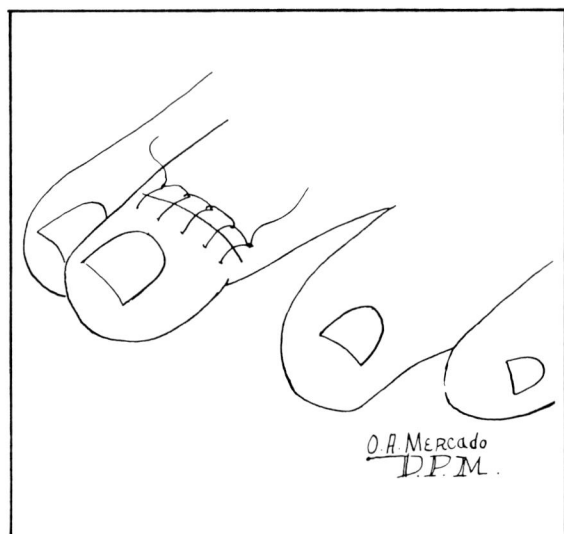

Fig. 4-4F

Heloma Molle

A heloma molle is a localized keratosis caused by intermittent pressure and rubbing between the head of the fifth proximal phalanx and the lateral aspect of the fourth proximal phalangeal base.

Sometimes, a bursal sac (or even a neuroma) is found in the fourth intermetatarsal area (Fig. 4-5A).

Our surgery aims at the correction of the problem by 1. resection of the hypertrophic lateral base of the fourth proximal phalanx; 2. a fifth toe arthroplastly; 3. resection of the bursal sac (neuroma, etc.) if present.

DIGITAL SURGERY

Technique

A lineal incision is made extending from the lateral aspect of the fourth metatarsal phalangeal joint unto the base of the fourth toe. Note that we avoid going into the interdigital space as the tissues here are usually macerated and not conducive to sound wound healing. Also, an incision into the interdigital space would not afford adequate exposure (Fig. 4-5B) for this procedure.

The incision is deepened, and the intermetatarsal area is explored for a possible mass. If one is found, it is resected in-toto. An incision is then made on the metatarsal phalangeal joint capsular ligament lateral to the tendon of Extensor Digitorum Longus (Fig. 4-5C).

The capsule is carefully underscored and the lateral aspect of the phalangeal base is exposed and resected (Fig. 4-5D and E). The capsule is then carefully closed with 3-0 Dexon. The wound is closed using a continuous lock suture with the material of choice.

An arthroplasty is then performed on the fifth toe. The wounds are dressed in the usual manner, healing is uneventful.

Precautions

Heloma Molle surgery is really not difficult and when performed well, it will yield consistently good results. Some points to keep in mind are:

1. Perform the fourth proximal phalangeal base osteotomy first, that way the toes can be manipulated without fear of disturbing the fifth toe surgery.
2. Get adequate exposure to the fourth phalangeal base to insure adequate removal of bone and exploration for any masses that may be found in the intermetatarsal space.

Heloma Molle Operation

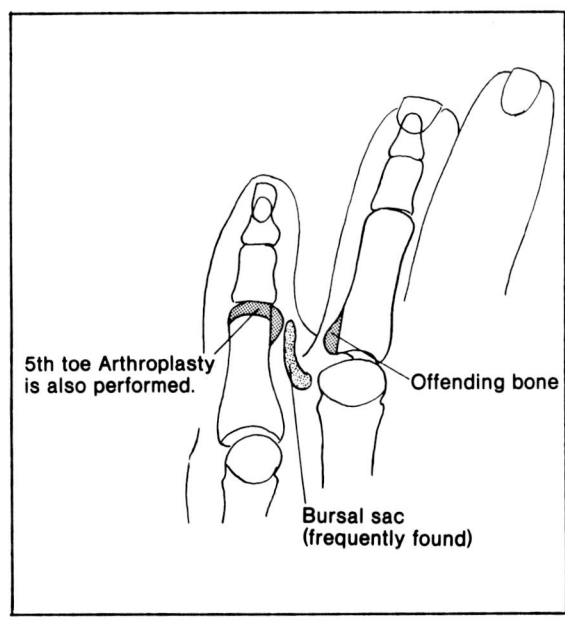

Fig. 4-5A

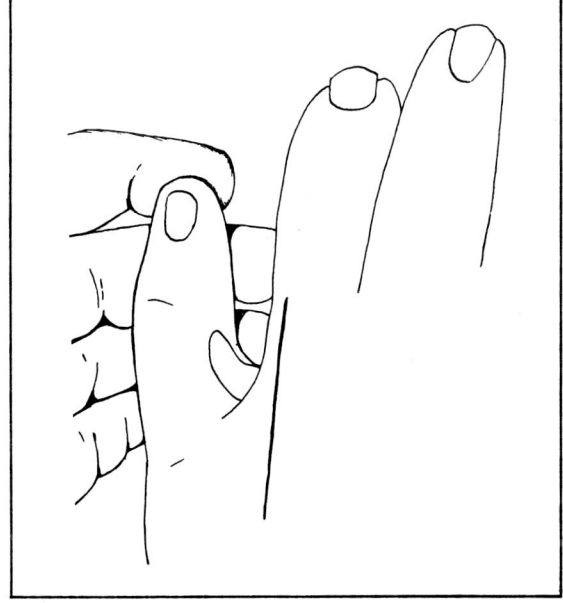

Fig. 4-5B

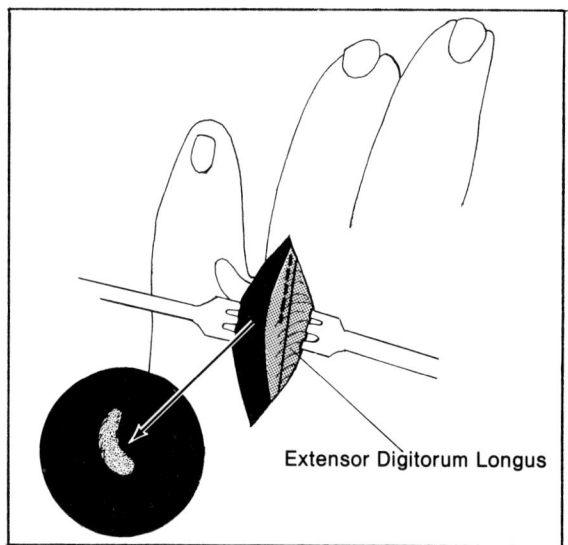

Fig. 4-5C

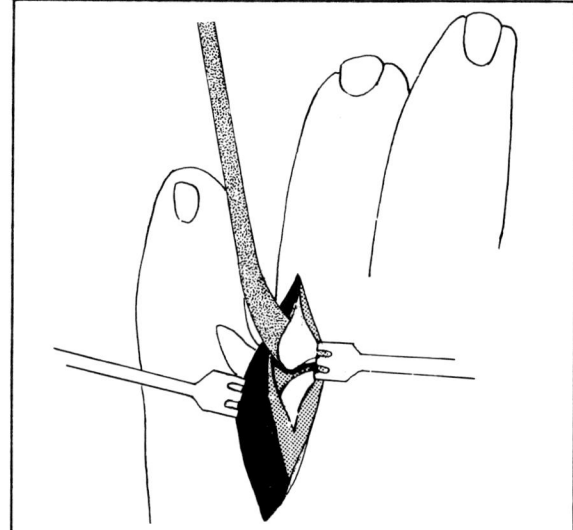

Fig. 4-5D

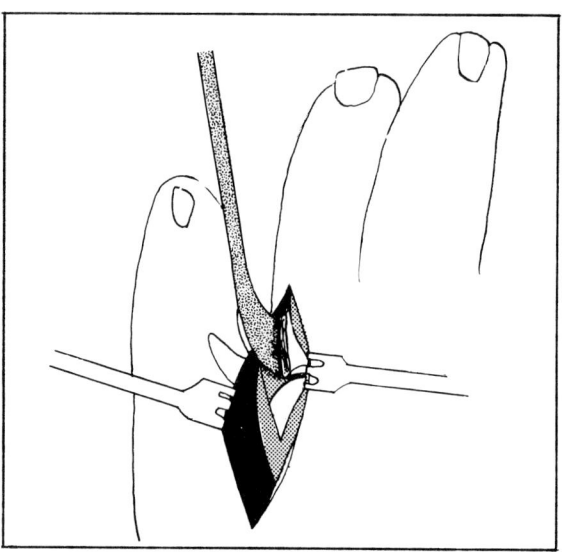

Fig. 4-5E

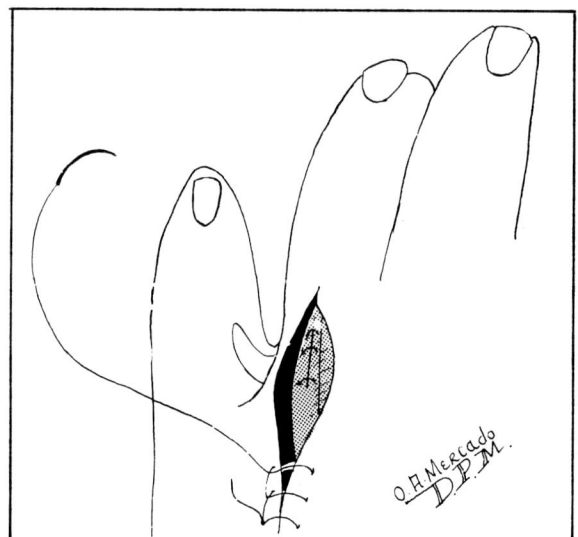

Fig. 4-5F

Distal Heloma Durum

The Distal Heloma Durum is as a rule found on the fifth toe, and it may or may not be associated with a Heloma Durum over the proximal interphalangeal joint. It usually occurs on the distal-lateral aspect of the toe, but sometimes it is found on the distal-medial aspect.

The cause of the Distal Heloma Durum is an enlargement of the distal phalangeal tip. I like to tell the students that the distal phalanx is shaped somewhat like a **Mexican sombrero,** and that the exostosis of a Distal Heloma Durum is caused by an enlargement on the **brim** of the sombrero (Fig. 4-6).

DIGITAL SURGERY

Distal Heloma Durum

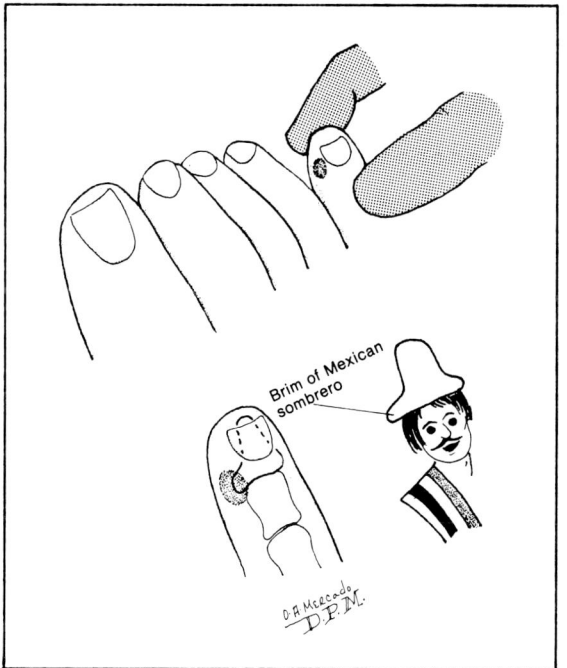

Fig. 4-6

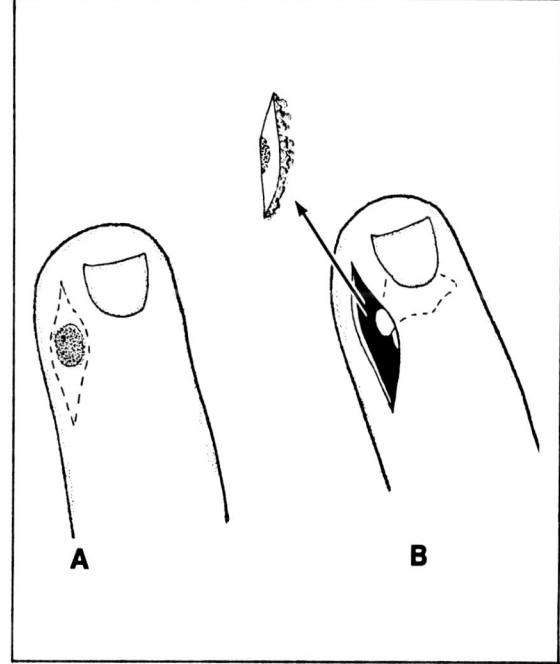

Fig. 4-7A-B

Our surgery aims at the removal of the exostosis by:
1. Simple Ostectomy, or
2. Bone Rasping (Osteotripsy)

Simple Ostectomy

The Simple Ostectomy technique, as can be seen in Fig. 4-7A-D is performed as follows:

Two semi-elliptical incisions are made surrounding the keratotic lesion, or most of the lesion in the case of a very large keratosis. The incisions are deepened to the bone and the keratosis is removed.

The tissues are underscored and the exostosis is exposed and resected. Care is taken to remove the exostosis even with the distal phalangeal shaft and avoiding injury to the articular cartilage. The wound is closed with simple sutures of 5-0 Nylon. Healing is uneventful.

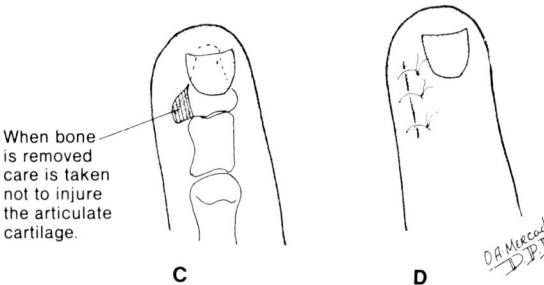

Fig. 4-7C-D

Bone Rasping Technique

Removal of an exostosis by rasping is not new in medicine. In fact, it is commonly used by Plastic Surgeons in rhinoplasties. In foot surgery, however, rasping techniques did not come into vogue until the middle sixties. The first man to write on the subject of rasping techniques for foot surgery, was **Morton Polokoff.** In his 1962 article entitled, "Raspostectomy of Exostoses and Hypertrophied Condyles with Files and Rasps", he stated that he had been teaching colleagues his rasping techniques since 1951.

Because of its relative simplicity to the surgeon and patient and its adaptability to foot surgery, the use of rasping techniques rapidly spread throughout the country: having as its principal advocator and teacher, **Edwin Prober.**

Osteotripsy

The term Osteotripsy did not come into general usage until the late sixties. It was suggested by **Saxon,** the Secretary Consultant of the American Podiatry Association Nomenclature Committee in 1964, to replace the more common term "Raspostectomy". **Osteotripsy** is now included as the acceptable term in the Standard Podiatric Nomenclature of Diseases and Operations.

Osteotripsy Technique for Distal Heloma Durum

A small incision is made on the distal aspect of the toe. The incision is deepened. A small periosteal elevator is then used to underscore the wound and free all of the tissues around the exostosis (Fig. 4-8A-B-C).

A small hand rasp, a power drill can also be used, is introduced into the wound and the exostosis is rasped smooth (Fig. 4-8D). Saline solution is then used to flush out the toothpaste-like residue created by the rasping (Fig. 4-8E).

After the wound is flushed, a **puckering** of the tissue over the area of the exostosis will be noted. This indicates that an adequate amount of bone has been resected (Fig. 4-8F). The wound is closed with a steri-strip or one simple suture. Healing is uneventful (Fig. 4-8G).

DIGITAL SURGERY

Bone Rasping Technique

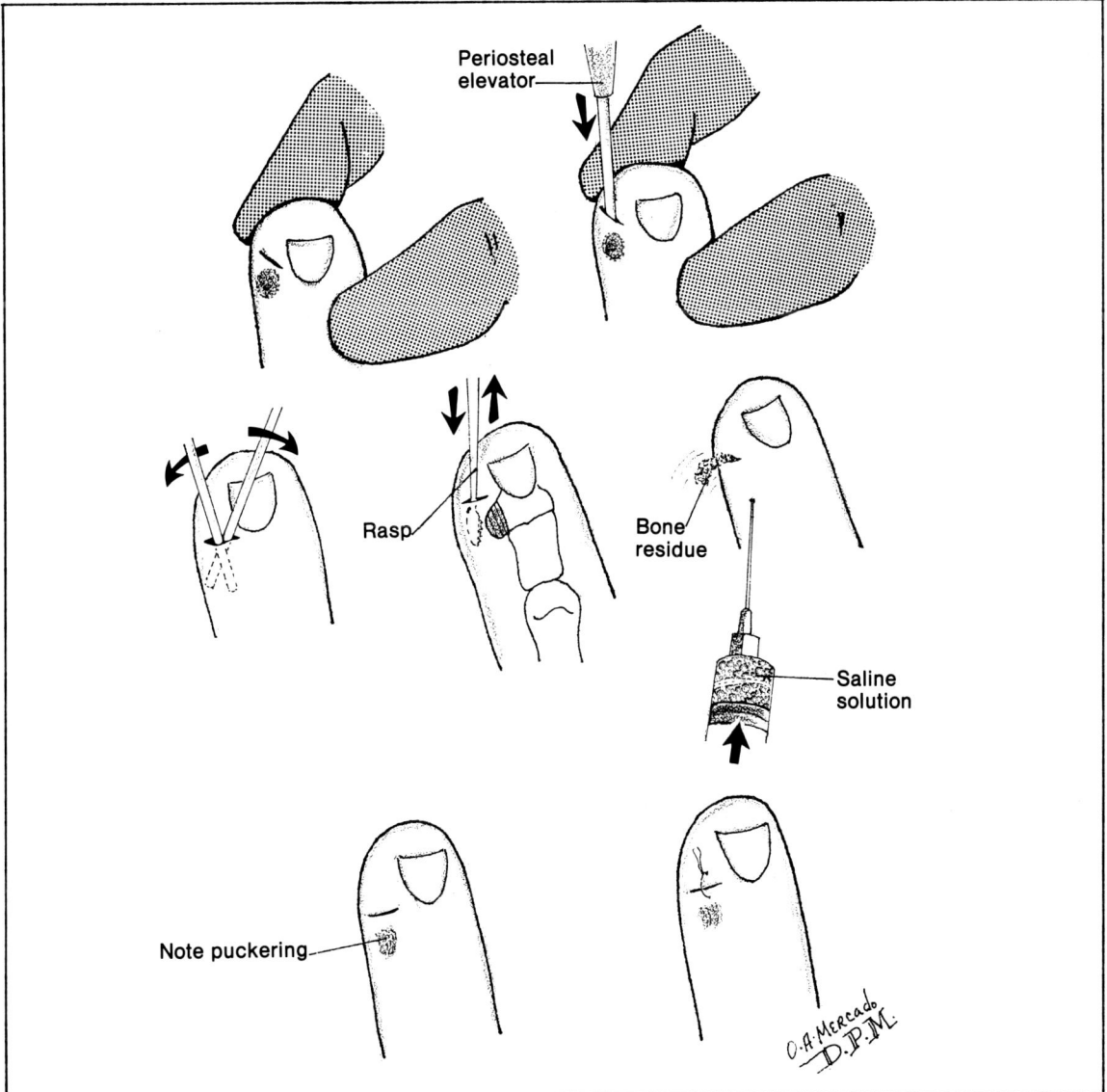

Fig. 4-8

Precautions

The osteotripsy technique for correction of a Distal Heloma Durum is a safe and excellent method for removing the offending Hyperostosis. However, the surgeon should remember to:

1. Remove enough bone to cause a puckering of the tissue over the area of the exostosis.
2. Flush the area clean.
3. Close the wound with a simple suture or a steri-strip.

Hyperkeratotic Lesions on the Hallux

Hyperkeratotic lesions found on the hallux are generally of two types:
1. The Pinch Callus
2. The Plantar Interphalangeal Joint Callus

It is important that the Surgeon evaluate the condition correctly to avoid the high percentage of surgical failures often found in this area.

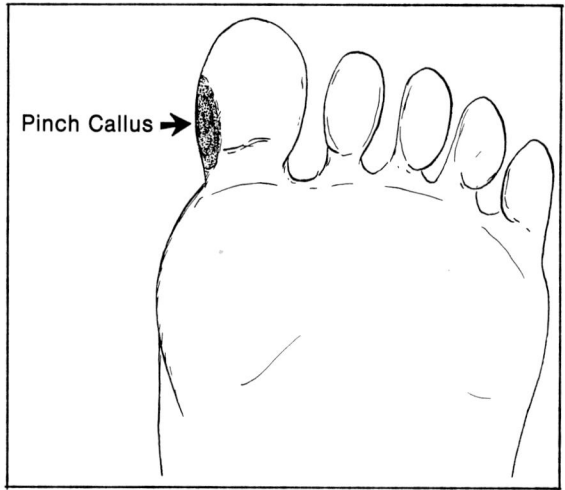

Fig. 4-9A

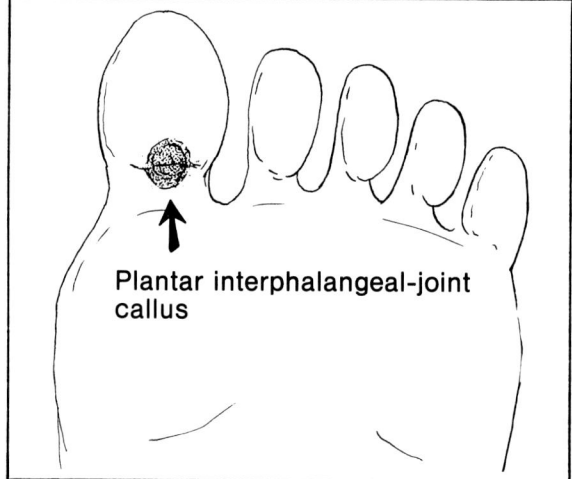

Fig. 4-9B

Pinch Callus

The Pinch Callus is usually found on the medial-plantar aspect of the hallux (Fig. 4-9A). It is usually the result of external pressure on the medial interphalangeal joint (Fig. 4-9C-D). Often it is found in the rotated great toe of Hallux Abducto Valgus.

When the condition is found associated with Hallux Abducto Valgus, and is of a mild nature, the derotation of the toe during Hallux Abducto Valgus Surgery will correct the problem.

When the condition is found in an essentially straight hallux, then surgery must be performed directly on the interphalangeal joint to alleviate the problem.

Occasionally, a Pinch Callus is present on a **rotated** hallux, **not associated** with Hallux Abducto Valgus. Our surgery then aims at the derotation of the hallux by performing a rotational osteotomy.

Pre-operative Evaluation

As stated before, the surgeon must first be certain that the Pinch Callus is caused by the hypertrophic interphalangeal joint, and not an accessory interphalangeal sesamoid.

A Pinch Callus will be found on the medial-plantar aspect of the hallux. An interphalangeal sesamoid will most often cause a circumscribed callus on the plantar interphalangeal joint area (Fig. 4-9B). X-rays will of course make the differential diagnosis easier. But, it is best to remember that sometimes when the interphalangeal sesamoid is small, it is very hard to visualize roentgenographically. Of course, it is possible to find a Pinch Callus and an Interphalangeal Joint Callus on the same patient.

DIGITAL SURGERY

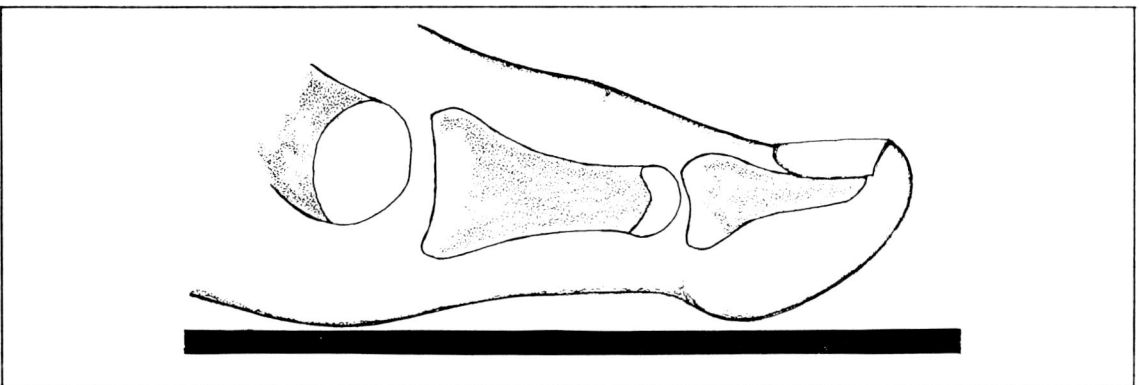

Fig. 4-9C

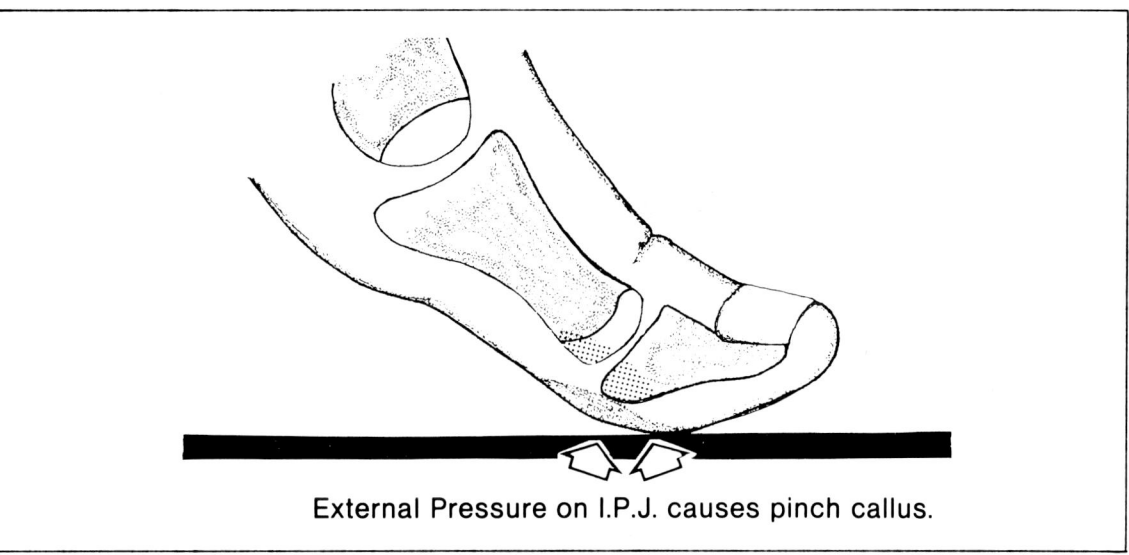

External Pressure on I.P.J. causes pinch callus.

Fig. 4-9D

Our surgical technique aims at the resection of the hyperostotic portion on the medial-plantar aspect of the interphalangeal joint (Fig. 4-10A shaded area).

An incision approximately 4 cm. in length, is made on the medial aspect of the hallux. The incision is deepened and retracted to expose the interphalangeal capsular ligament. The ligament is incised and carefully retracted to expose the hyperostotic base of the distal phalanx and head of the proximal phalanx (Fig. 4-10B).

With a small osteotome, the hypertrophic bone is excised (Fig. 4-10C). The bone is then rounded with a curved bone forceps, and rasped smooth. It is essential that **enough bone** is resected as failure to do so will result in an inordinate amount of surgical failures.

The capsule is carefully closed with 3-0 Dexon. The wound is then closed with a continuous lock suture with the material of choice. The wound is dressed in the usual manner, healing is uneventful (Fig. 4-10D).

Surgical Technique for Straight Hallux

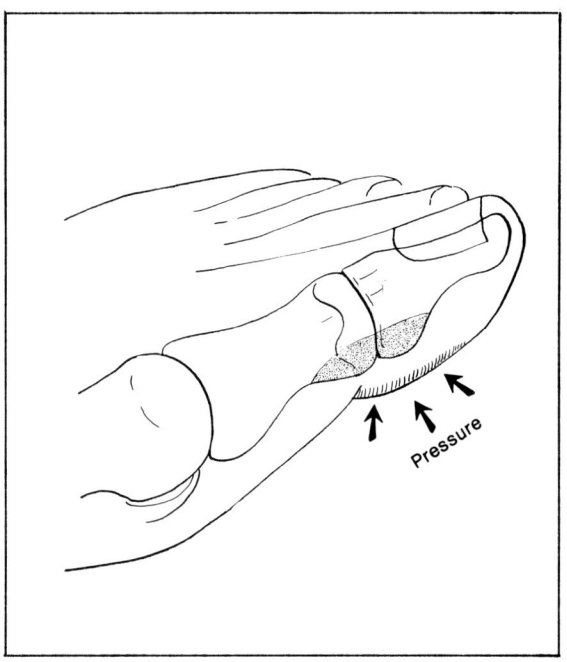

Fig. 4-10A

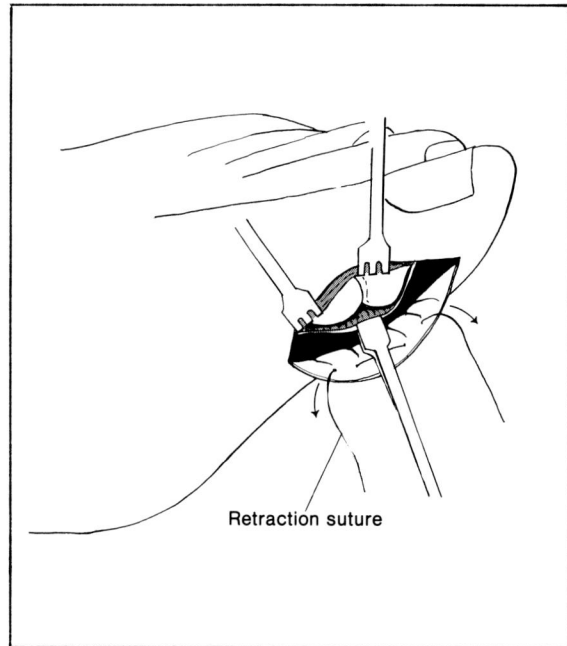

Fig. 4-10B

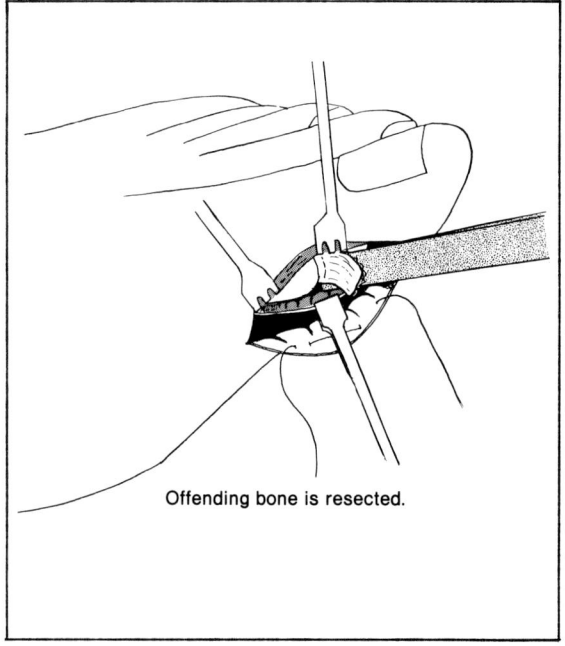

Fig. 4-10C

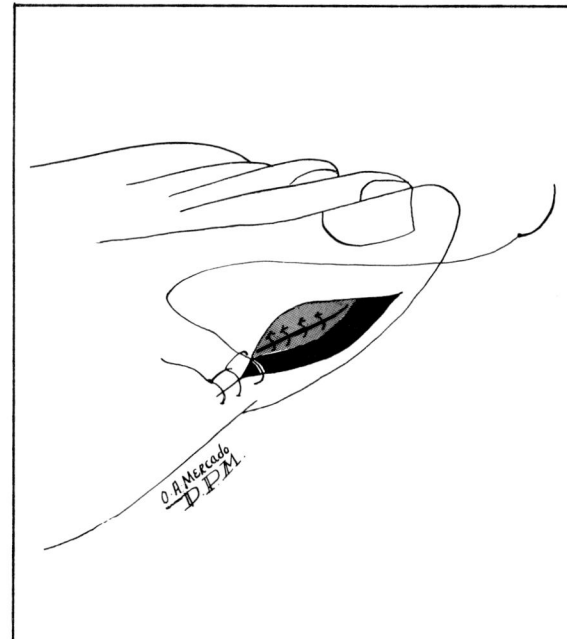

Fig. 4-10D

Technique for a Rotated Hallux

When a pinch callus is present on a **rotated** hallux, not associated with Hallux Abducto Valgus, treatment becomes difficult. If an ostectomy is performed on the medial-plantar aspect of the interphalangeal joint, as would be done on a straight toe, the chances of the pinch callus **recurring** are almost certain. Fortunately, rotated hallucial segments are **rare** (Fig. 4-11A).

The technique that we recommend is as follows: a lineal incision is made on the medial aspect of the interphalangeal joint (Fig. 4-11B). The incision is deepened and retracted so as to expose the distal shaft and head of the proximal phalanx. The extensor hallucis longus tendon is retracted dorsally and lateralwards exposing the periosteum and capsular tissue.

The periosteum is carefully incised and retracted so as to expose the anatomical neck area of the proximal phalanx. An Osteotomy is performed, transecting the anatomical neck. The hallux is then carefully **derotated** into a normal position. The Osteotomy is fixated with two small, criss-crossing Kirschner wires (Fig. 4-11D, 12-A, B, C).

The capsule and periosteum are closed with 3-0 Dexon. The wound is sutured with the material of choice. The correction is maintained with an above the ankle plaster of paris cast. The cast and k-wires are removed in 3 weeks. Healing is uneventful.

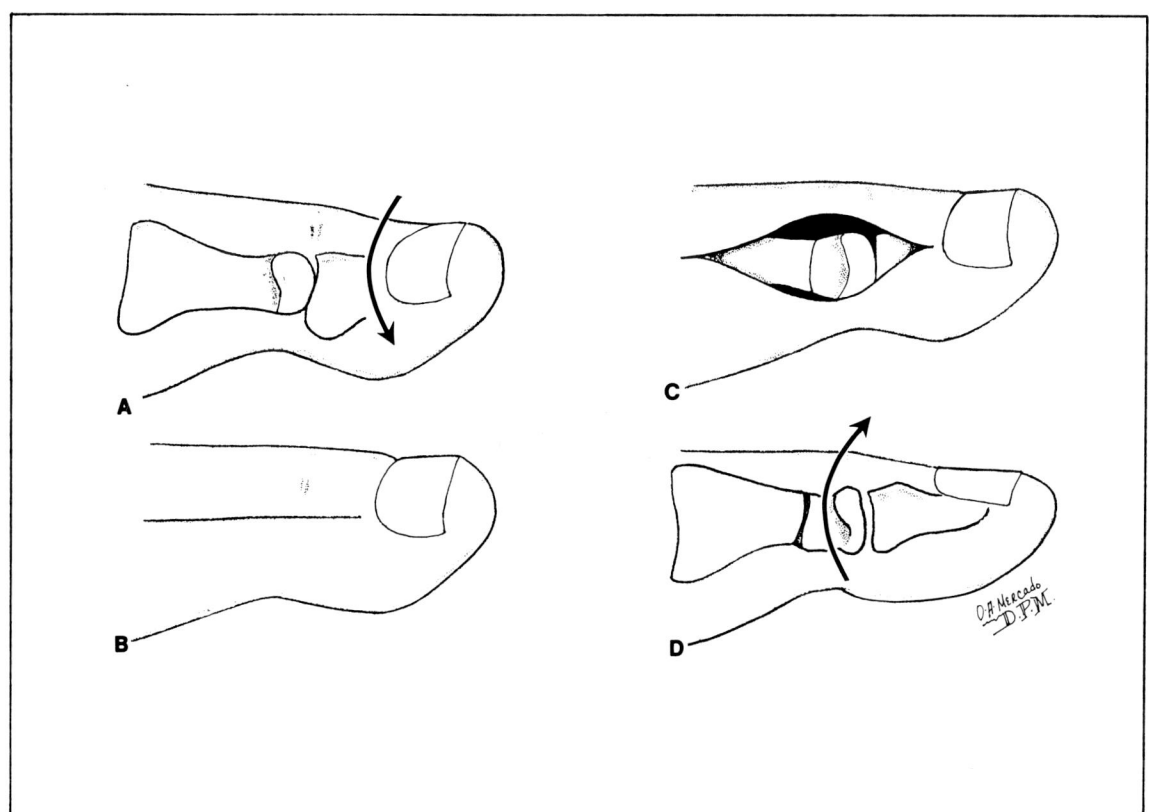

Fig. 4-11

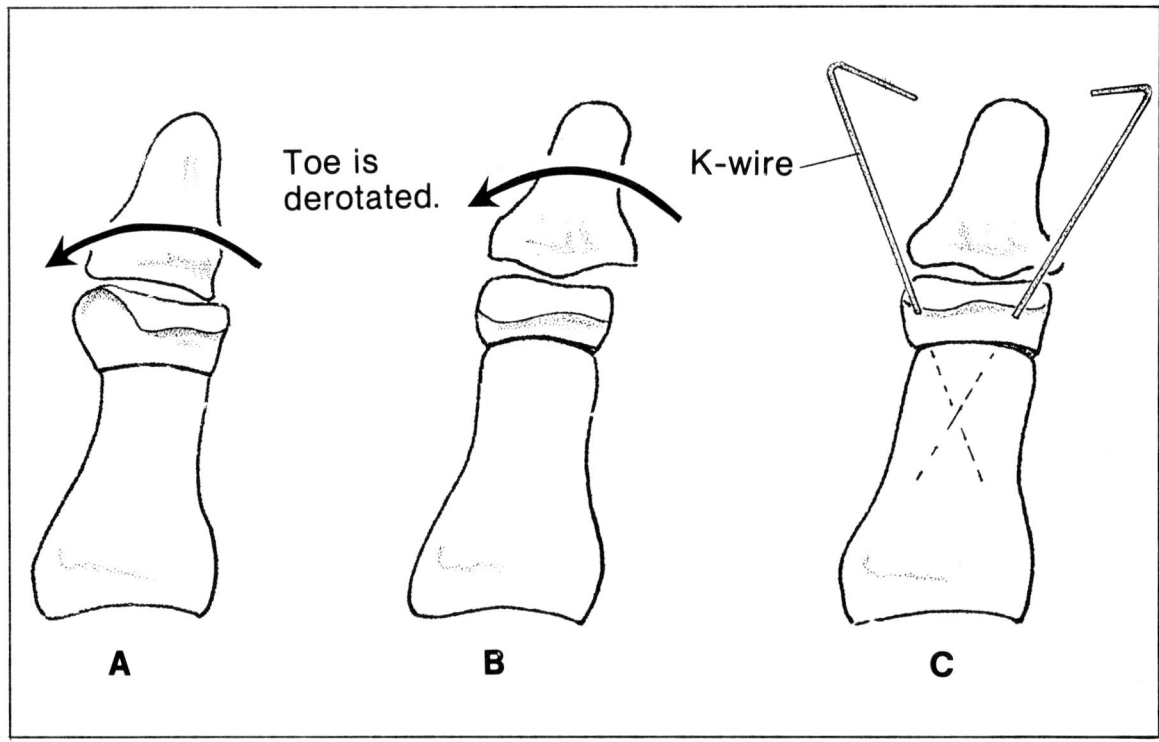

Fig. 4-12

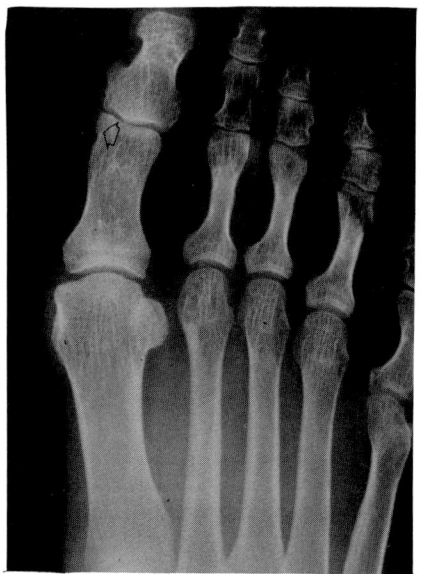

Fig. 4-13A. Previous ostectomy (see arrow) was unsuccessful because hallucial rotation.

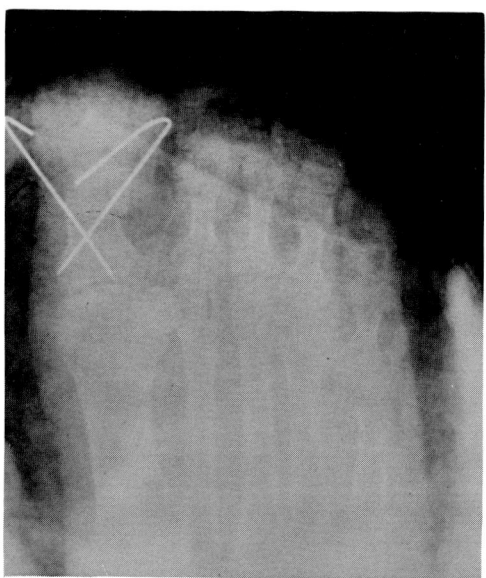

Fig. 4-13B. Osteotomy (dotted line) is fixated with K-wires. The wires are bent and incorporated in the dressing.

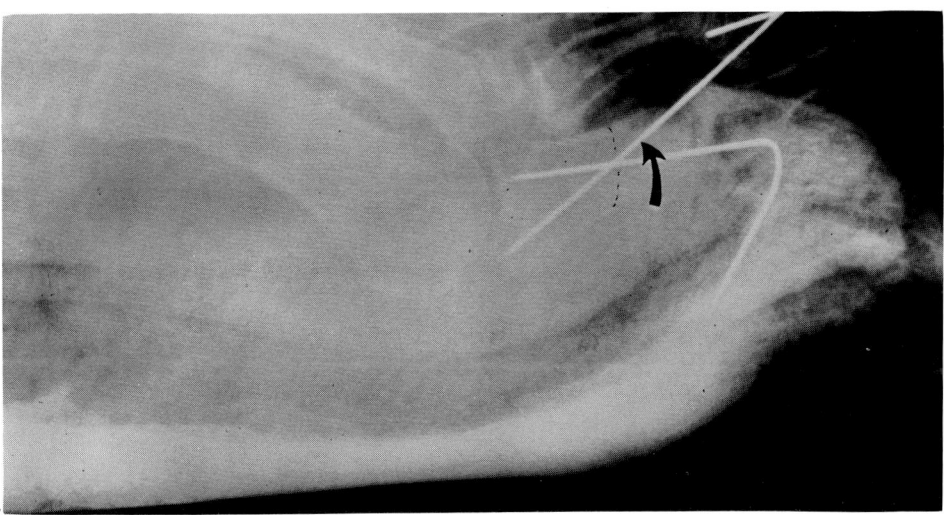

Fig. 4-13C. Lateral view of fixation.

Plantar Interphalangeal Joint Callus

The Plantar Interphalangeal Joint Callus is usually found as a well circumscribed keratotic lesion on the plantar aspect of the hallux.

It is usually caused by an **interphalangeal sesamoid** or an excessive accumulation of fibro-cartilagenous tissue (Fig. 4-14A) which receives undue pressure during the propulsive (toe-off) stage of locomotion.

Pre-operative Evaluation

The differential diagnosis between a Pinch Callus and Interphalangeal Joint Callus must be made. Dorsal-plantar and oblique x-rays are essential. However, the Surgeon must be aware that sometimes the interphalangeal sesamoid is very small or that even a true sesamoid per se, does not exist, but rather an excessive accumulation of fibro-cartilagenous tissue which is not visible on x-rays.

Technique

Our surgical approach is similar to the Pinch Callus, an incision approximately 4 cm. long is made on the medial aspect of the hallux. The incision is deepened and retracted. The interphalangeal capsular ligament is underscored and the plantar aspect is retracted to reveal the Flexor Hallucis Longus tendon.

The tendon is underscored and retracted. The interphalangeal sesamoid will be found laying on the tendon in between the tendon and the capsular ligament (Fig. 4-14B). The sesamoid is grasped with a thumb and finger forceps, and carefully retracted. Care is taken not to injure the tendon. Sometimes the sesamoid is extremely wide and large. It is important to remove the sesamoid in-toto (Fig. 4-14C) as well as any fibro-cartilagenous tissue found.

The wound is closed in the usual manner, healing is usually uneventful.

Precautions

The most important precautions are:
1. Proper differential diagnosis.
2. Complete removal of sesamoid and/or fibro-cartilagenous tissue.

Interphalangeal Sesamoid

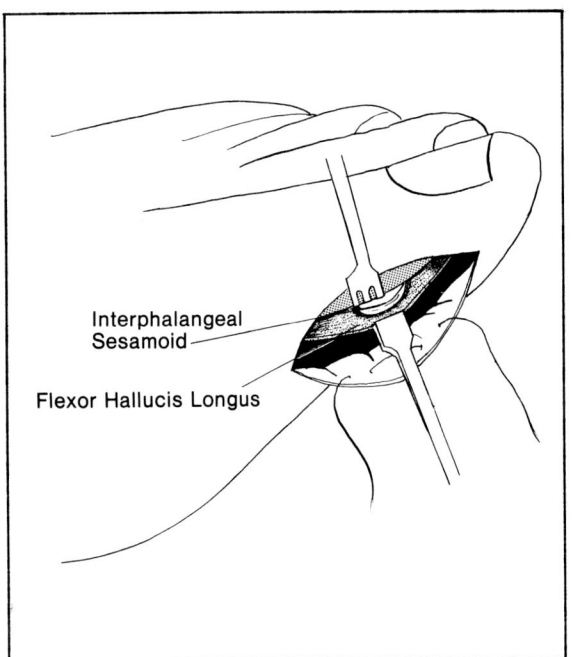

Fig. 4-14A

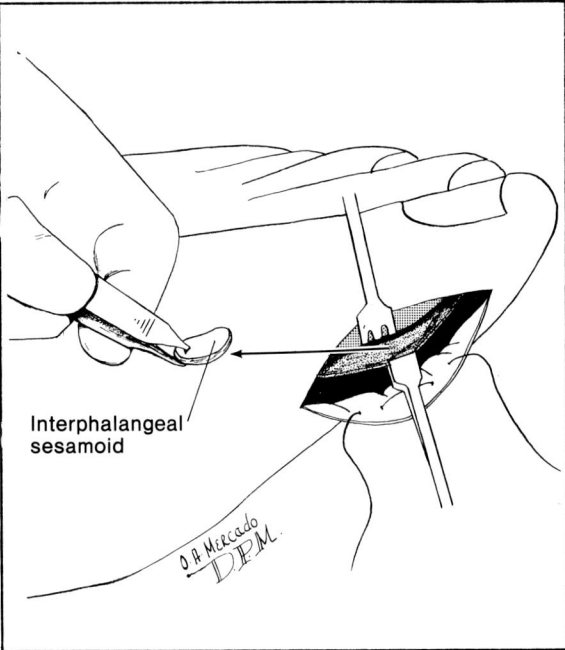

Fig. 4-14B

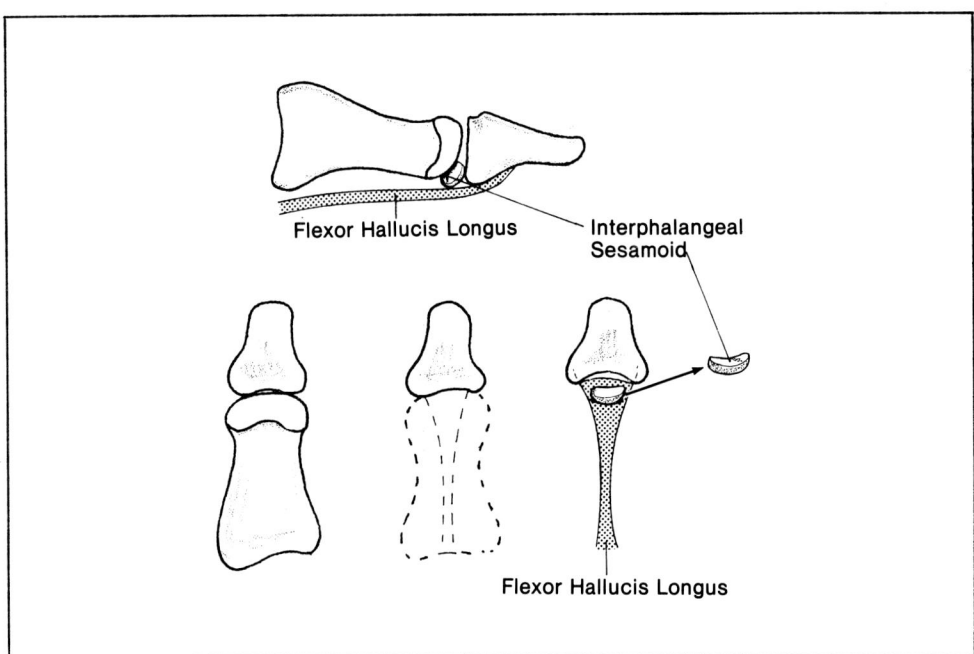

Fig. 4-14C

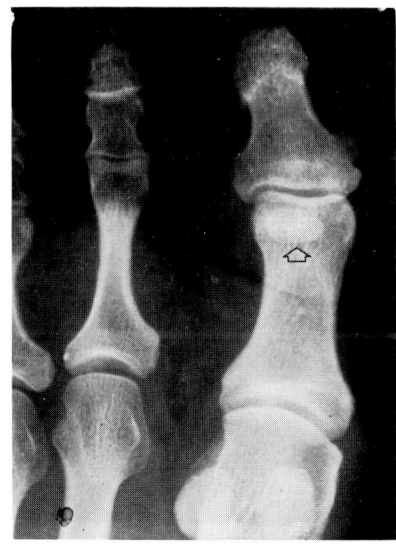
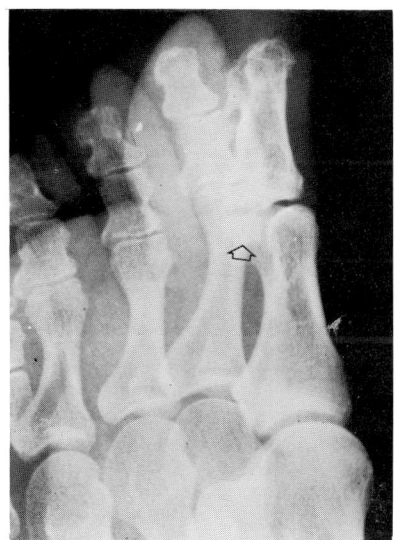

Fig. 4-15A. Dorsal plantar view. Arrow points to interphalangeal sesamoid.

Fig. 4-15B. Oblique view of interphalangeal sesamoid.

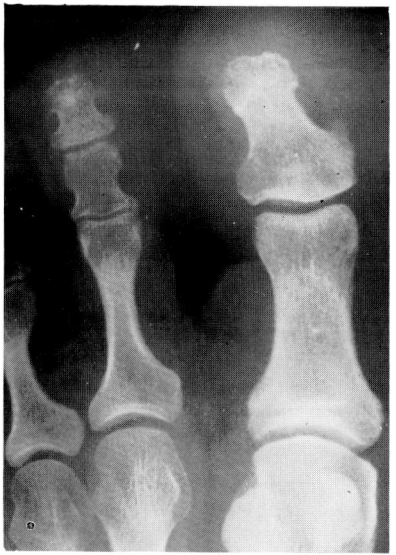
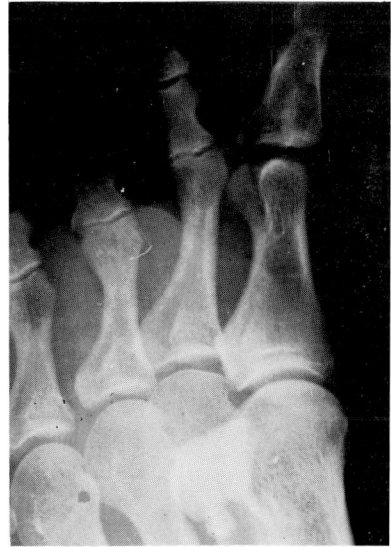

Fig. 4-15C. Post-operative dorsal plantar view.

Fig. 4-15D. Post-operative oblique view.

Deviated Toe

Deviated toes are usually caused by an anatomical malformation of the middle phalanx. The distal articulate facet is markedly deviated, usually towards the medial aspect, causing the toe to rub against its adjoining member and the shoe (Fig. 4-16A).

Our surgery aims at the realignment of the deviated toe by:
1. Angulated ostectomy of middle phalanx
2. Resection of the middle phalanx

Angulated Ostectomy

Our approach is the same as for a hammer toe correction. A transversed incision is made on the tendon and capsule immediately over the middle phalangeal head. The tendons are underscored and retracted. The collateral ligaments on the head of the middle phalanx are cut and the malformed phalangeal head is exposed.

An angulated ostectomy is performed (Fig. 4-16B) and the bone is rasped smooth. The toe is held in a corrected position and the tendons are sutured with 3-0 Dexon. The skin is sutured with 5-0 Nylon. Healing is uneventful.

Resection of Middle Phalanx

Sometimes the deviation of the toe is so marked that the only way to correct the deformity is to **remove** the entire middle phalanx. The malformed middle phalanx in these cases is usually stunted, so that their removal will not constitute a great loss, nor will it create an unmanageable amount of excess tissue (Fig. 4-16D).

Our approach is the same as for the angulated ostectomy. The middle phalanx is easily removed once the collateral ligaments at its **head** and **base** are cut. The toe is held in a corrected position and the tendons are sutured snugly with 3-0 Dexon.

The skin is then carefully sutured with 5-0 Nylon using a combination of simple, horizontal and mattress sutures. There is usually a good deal of **swelling** in these cases post-op, but if the patient is warned before the surgery, they will be expecting it.

Precautions

Resection of the middle phalanx for a deviated toe is **not** a common procedure. However, if the surgeon takes time to explain to the patients the reasons for the surgery and the reasonable results they can expect, then the procedure will yield consistently good results.

DIGITAL SURGERY

Deviated Toe

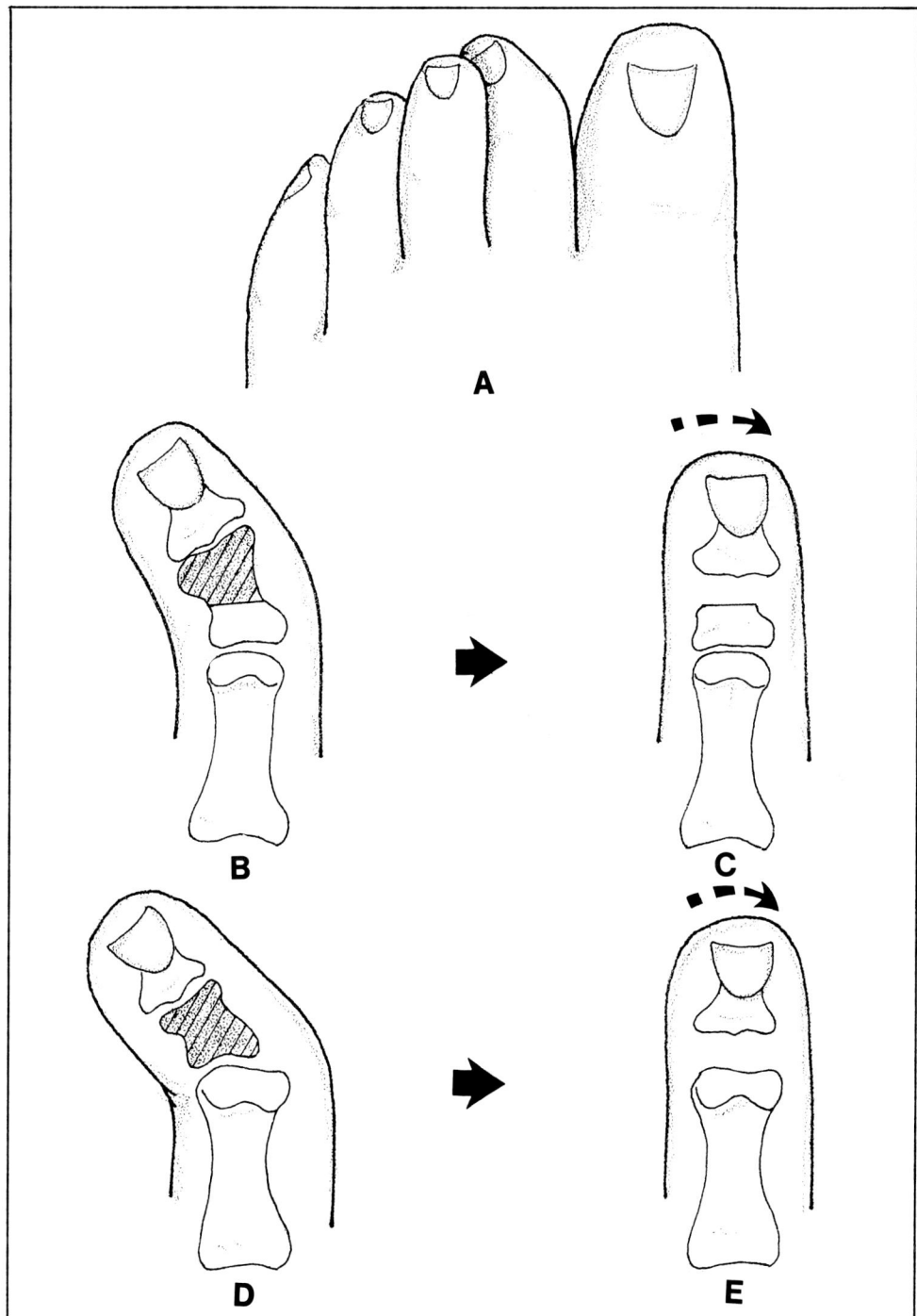

Fig. 4-16

CONGENITAL DEFORMITIES

Overlapping Fifth Toe

An overlapping fifth toe is a congenital deformity which is usually bilateral. The problem is caused by a contracted Extensor Digitorum Longus tendon which causes dorsal tilting and overlapping of the fifth toe on the fourth (Fig. 4-17A).

As time passes, the skin at the base of the toe becomes **taut** and the dorsal metatarsal phalangeal joint capsule becomes contracted thus helping to exaggerate and maintain the condition.

For our purpose here, we will classify the overlapping fifth toe into **two categories:**

A. Simple Overlapping Fifth Toe
B. Severe Overlapping Fifth Toe

Simple Overlapping Fifth Toe

A simple overlapping fifth toe is usually seen in young children. Our surgery aims at:

1. Tenotomy of Extensor Digitorum Longus
2. Z-plasty Skin Release
3. Dorsal Capsulotomy of the metatarsal phalangeal joint capsule
4. Plantar skin wedge resection
5. Repositioning of the toe

Technique

An incision is made immediately over the tendon of Extensor Digitorum Longus at the level of the metatarsal shaft. The fifth toe is planti-flexed and the contracted tendon is cut (tenotomized). A Z-incision is made at the base of the toe. Through this incision the contracted capsular ligament of the metatarsal phalangeal joint is cut (Fig. 4-17B).

Two transversed semi-elliptical incisions are made on the plantar aspect of the toe, and the wedge thus formed is resected. It is important to resect **only** the skin. There are fragile vessels in this area and we do not want to interfere with them. The fifth toe is planti-flexed to the desired position and the wedge is closed using a horizontal mattress suture with the material of choice (Fig. 4-17C). The wounds on the top of the foot are sutured, taking care to use only one suture on the Z-plasty skin release incision. Wound healing is uneventful and the results are predictably good (Fig. 4-17D).

DIGITAL SURGERY

Simple Overlapping Fifth Toe

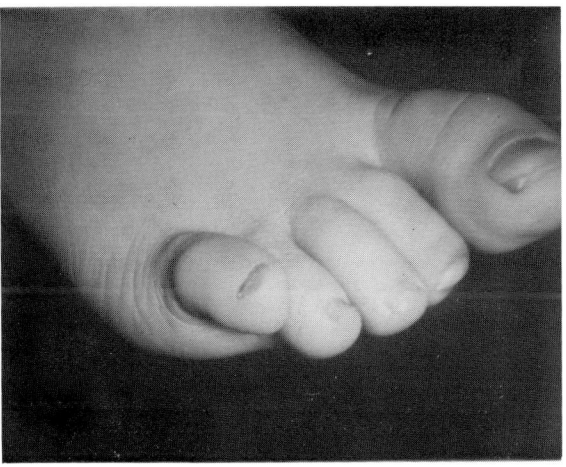

Fig. 4-17A. Pre-operative overlapping fifth toe.

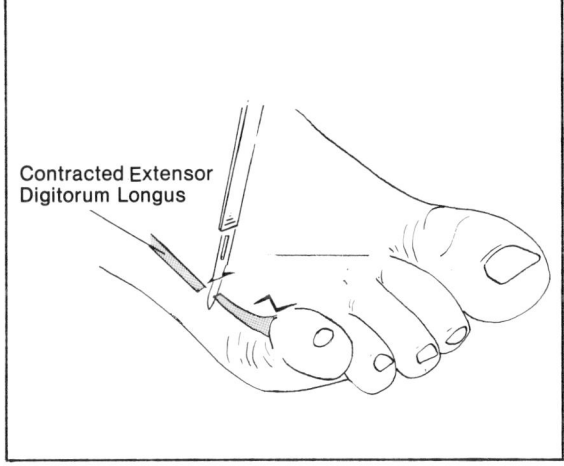

Fig. 4-17B

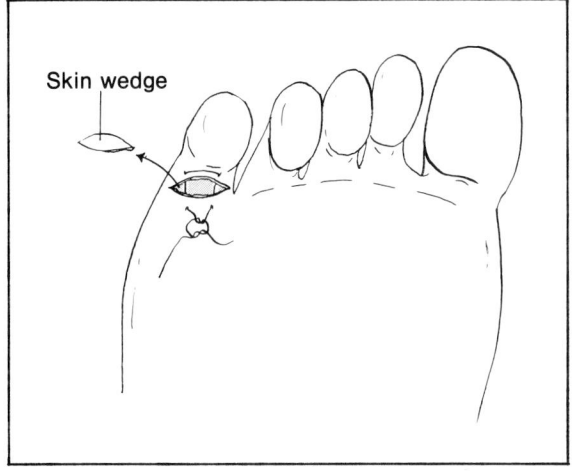

Fig. 4-17C

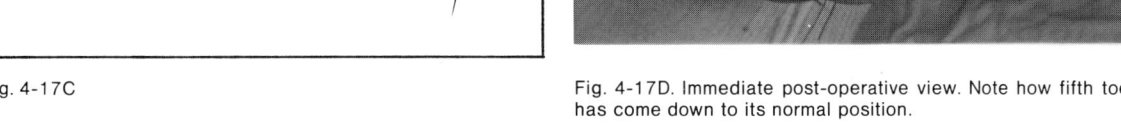

Fig. 4-17D. Immediate post-operative view. Note how fifth toe has come down to its normal position.

Severe Overlapping Fifth Toe

Severe overlapping fifth toes are usually seen on adolescents and adults. They are the end result of uncorrected simple overlapping fifth toes.

In a severe overlapping fifth toe, we have a **marked contraction** of the Extensor Digitorum Longus tendon; the dorsal metatarsal phalangeal joint capsule; the collateral ligaments; and the tendon of Abductor Digiti Quinti (Fig. 4-18A).

Our surgery aims at:

1. Tenectomy of Extensor Digitorum Longus
2. Y-shaped skin release
3. Dorsal Capsulotomy of the metatarsal phalangeal joint capsule
4. Release of contracted collateral ligaments
5. Tenotomy of Abductor Digiti Quinti
6. Plantar skin wedge resection
7. Repositioning of the toe

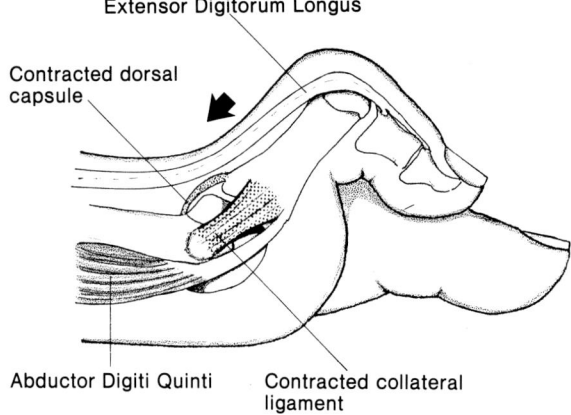

Fig. 4-18A

Technique

The plantar and dorsal incisions are carefully marked with a surgical pen. The dorsal incision extends from the metatarsal shaft and bifurcates around the base of the toe thus forming a **Y-shaped** incision (Fig. 4-18C).

The incision is carefully deepened and the superficial vessels are ligated to prevent post-operative hematoma. The incision is underscored exposing the contracted tendon and Hood Ligament (Fig. 4-18F). The Hood Ligament is incised and the contracted tendon is exposed and a section of it is resected (tenectomy) as seen in Fig. 4-18G.

The contracted tendon of Abductor Digiti Quinti is exposed next and a tenectomy is performed (Fig. 4-18H and I). An incision is made on the joint capsule. The capsule is carefully underscored and the contracted collateral ligaments, found inside of the capsule, are released (Fig. 4-18J).

The metatarsal head is delivered outside of the wound to ascertain that all contracted tissues have been released. Sometimes adaptive changes will be found on the head due to the dorsal displacement of the proximal phalanx (Fig. 4-18K).

DIGITAL SURGERY

A plantar wedge of skin is then resected from the previously marked area (fig. 4-18D and L). Care is taken to remove **only** the skin as there are fragile vessels in this area and we do not want to embarrass the vascular circulation to the toe (Fig. 4-18L and M). The fifth toe is then held in a corrected position and the plantar incision is closed with simple sutures of 5-0 Nylon.

The dorsal capsule and tissues are **loosely** sutured with 3-0 Dexon. The wound is closed with simple sutures of 5-0 Nylon (Fig. 4-18O). The toe is bandaged in a plant-flexed position to maintain the correction. Healing is usually uneventful.

Precautions

Overlapping fifth toe surgery will yield consistently good results if performed as described here. However, the surgeon should keep the following points in mind:

1. Inform the patient that an overlapping fifth toe does **not** purchase the floor as do the other toes (Fig. 4-18B).
2. Even in the best of surgeries, the toe **will not** be able to purchase the floor post-operatively. Essentially we are bringing the toe down so that it **will not** rub against the shoe.
3. Take care to release **all** of the contracted tendons, capsule and collateral ligaments.

Severe Overlapping Fifth Toe

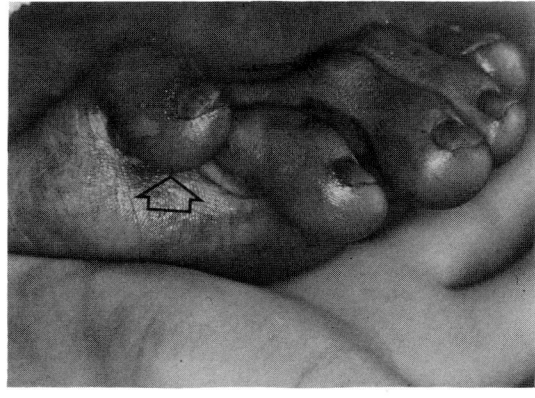

Fig. 4-18B. When the foot is loaded the fifth toe will not **purchase.**

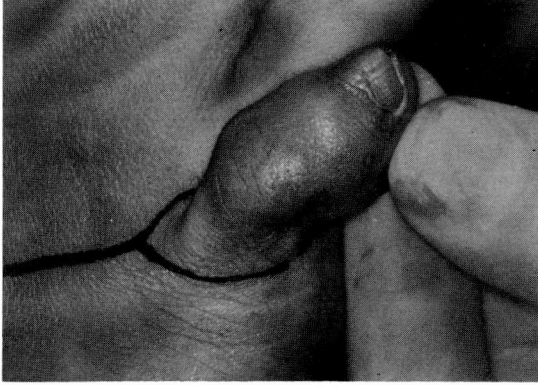

Fig. 4-18C. The dorsal *y-shaped* incision is clearly outlined.

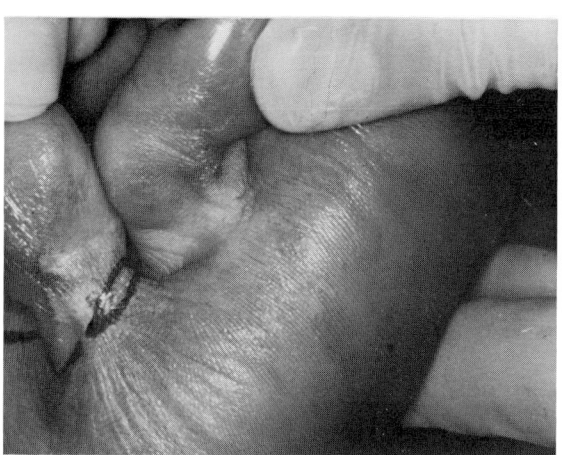

Fig. 4-18D. The plantar wedge incision is marked with a surgical pen.

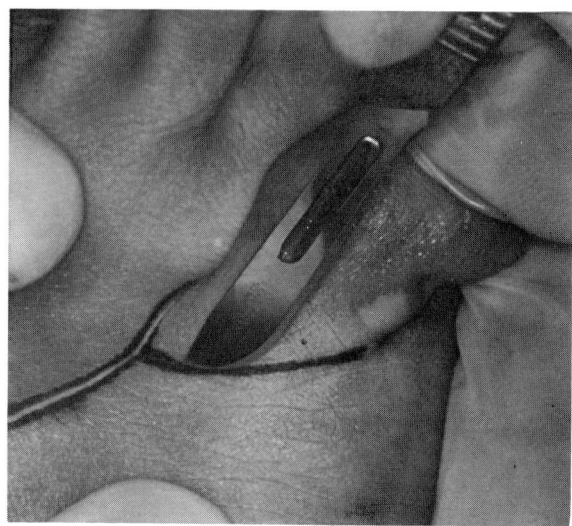

Fig. 4-18E

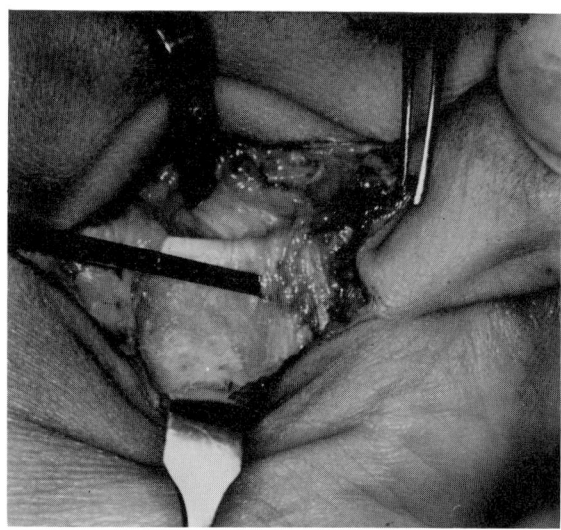

Fig. 4-18F. Small periosteal elevator points to contracted **Hood Ligament.**

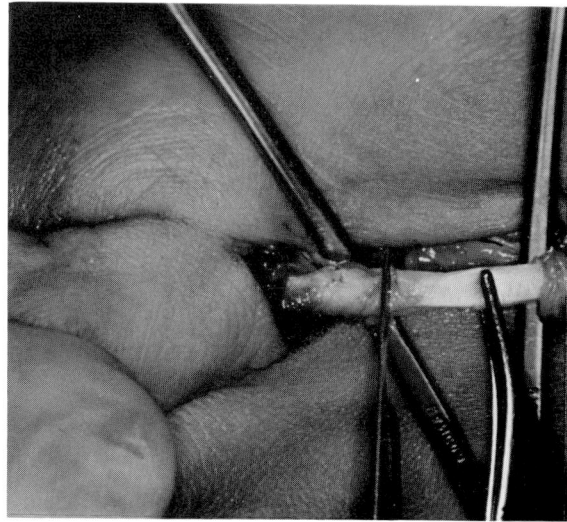

Fig. 4-18G. A tenectomy is performed on the contracted extensor digitorum longus tendon.

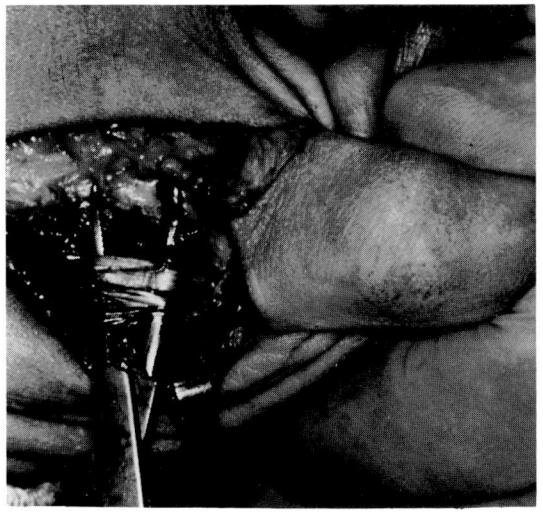

Fig. 4-18H. The **contracted** tendon of abductor digiti quinti is exposed.

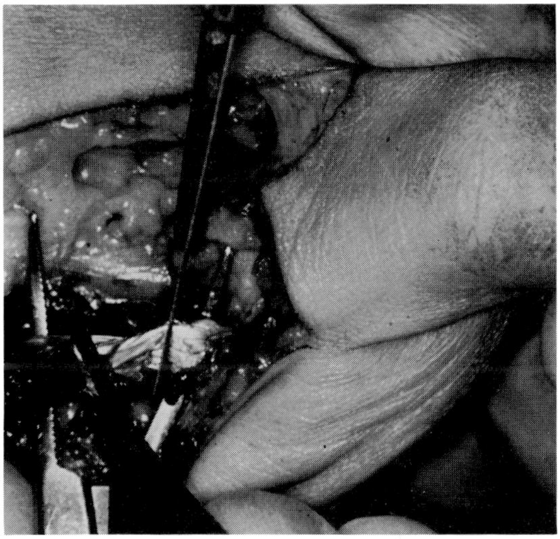

Fig. 4-18I. . . . and a section is removed (tenectomy).

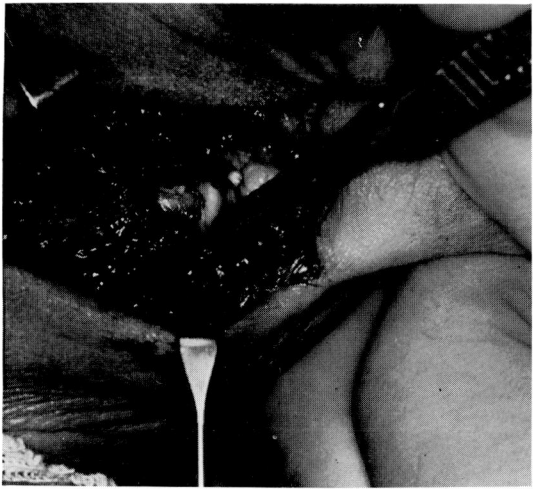

Fig. 4-18J. An incision is made on the joint capsule and the contracted collateral ligaments are released.

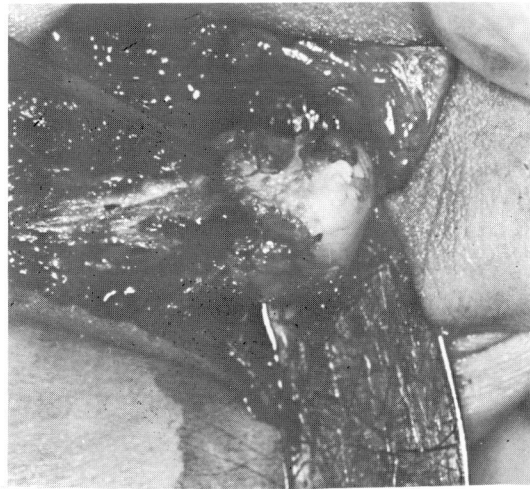

Fig. 4-18K. Note adaptive changes on the metatarsal head — caused by the dorsal displacement of the proximal phalangeal base.

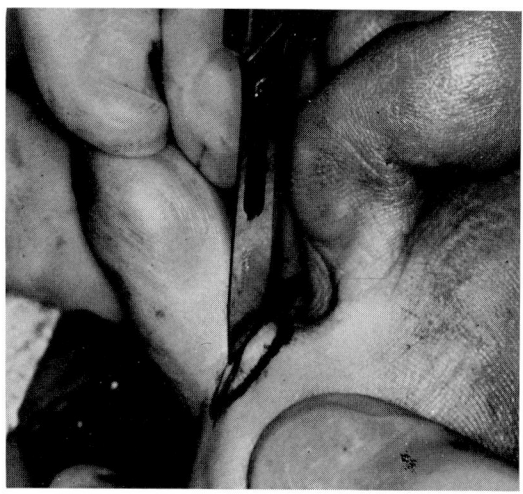

Fig. 4-18L. Only the skin is resected as there are fragile vessels in this area and we do not want to interfere with them.

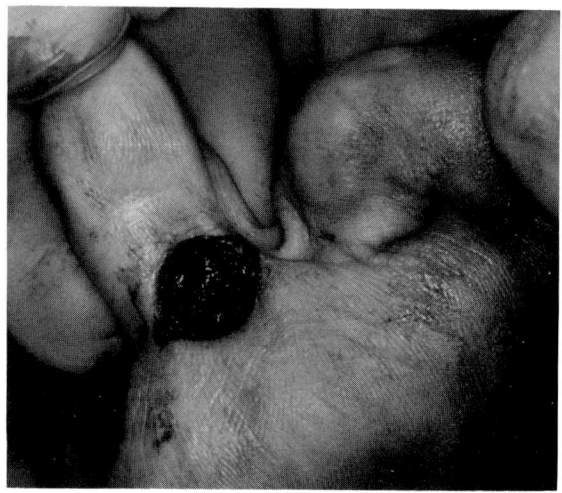

Fig. 4-18M. The plantar skin wedge is resected.

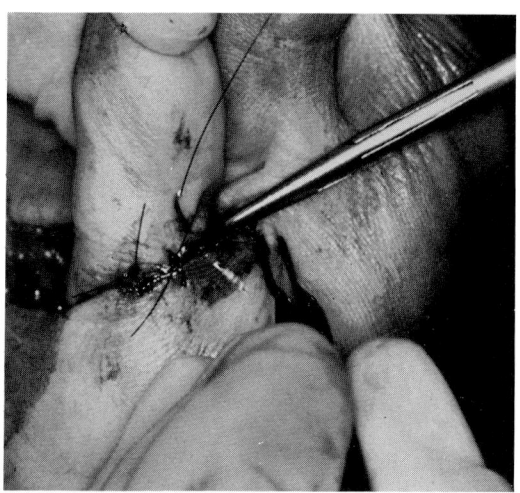

Fig. 4-18N. The plantar skin is sutured — this will help to maintain the correction.

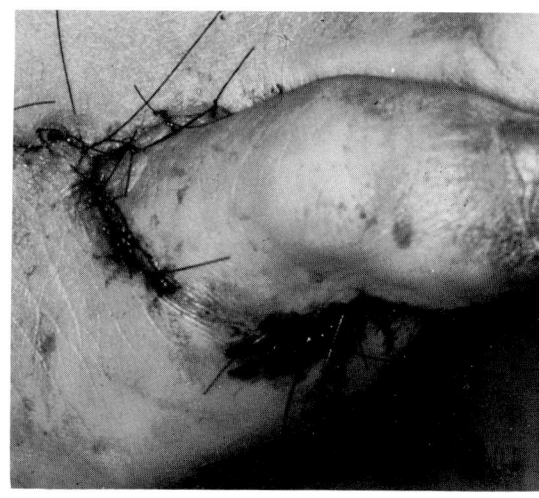

Fig. 4-18O. The wound is sutured with 5-0 nylon. Note the corrected position of the toe (compare with Figs. 4-18B and C).

DIGITAL SURGERY

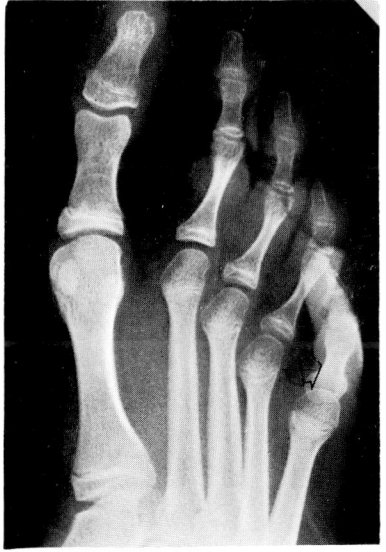 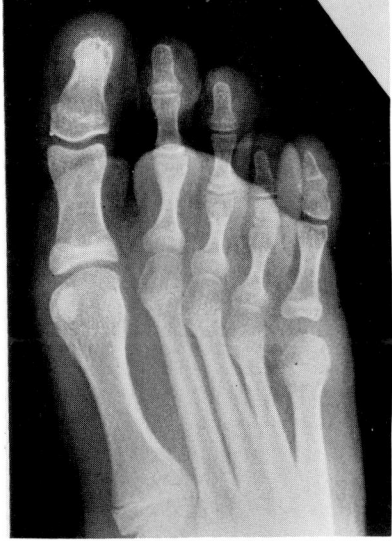

Fig. 4-18P. Pre-operative x-rays of patient seen in Figs. 4-18B-O.

Fig. 4-18Q. Post-operative x-ray. Note excellent alignment of phalanges.

Syndactalism

Syndactalism **(webbed toes)** is a congenital condition which occurs between two or more toes and is usually bilateral (Fig. 4-19A). It presents a surgical problem that, unless it is evaluated properly, can lead the surgeon into a dark pitfall.

The problem with webbed toes is that they are usually **not symptomatic** and are more of a bother to the parents than to the child. Also, the separation of two toes, in the minds of a lay person or even an uninitiated surgeon, just does **not** appear to be a formidable job.

The surgeon should evaluate the condition to see if the webbed toes are bothering the child. If they are, then they should be corrected. If the problem is one of **cosmesis,** then the parents should be forewarned of the difficulty of the operation. The vascularity in the area is fragile and often **anomalous.** Also, no matter how the incisions are placed for the flaps, there is never enough skin to cover all the denuded area and the surgeon must rely on secondary intention healing or rotational skin grafting.

Technique

It is best to outline the lines of incision on the foot with a marking solution or pen. This will make the placing of the incisions easier and more accurate. The first incision is made on the dorsum of the second toe just lateral to the mid-line of the toe. Two transversed incisions are then made, one distal and one proximal to complete the flap (Fig. 4-19B). When making the proximal end of the flap, the surgeon must decide how much separation he wants to obtain and how far down he wants the cleft of the toes to lie. Remember that the cleft in-between the second and third toes is more distal than the cleft in-between the first and second or third and fourth.

A somewhat triangular incision is then made at the base of the toes. The purpose of this triangular incision is to create a flap which will be **rotated** and used to cover the denuded interdigital space created when the dorsal and plantar digital flaps are brought around the toes. Note that the anchor **(nutrient end)** of the rotational flap is at the base of the third toe. It is important to make the anchor portion wide enough to insure adequate attachment of the rotational flap and viability.

Once the dorsal flaps incisions are made, the plantar incisions are made as follows: a lineal incision is made on the plantar of the third toe. Two additional incisions are made to create a plantar flap (Fig. 4-19C). The distal incision is usually difficult because of the bulbousity of the toe in this area.

Once the flaps are incised, the skin and **only** the skin is underscored, taking care to preserve the underlying vascularity. The flaps are handled with extreme care and the separation of the toes is accomplished by carefully cutting through the interdigital space. A lot of vessels can be preserved by retracting them medially or laterally. There is a network of vessels at the base (cleft) of the toes which should be preserved.

Once the separation is accomplished, the dorsal flap is brought down and around the third toe. You will immediately notice that the flaps will not meet the margins of the skin. They **do not** have to meet. To try and stretch the skin and suture it too tightly will lead to an **ischemic** toe!

The rotational flap is brought around and into the interdigital space to cover as much of the denuded tissue in this area as possible. The rotational flap is trimmed, if necessary, and sutured loosely in place with 5-0 Nylon (Fig. 4-19D and E).

The dorsal and plantar flaps are also sutured loosely in place (Fig. 4-19F and G). The wounds are carefully dressed with vaseline gauze, sterile 3x3 and kling bandages, making sure that the tip of the toes are visible so that the color and capillary filling time can be checked post-operatively.

Precautions

1. Explain to the patient's parents the inherent problems with the procedure.
2. **Do not** try to stretch the flaps to meet the skin margins.
3. Suture the flaps **loosely.**
4. Preserve the vascularity as much as possible.
5. When there are three or more toes involved, separate only two and allow sufficient time (six months or more) in between surgeries.
6. If there is any **bone** work required along with the separation of the toes, separate the toes only. After six months or more, the bone work can be performed.

DIGITAL SURGERY

Separation of Webbed Toes

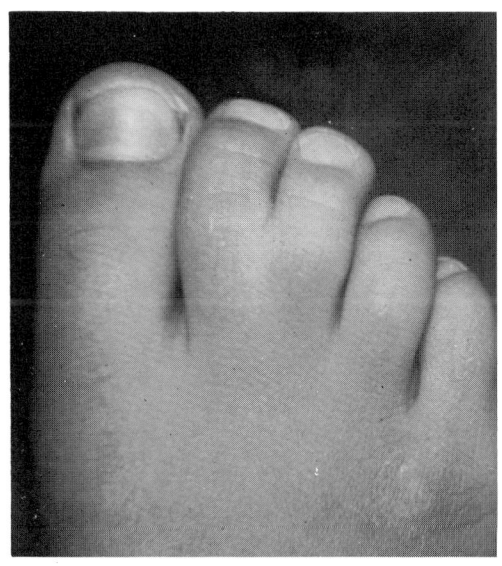

Fig. 4-19A

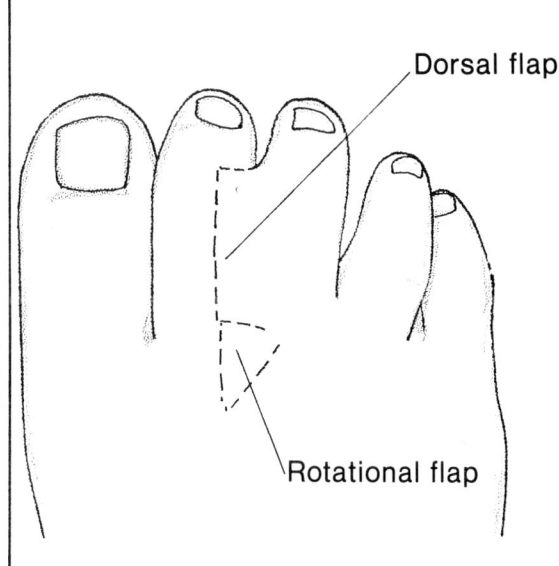

Fig. 4-19B

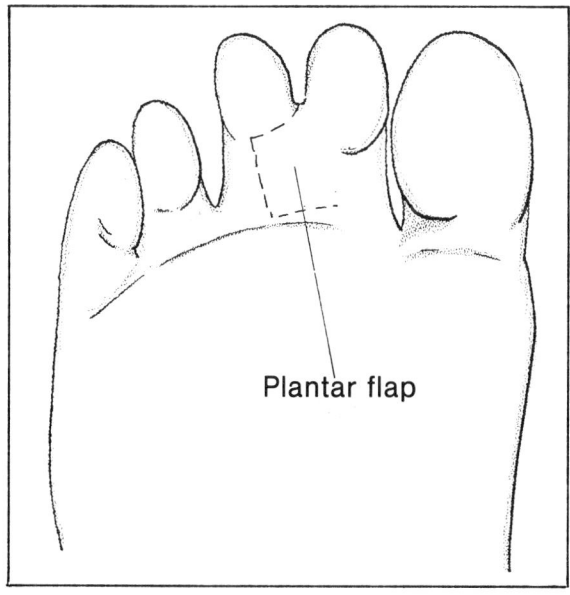

Fig. 4-19C

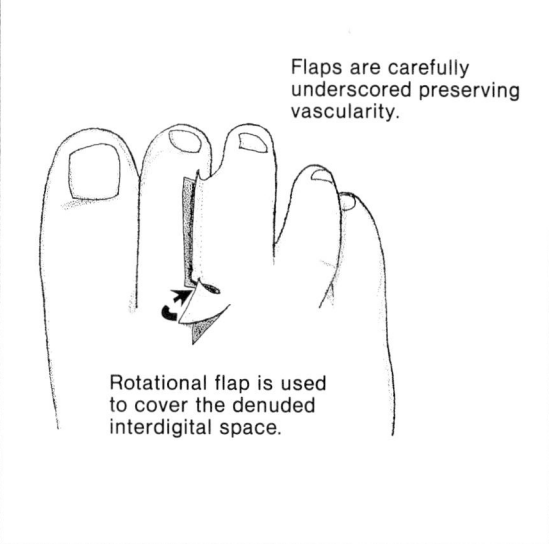

Fig. 4-19D

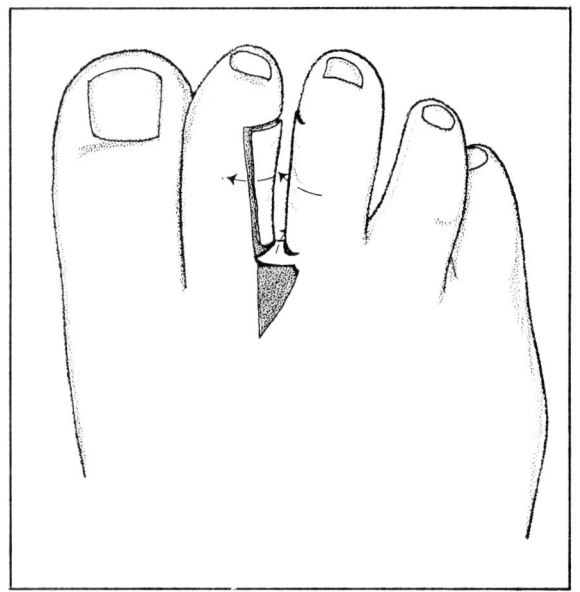

Fig. 4-19E

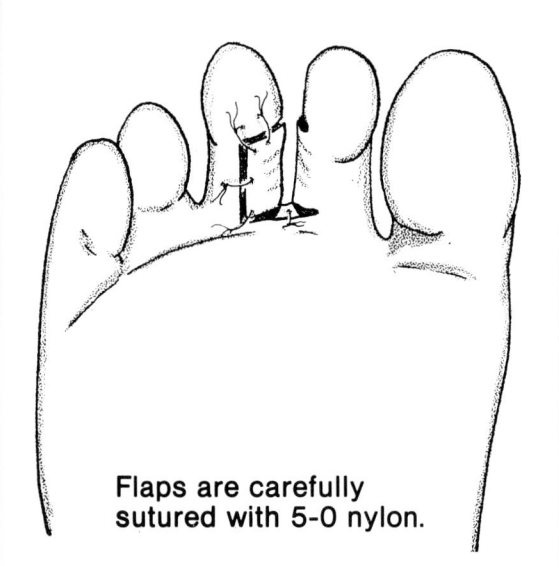

Flaps are carefully sutured with 5-0 nylon.

Fig. 4-19F

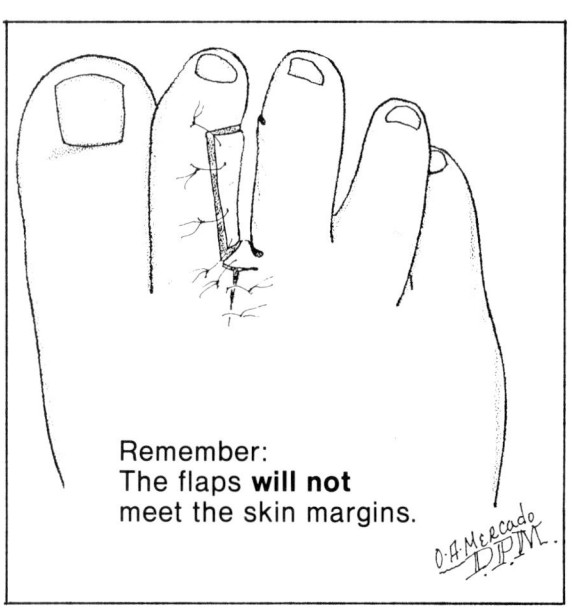

Remember:
The flaps **will not** meet the skin margins.

Fig. 4-19G

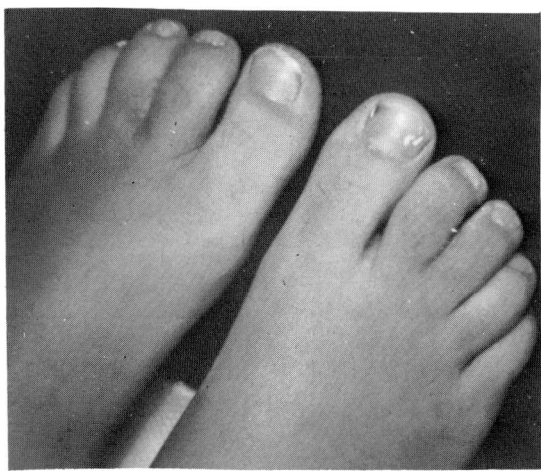

Fig. 4-19H

DIGITAL SURGERY

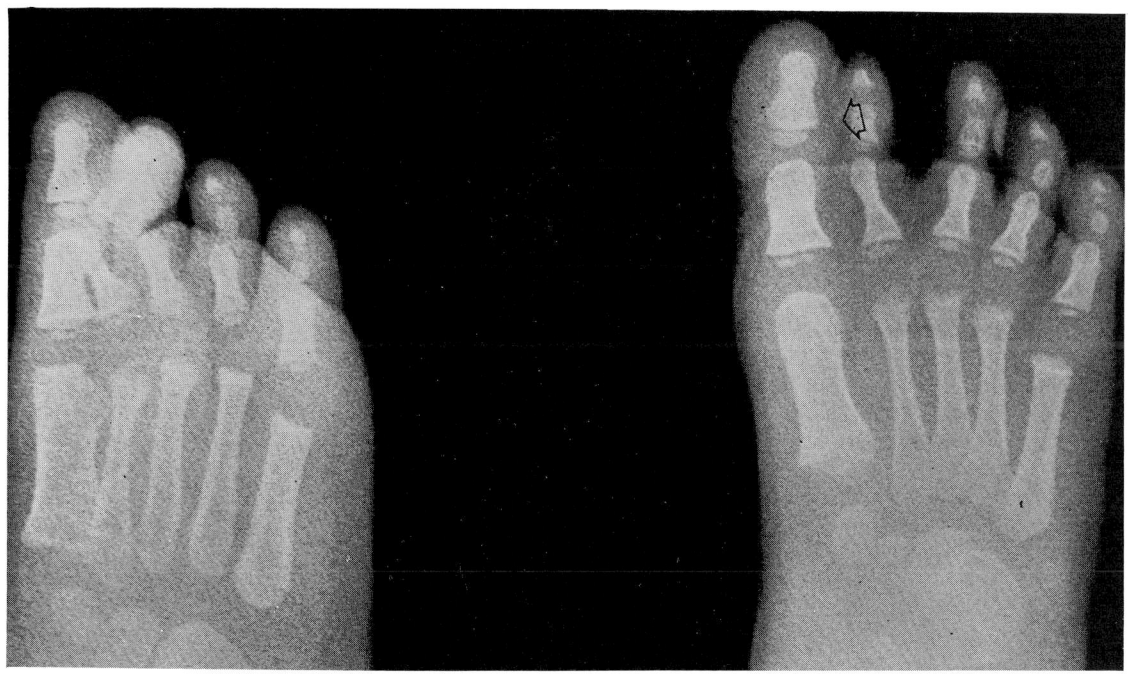

Fig. 4-20A. Pre-operative x-rays — syndactylism of first and second toes (oblique and D.P. views).

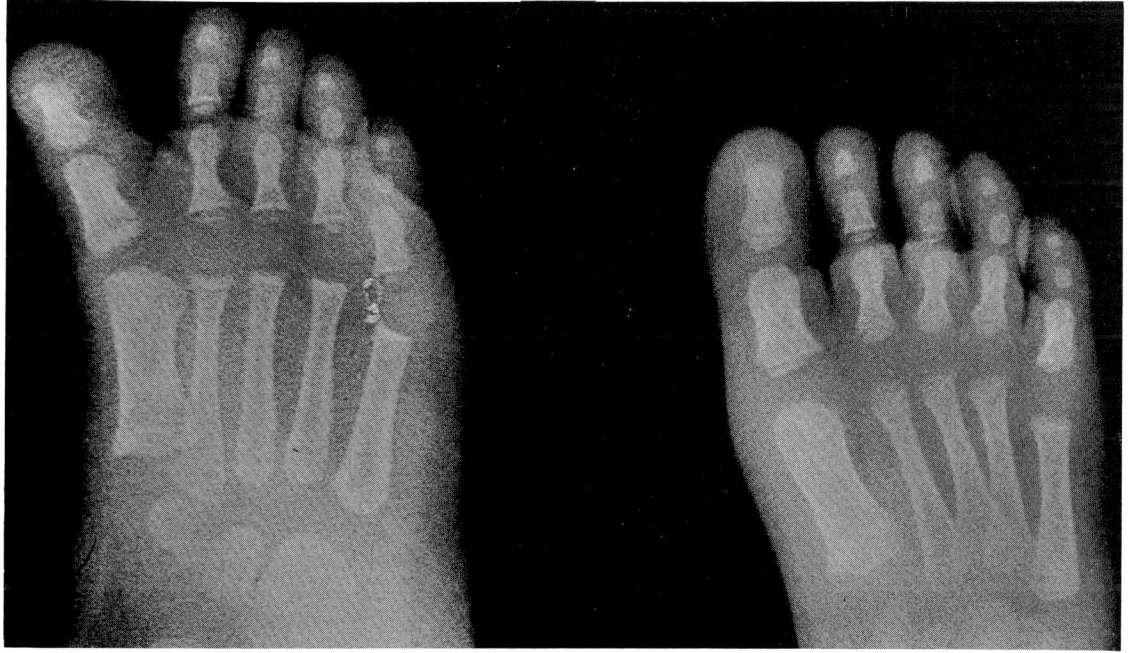

Fig. 4-20B. Post-operative x-rays shows separation of first and second toes (oblique and D.P. views).

Polydactalism

Polydactalism **(supernumerary toe)** is a congenital deformity usually occurring bilaterally. As in the case of syndactalism, the surgeon must proceed with extreme care in planning his surgical approach. The supernumerary toe is to be removed in such a way as to leave behind a functioning, as well as a **normal looking** foot.

If the polydactalism is further complicated by syndactalism, then the supernumerary toe is removed first and at later time the syndactalism can be corrected. Surgery of the really **malformed** foot will sometimes require three, four or more stages until the desired result is accomplished.

Technique

After the patient and x-rays have been properly evaluated (Fig. 4-21A), a wedge consisting of two semi-elliptical incisions is made surrounding the supernumerary toe (Fig. 4-21C).

The incisions are deepened to the bone and the supernumerary toe along with its middle and distal phalanx is resected in-toto. Since the polydactalism is sharing the proximal phalanx along with the fifth toe, no attempt is made to remodel this bone (Fg. 4-21B).

The skin margins are underscored and sutured using a continuous lock suture with the material of choice (Fig. 4-21D). The foot is dressed in the usual manner, healing is uneventful.

Precautions

The most important precaution the surgeon can follow is to avoid doing too much work at one time and above all, to **plan** his surgery well.

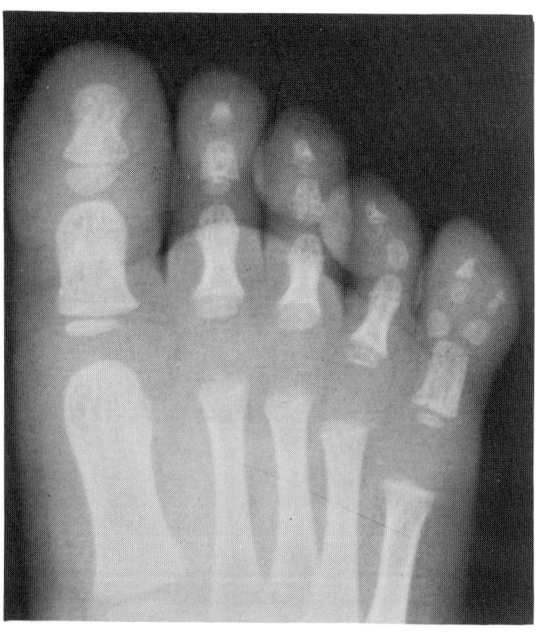 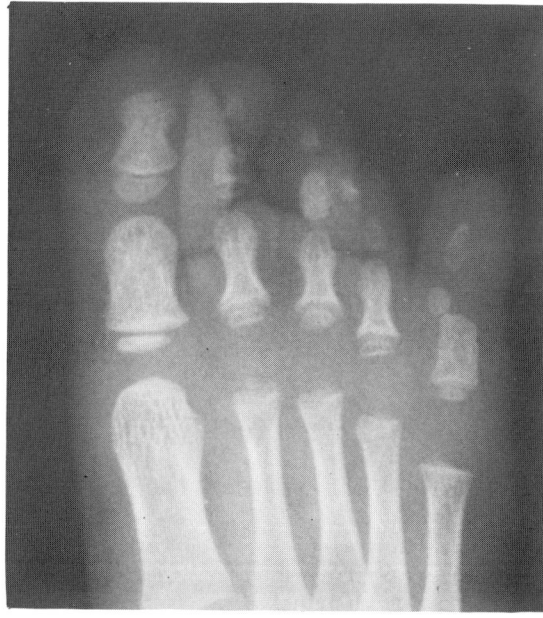

Fig. 4-21A. Pre-operative x-ray reveals a supernumerary toe consisting of a middle and distal phalanx, sharing the proximal phalanx with the fifth toe.

Fig. 4-21B. Post-operative x-ray shows resection of supernumerary toe.

DIGITAL SURGERY

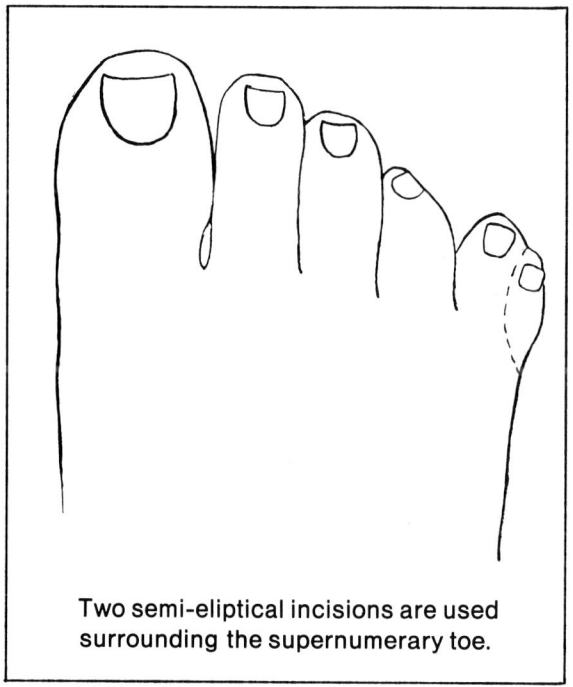

Two semi-eliptical incisions are used surrounding the supernumerary toe.

Fig. 4-21C

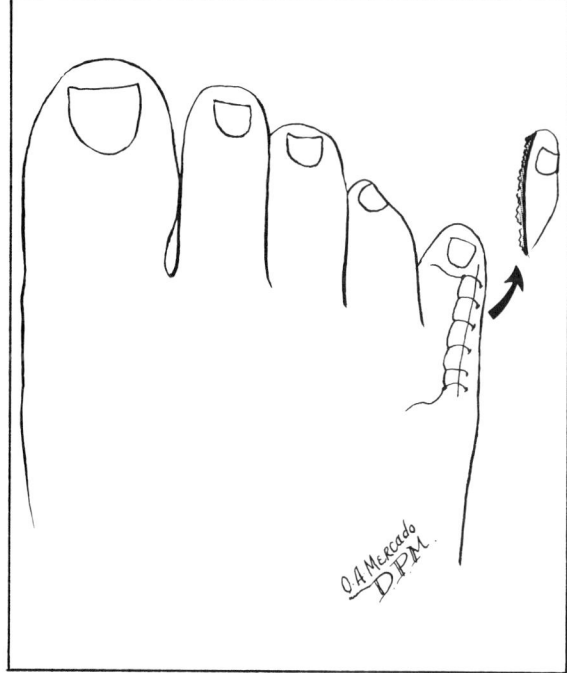

Fig. 21-D

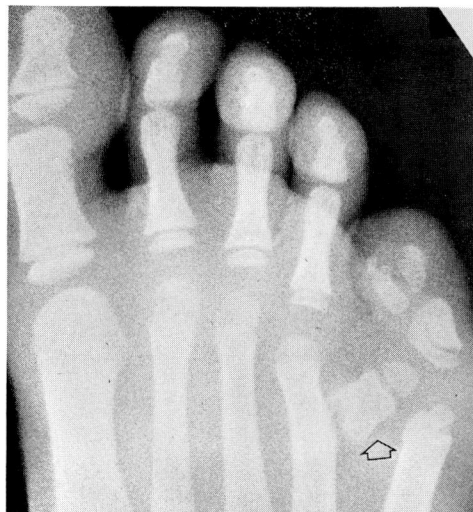

Fig. 4-22A. Pre-operative x-ray reveals supernumerary metatarsal (see arrow) and distal phalanges.

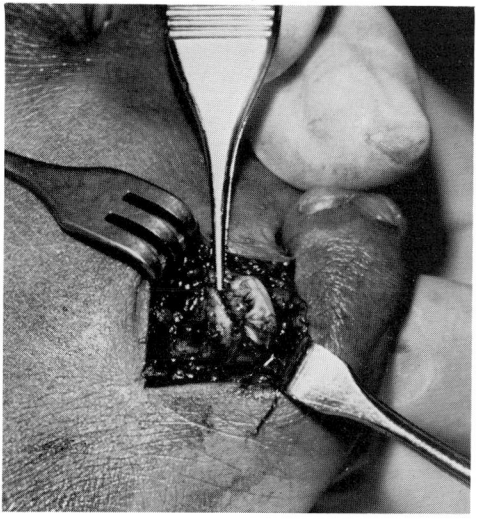

Fig. 4-22B. Supernumerary metatarsal is exposed and . .

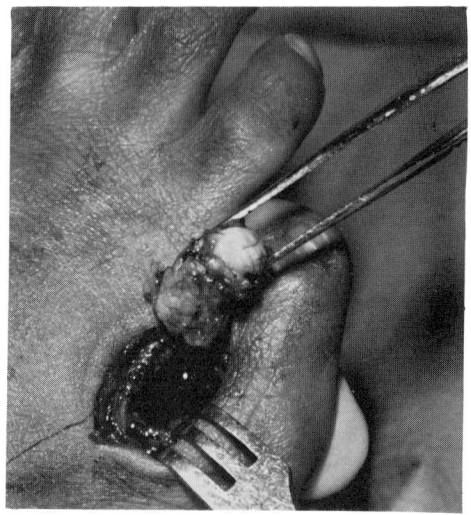

Fig. 4-22C. . . . resected in-toto.

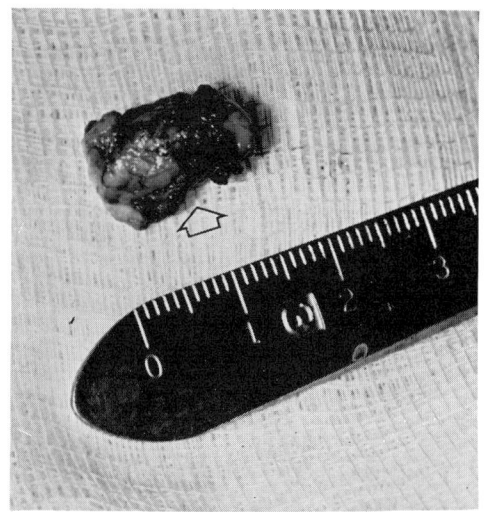

Fig. 4-22D. Compare resected supernumerary metatarsal with pre-operative x-ray (Fig. 4-22A). Arrow is in the same position.

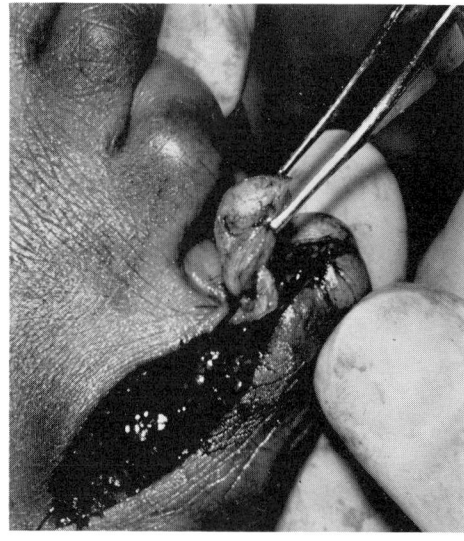

Fig. 4-22E. Supernumerary toe is resected.

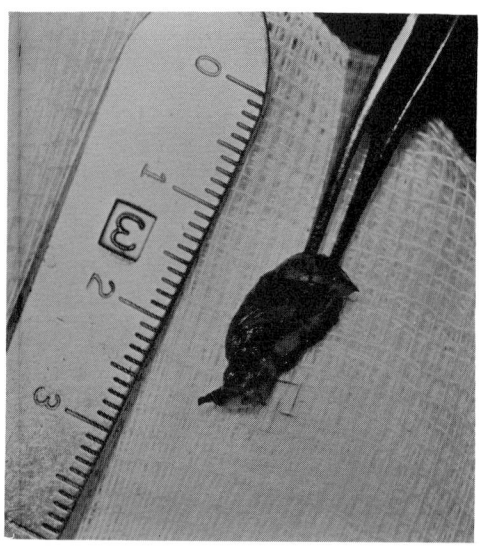

Fig. 4-22F. Close-up of resected supernumerary.

DIGITAL SURGERY

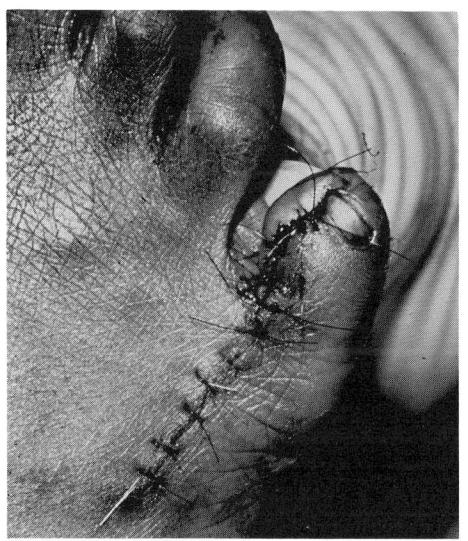

Fig. 4-22G. Wound is sutured with 5-0 nylon.

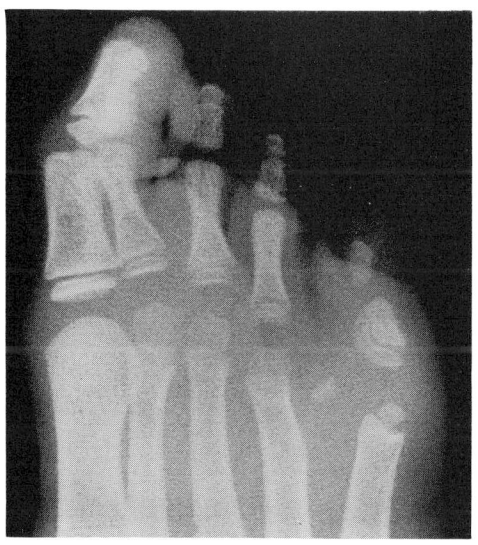

Fig. 4-22H. Post-operative x-ray shows resection of supernumerary metatarsal and phalanges.

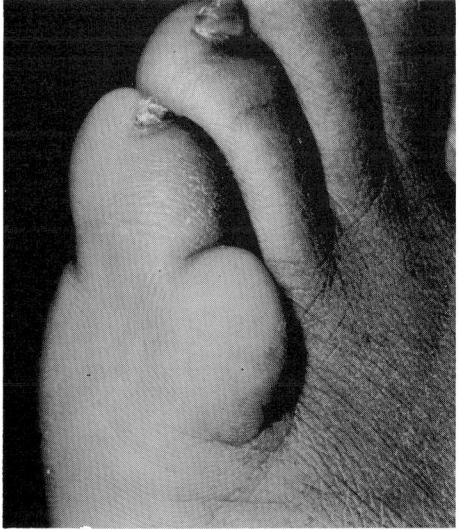

Fig. 4-23A. Supernumerary toe over fifth.

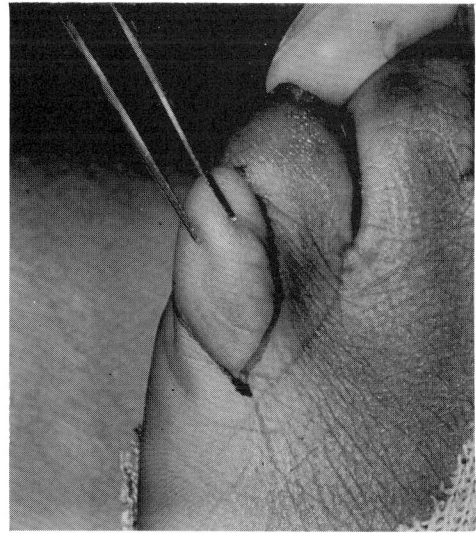

Fig. 4-23B. The incision line is carefully marked.

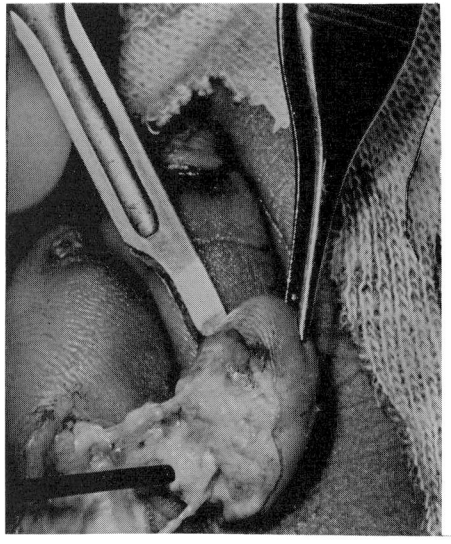

Fig. 4-23C. Supernumerary toe is resected. Vessels are ligated. Pointer shows accessory phalanx.

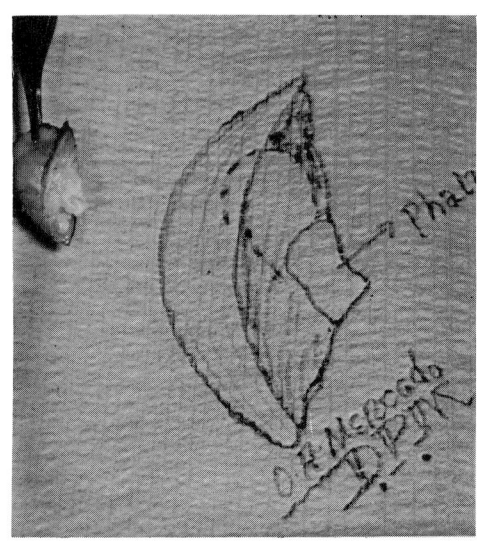

Fig. 4-23D. Drawing shows outline of phalanx.

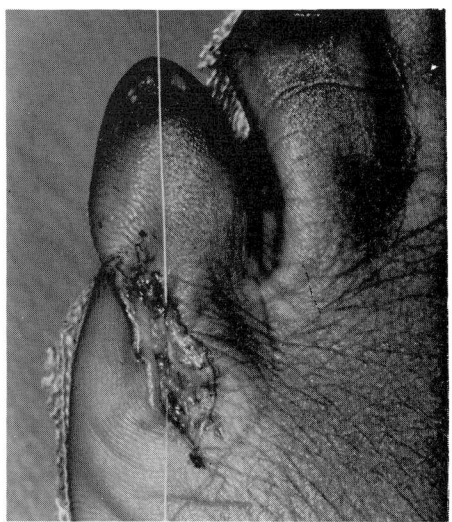

Fig. 4-23E. Sub-cutaneous tissues are closed with 4-0 Dexon.

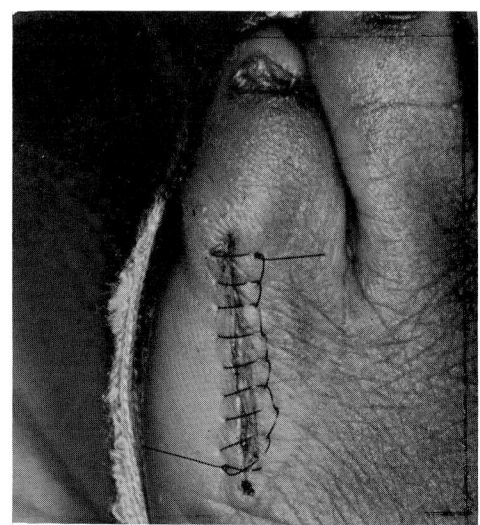

Fig. 4-23F. The wound is closed with a continuous lock suture of 5-0 nylon.

CHAPTER 5 — PRINCIPLES OF BONE SURGERY

    I. Anatomy of Bone
- A. Cortical and Cancellous bone healing
- B. Clinical Significance

    II. Performing the Osteotomy

    III. Fixation of Bone
- A. External Fixation
- B. Internal Fixation
    1. Stainless Steel Materials
    2. Bone Pegs—**starting a bone bank**

CHAPTER 5

PRINCIPLES OF BONE SURGERY

Most of the surgery performed on the foot takes place in bone tissue. Therefore, it will behoove us to review: (1) the anatomy of bone; (2) the difference between **cortical** and **cancellous** bone healing and its clinical significance; (3) how an osteotomy is performed; (4) methods of fixation.

Anatomy of Bone

Any long bone (fig. 5-1A) is composed of a **base**, a **shaft** and a **head**. The base and head are composed of **cancellous bone**. The shaft is composed of compact or **cortical bone**. By having a springy head, a hard shaft and a resilient base, Mother Nature has created her own way of absorbing shock and distributing weight. In my mind, the metatarsals have always reminded me of miniature **shock absorbers** (fig. 5-1B).

PRINCIPLES OF BONE SURGERY

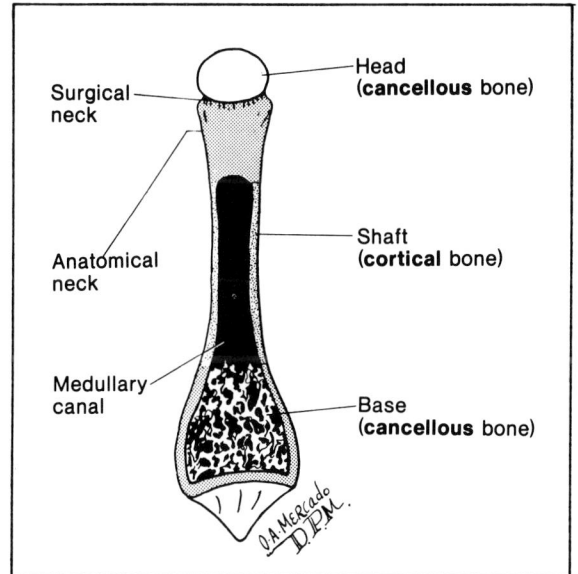

Fig. 5-1A

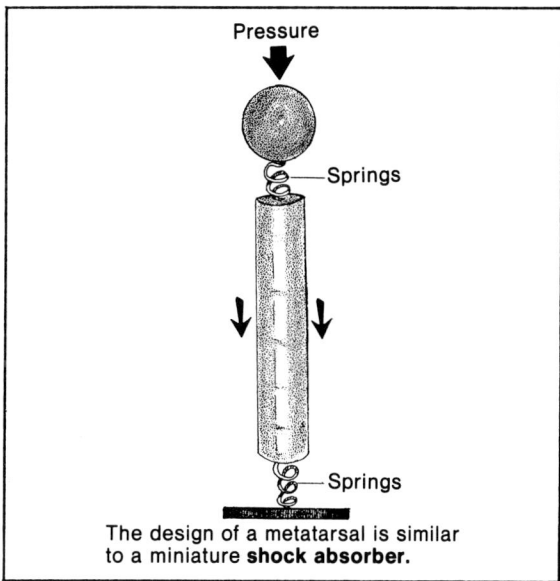

The design of a metatarsal is similar to a miniature **shock absorber.**

Fig. 5-1B

Vascularity of Bone

In school we learn our anatomy from dried-up bones and there is tendency to think of bones as being dry and dead. Nothing could be further from the truth. In reality, bone is eminently viable. A French physiologist once said, "If you scratch bone, it bleeds; if you cut-it, it heals; but, if you burn it, it dies". The surgeon should remember these words when he performs osteotomies, particularly with power equipment.

Our illustration in fig. 5-2A, reveals a cross section of a metatarsal shaft. First, we see the covering of the bone which is known as the **periosteum.**

The periosteum has small **nutrient vessels,** each of which enter the bone (along with nerves and veins) by way of a tiny hole or opening. This small opening leads into a tunnel-like canal known as **Volkman's canal,** the transversed nutrient canals of bone.

Volkman's canals connect with other tunnel-like canals which transverse the bone longitudinally. These longitudinal nutrient canals are known as the **Haversian canals.** In the center of our cross-section, we can see three Haversian canals, two of which are being connected by a Volkman's canal.

At the top of the bone, the Haversian canals are seen as small openings in the center of a series of concentric rings. These concentric rings are made up of still smaller holes known as **lacunae,** which means crib. Each of these lacunae contain, actually craddle, an **osteocyte,** the bone forming cell.

The concentric rings are called **lamellae,** meaning a lamina or page. To give you an idea of how they are arranged, if you were to roll-up a number of loose pages into a tube, the hole in the center of the tube would be the equivalent of the Haversian canal, the pages would be the lamellae (see fig. 5-2B).

In the bone, the unit formed by the Haversian canal, the lamellae, the lacunae and their ostocytes are referred to as the **Haversian System.** The inside of our cross-section is known as the **endosteum,** the lining of the **medullary canal.**

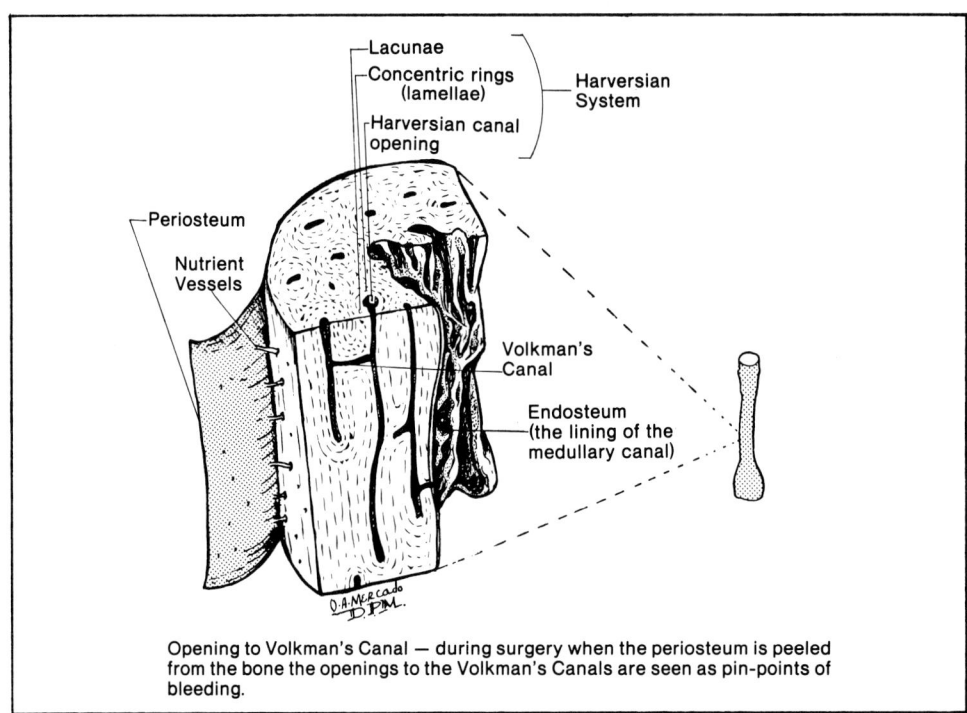

Fig. 5-2A

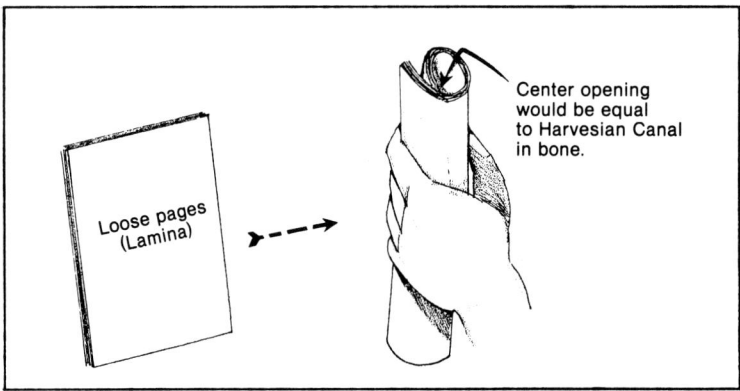

Fig. 5-2B

Cartilage Nutrition

Cartilage has no circulation of its own. It depends entirely on the subchondral bone for its nutrition. The surgeon should always keep this point in mind when performing osteotomies near the articular facets; it is important to allow sufficient bone between the cartilage and the osteotomy site to insure **cartilagenous viability.**

Healing of Bone

Cancellous bone heals from side to side; there is little or no proliferation; healing is **enhanced** by compression.

Cortical bone, on the other hand, heals by; first, having **periosteal proliferation** around the shaft; next, the ends of the bone exhibit lack of osteophytic activity **((empty lacunae);** the periosteal proliferation continues until a large **callus** is formed around the shaft. This callus formation is a **classic sign** of cortical bone healing; finally, the bone undergoes **reabsorbtion** (remodeling of the callus tissue).

The main difference between cancellous and compact bone is in the number of osteocytes they contain. In cancellous bone, the osteocytes are the same as in compact bone, but they are farther apart. Consequently there are less of them in a given area. In compact bone, the osteocytes are closer together, actually **compacted;** resulting in a greater number of osteocytes.

Perhaps we can use an analogy here to better illustrate the difference between cancellous and compact bone healing. Let us take a square block area from, lets say, a ghetto section in Chicago. The area would be teaming with thousands of people who have been compacted into tight living quarters. If we then went to the plains of Nebraska, and took a square block section, we would possibly have a few farmers with plenty of room around them.

Let us now suppose that a car accident occurs in the middle of one of our imaginary blocks. In our Nebraska block sometime may elapse before the farmers discover the accident. In time, however, the accident would be quickly and neatly taken care of.

If the accident were to happen in the middle of our city block ... well, we would surely have a great number of people involved. More people would react than necessary, resulting in a chaotic scene which would certainly prolong the cleaning up of the accident. In time, however, things would get back to normal.

In **cancellous bone,** then, there are less osteocytes, so the reaction is neat and predictable. If you compress the bone, the osteocytic activity will be increased and healing will be enhanced.

In **compact bone,** with its greater number of osteocytes, there will be an over reaction of osteocytic activity. Actually more osteocytes than needed will become involved, thus leading to the classic callus formation associated with cortical bone.

Clinical Significance

Figure 5-3A is an x-ray of a 20 year old female patient who complained of a painful Intractable Plantar Keratosis under the second metatarsal head. The x-ray revealed an elongated second metatarsal shaft.

We decided to shorten the second metatarsal shaft in order to realign the metatarsal parabola, thus redistributing the weight more evenly on all the metatarsal heads. The procedure performed was a peg and hole technique, an operation which was devised at Franklin Boulevard Community Hospital a number of years ago to provide shortening of a metatarsal ray (see Chapter 6 — Fig. 6-15).

In the peg and hole technique the metatarsal is cut transversely at the junction of the middle and distal one third of the metatarsal shaft, right on **cortical bone.** The distal end of the shaft is then retracted dorsally and a peg is fashioned from the shaft. Incidentally, the size of the peg will depend on the amount of shortening desired.

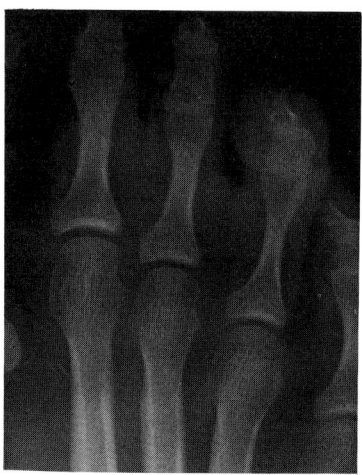

Fig. 5-3A. Pre-operative x-ray view elongated 2nd. metatarsal.

The medullary canal on the proximal end of the shaft is carefully reamed out. The previously fashioned peg in the distal end of the metatarsal is then inserted into the reamed out medullary canal, thus shortening the metatarsal ray.

The tight fit of the peg inside the medullary canal will be sufficient to fixate the osteotomy. The wound is closed layer by layer in the usual manner and an above the ankle walking cast is applied for three weeks.

The x-ray seen on Fig. 5-3B was taken three weeks after surgery at the time the cast was removed. On close inspection you will note that there is **little,** if any, periosteal proliferation present. The ends of the osteotomy appear white — viable. The empty lacunae, lack of osteophytic activity, is not yet evident.

John Chanley, the renowned British orthopedist, did a great deal of research on **bone healing** and he found that clinical healing occurs in twenty-one days. I have followed the theories of Dr. Chanley and found that they augment our work tremendously. An osteotomy that is well executed and fixated does **not** need more than three weeks in a cast. My patients, even triple arthrodesis cases, are out of a cast and ambulating at the end of three weeks while other surgeons would have kept the same patient in a cast for six or more weeks.

The x-rays in Fig. 5-3C, taken two months after the surgery, reveals the beginning of periosteal proliferation around the osteotomy site. Also, there is a definite lack of osteophytic activity — **empty lacunae** — at the ends of the osteotomy site. The x-ray taken six months after the surgery (fig. 5-3D) reveals the callus formation around the osteotomy line, the classic sign of cortical bone healing. This callus formation around the metatarsal osteotomy site caused a lump under the skin which became irritating to the patient. Indeed, it was this complication that cause us to look for a different method of shortening a metatarsal ray.

At the end of a year, (fig. 5-3E), the bone callus is reabsorbed and the metatarsal shaft returns to its normal appearance. Note that the metatarsal **parabola** has been reestablished; the patients painful Intractable Plantar Keratosis disappeared, and she was happy with the results. However, the important point is that, because of the location of the osteotomy, the patient under went a longer period of discomfort and recuperation.

PRINCIPLES OF BONE SURGERY

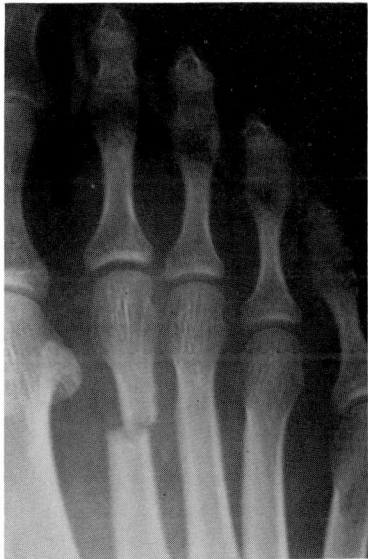

Fig. 5-3B. Three weeks post-operative x-ray (Mercado peg and hole technique was performed). There is little, if any, proliferation present.

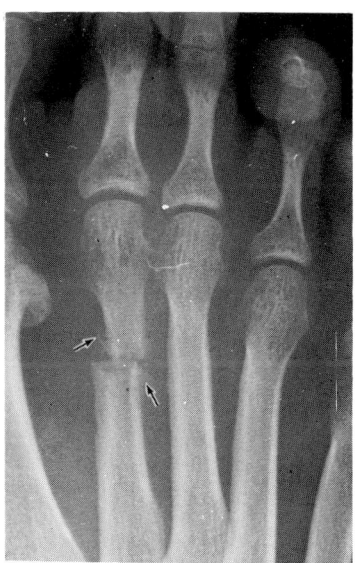

Fig. 5-3C. Two months after surgery the beginning of periosteal proliferation (arrows) is seen. Also note lack of osteophytic activity — empty Lacunae — at the ends of the osteotomy site.

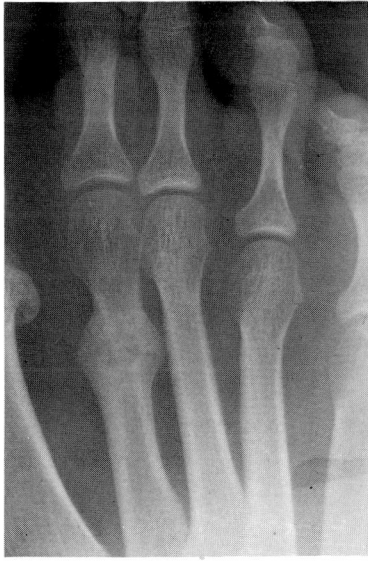

Fig. 5-3D. Six months after surgery, the classic sign of cortical bone healing — callus formation — is seen.

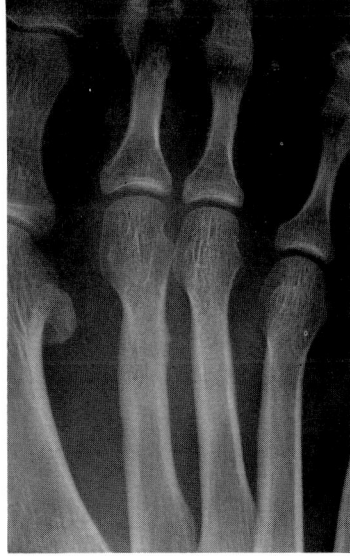

Fig. 5-3E. At the end of a year, the bone callus has been reabsorbed. The shaft returns to its normal appearance (compare with Fig. 5-3A).

Clinical Application

Utilizing the knowledge of bone healing that we have gathered over the years, we were able to devise a technique for metatarsal bone shortening (Chapter 6 — Fig. 6-12A-F) where the osteotomy is performed at the anatomical neck (cancellous bone) and healing takes place without periosteal proliferation.

In figure 5-4A, we see the x-ray of a twenty year old female patient who was suffering with an Intractable Plantar Keratosis under an elongated second metatarsal head. A **Mercado-Smith Osteotomy** was performed removing 3mm. of bone from the anatomical neck area. The metatarsal head was fixated with a small Kirschner wire (fig. 5-4B). A cast was applied and in three weeks it was removed along with the Kirschner wire.

Because the osteotomy was placed in cancellous bone, the metatarsal shaft was shortened without periosteal proliferation. The x-ray in figure 5-4C shows the patient four months after the surgery, note the reestablished parabola; the Intractable Plantar Keratosis disappeared and the patient was happy with results. More important, the recuperation time of the patient was shortened considerably.

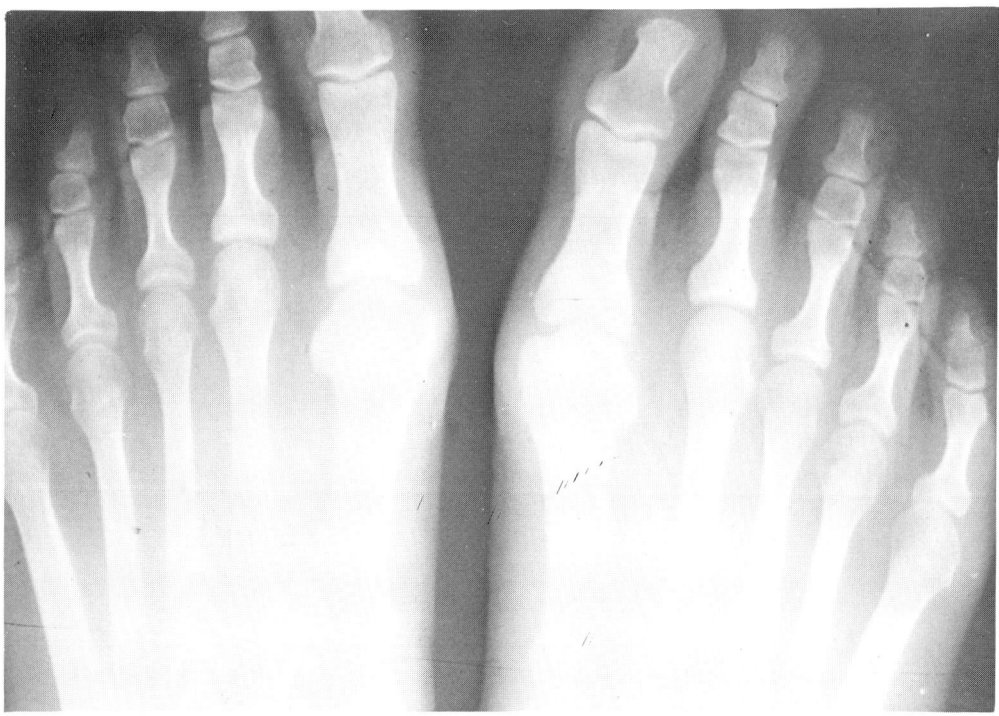

Fig. 5-4A. Pre-operative x-ray view. Note elongated 2nd. metatarsal shaft.

PRINCIPLES OF BONE SURGERY

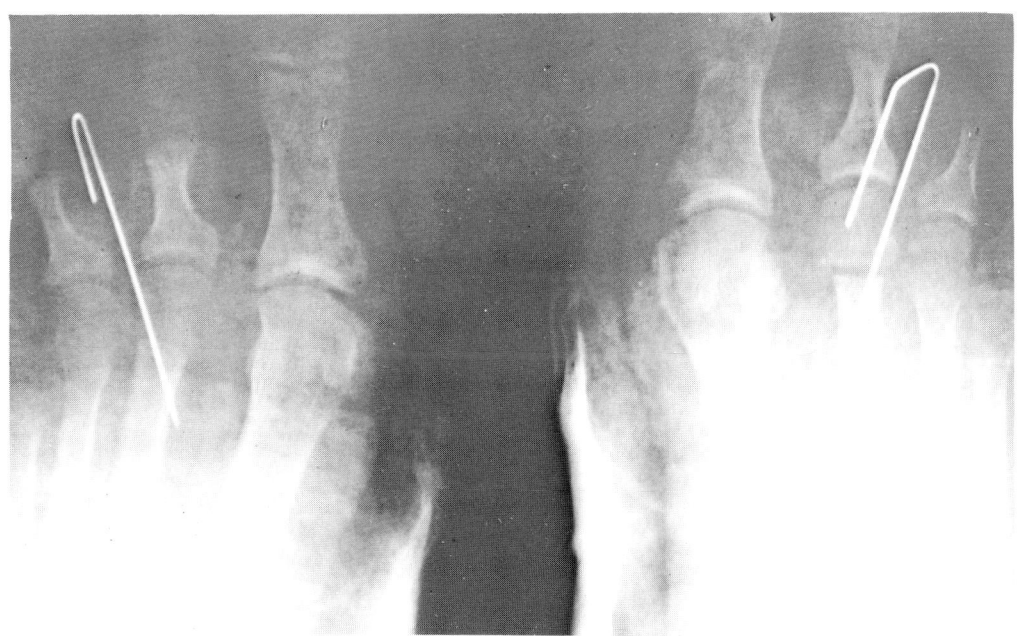

Fig. 5-4B. Post-operative x-ray. A Mercado-Smith Osteotomy was performed — shortening the 2nd. metatarsal by 3mm.

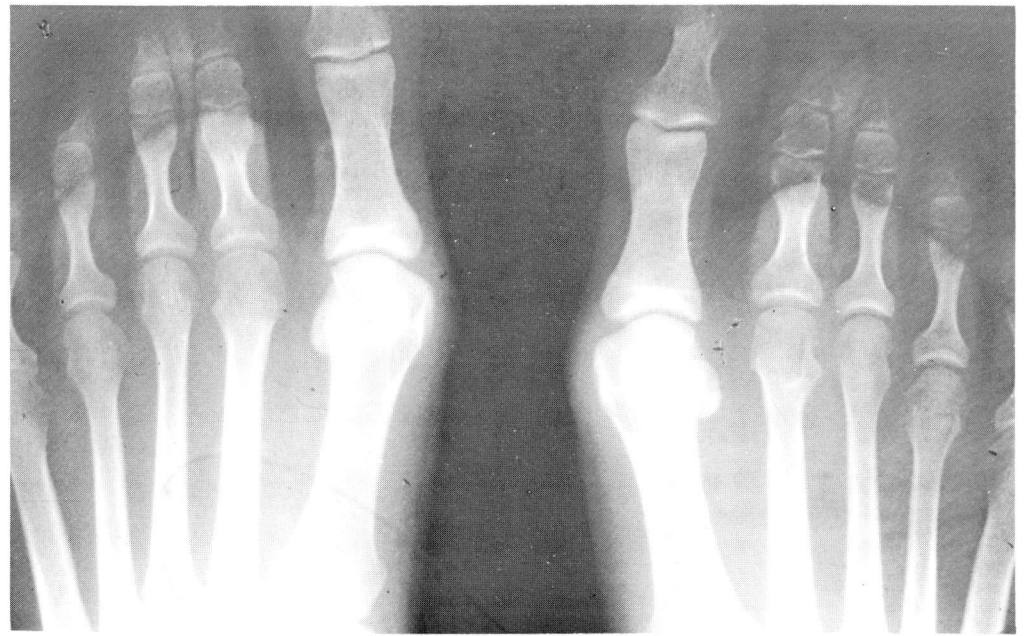

Fig. 5-4C. Four months post-operative x-ray. The parabola has been reestablished. Since osteotomy was placed in cancellous bone there is no periosteal proliferation.

Choosing the Osteotomy Site

The intelligent surgeon will take advantage of what is almost a **law** in bone healing physiology and plan his osteotomy, whenever possible, through cancellous bone.

In figure 5-5, we have illustrated a metatarsal with several cross-sections to reveal the types of bone found in the head, shaft and base. Note that at the level of the anatomical neck — where the shaft ends and the head begins — we have cancellous bone; but, just a couple of millimeters proximally, we are into cortical bone.

The importance of selecting the proper site for the osteotomy can be readily seen in the x-ray of Figure 5-6. This x-ray belongs to a patient who complained of a painful keratosis under the heads of the 2nd, 3rd. and 4th. metatarsals. On examination the heads were found to be **planti-flexed.**

The surgery decided on was an osteoclasis to the inner three metatarsals. This technique would elevate the metatarsal heads while preserving the parabola (Chapter 6 — Fig. 6-16A-J).

What makes this case so interesting is that a motion picture was made at the time of the surgery — so that an actual **visual record** exists. On review of the film, it was noted that the osteoclasis on the **2nd. metatarsal head** was performed right at the level of the anatomical neck — on cancellous bone.

On the **3rd. metatarsal head,** the osteotomy was performed about one millimeter **proximal** to the anatomical neck — on cortical bone.

The osteoclasis on the **4th. metatarsal head,** was performed two millimeters or more into cortical bone. Remember, we are talking about performing an osteotomy two millimeters away from cancellous bone. The result of this **minute digression** from the ideal osteotomy site can be seen in the x-ray taken two months after the surgery (Fig. 5-6).

On the 2nd. metatarsal head where the osteotomy was performed at the correct site, the anatomical neck, there is little or no proliferation. Healing was quick and uneventful.

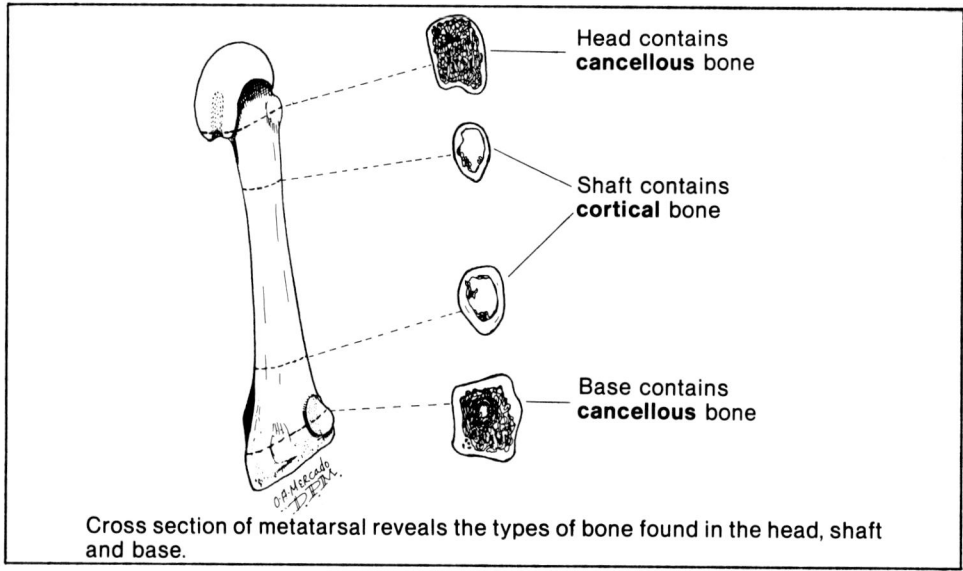

Cross section of metatarsal reveals the types of bone found in the head, shaft and base.

Fig. 5-5

PRINCIPLES OF BONE SURGERY

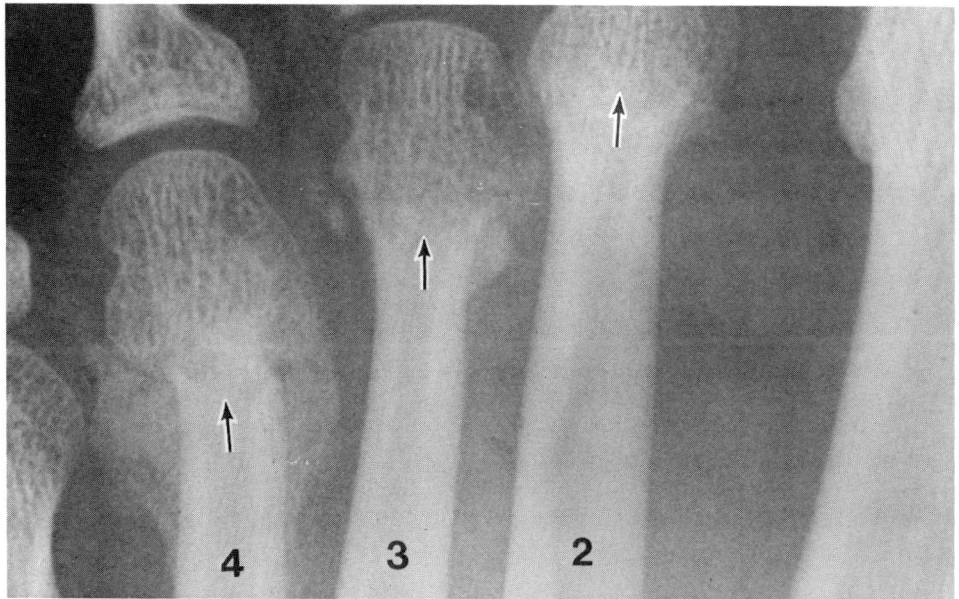

Fig. 5-6. An osteoclasis was performed on the inner three metatarsal (see arrows for osteotomy lines). See text for explanation.

Periosteal proliferation, however, is seen on the 3rd. metatarsal head around the osteotomy site — here we were one millimeter or so off the mark.

On the 4th metatarsal head, where we were off the mark by two small, **but significant,** millimeters, there is a remarkable amount of proliferation and callus formation.

The patient healed and the plantar keratosis was relieved, however, he went through months of extra healing time and discomfort and all because of a two millimeter indiscretion!

In figure 5-7A, we see a pre-operative x-ray of a hallux valgus. Upon careful examination you will note that the underlying problem is that of a laterally deviated articular facet. The technique of choice to correct the problem is a **Reverdin operation** (see Chapter 7).

The Reverdin operation calls for a wedge shaped osteotomy which is placed on the metatarsal head — in cancellous bone. Note that the wedge is placed at least one centimeter proximal to the joint line to insure cartilagenous viability. Three months later (Fig. 5-7B) the bone has healed so well that it is almost impossible to tell where the osteotomy line was placed.

A different type of wedge osteotomy was performed on the patient whose x-rays we see in figure 5-8A. A Closing Wedge Osteotomy was used to correct the metatarsus primus varus. The osteotomy is performed on cancellous bone — taking care to stay at least one centimeter from the metatarsal-cunneiform joint line to insure cartilagenous viability. One year later (Fig. 5-8B) the osteotomy line is completely healed **without** periosteal proliferation.

In cases where there is a very large intermetatarsal angle (Fig. 5-9A), the wedge needed to correct the metatarsal primus varus often goes slightly into cortical bone. This will result in some periosteal proliferation (arrow — Fig. 5-9B) which in time is reabsorbed.

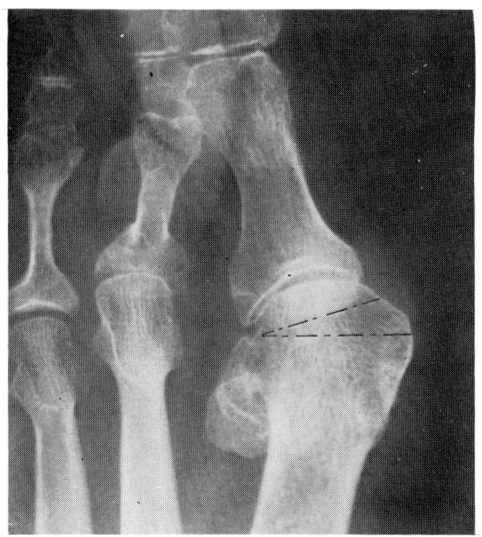

Fig. 5-7A. Pre-operative x-ray. Dotted line shows location of Reverdin Operation — note that it is in cancellous bone.

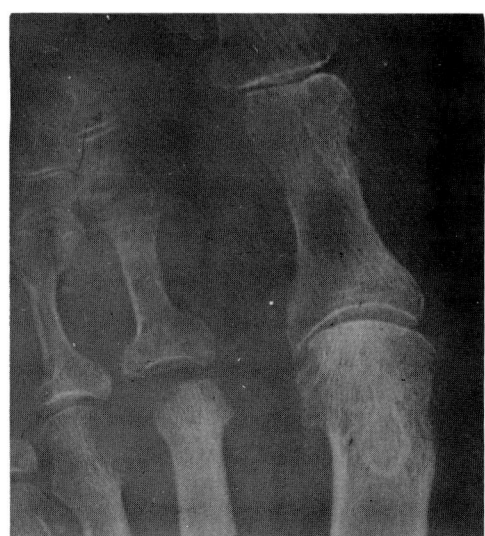

Fig. 5-7B. Three months after surgery, osteotomy line is almost invisible — since it was located in cancellous bone.

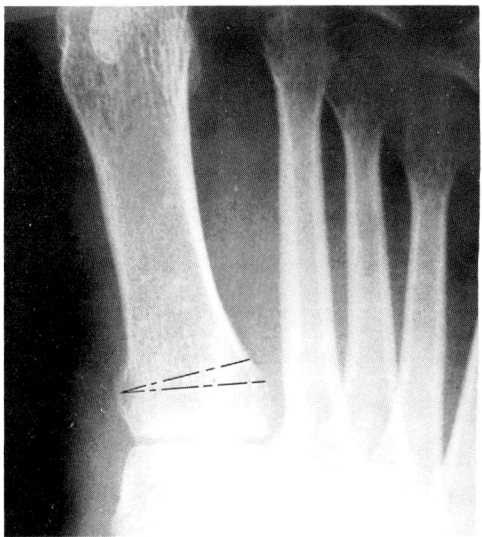

Fig. 5-8A. Pre-operative x-ray. Dotted line shows location of Closing Wedge Osteotomy — note that it is in cancellous bone.

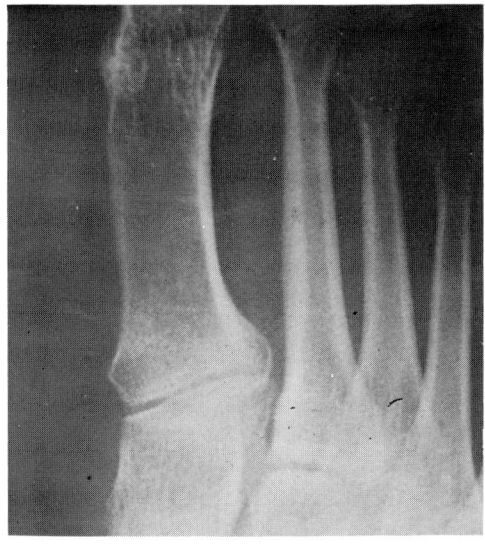

Fig. 5-8B. One year after surgery, the osteotomy line has healed without periosteal proliferation.

PRINCIPLES OF BONE SURGERY

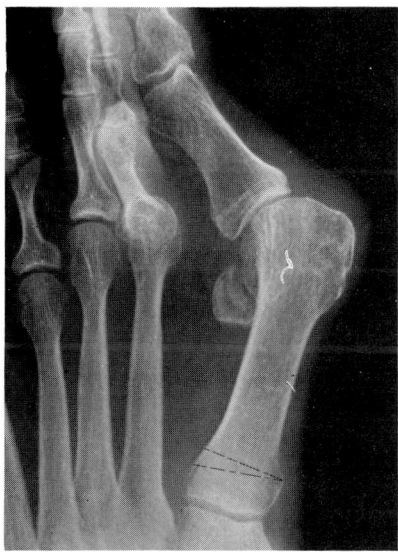
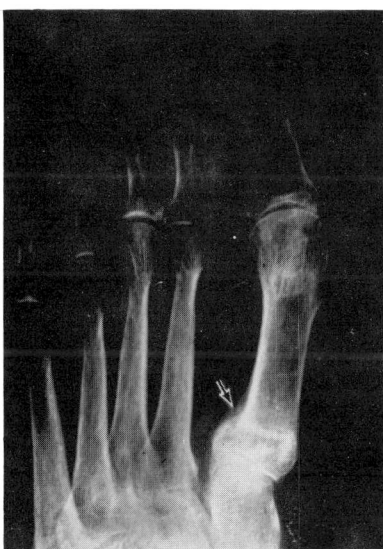

Fig. 5-9A. Pre-operative x-ray. Note large I.M. angle, dotted line shows location of Closing Wedge Osteotomy.

Fig. 5-9B. Because of the great I.M. angle the distal osteotomy line went into cortical bone – resulting in periosteal proliferation (arrow) which is reabsorbed in time.

Utilizing the Laws of Bone Healing

Bone is a wondrous material to work with. Once the surgeon understands it, he can do **almost** anything with it. To illustrate this point, lets use the case of a 33 year old male from Central Indiana who was referred to our service. He had had hallux valgus surgery one year before the x-ray in figure 5-10A was taken.

The patient complained that his "bunions" were worse than before the operation. He had excruciatingly painful transfer lesions under the 3rd. metatarsal head which severely limited his ability to walk.

The first surgery failed, as can be clearly seen in the x-rays, because the **wrong** techniques were performed. A simple bunionectomy was used when what was really needed was a Reverdin operation to realign the laterally displaced articular facet. Also, a complete metatarsal head resection was performed — totally destroying the metatarsal parabola. Complete metatarsal head resections are **no longer** used in foot surgery, except when the bone is **diseased** (i.e. Rheumatoid Arthritis, Freiberg's Infraction) or in **trauma** where the head cannot be repaired.

After careful study, it was decided to perform the following surgery:
1. A **Reverdin operation** to realign the laterally deviated articular facet of the 1st. metatarsal.
2. The **transfer** of the 3rd. metatarsal head to the 2nd. metatarsal shaft.
3. The shortening of the 4th. metatarsal ray by a **Suppan Cap Technique** — thus reestablishing the metatarsal parabola.

Incidentally, we decide on the proper parabola by tracing the patients x-ray on a piece of paper; copies are made of the tracing and then we do **paper cut-outs** until the desired parabola is obtained; these measurements are then used when we do the actual surgery.

The x-ray in figure 5-10B shows the patient immediately after the surgery — the cast is still on. The Reverdin osteotomy can be clearly seen. Notice how the articular facet is now realigned to articulate totally with the base of the proximal phalanx. This joint will now function normally and the hallux will not have the tendency of shifting lateralwards into a valgus position.

Kirschner wires were used to fixate the transferred 3rd. metatarsal head to the 2nd. shaft; and for the shortening of the 4th. metatarsal head. Also note that the 3rd. metatarsal head was removed at the level of the **cancellous bone.**

In figure 5-10C we see an x-ray taken three months after the surgery. The patient was back to **all** normal activities — with the reestablished parabola; his transfer lesion was completely eliminated. Note that the site where the Reverdin operation was performed has completely healed. The 2nd. metatarsal head, which used to be the 3rd. metatarsal head, has healed and is viable.

On the 3rd. metatarsal shaft, since the head was removed on cancellous bone, there is **no** proliferation. The Suppan Cap performed on the 4th. metatarsal head has also healed well with no evidence of periosteal proliferation.

Another case is illustrated in figure 5-11B. Here, a total 2nd. metatarsal head resection also resulted in a transfer lesion.

After doing the paper cut-outs, to establish an adequate metatarsal parabola, the surgery was performed — transferring the 3rd. metatarsal head to the 2nd shaft and performing a Mercado-Smith Osteotomy (Chapter 6 — Fig. 12A-F) to shorten the 4th. metatarsal ray.

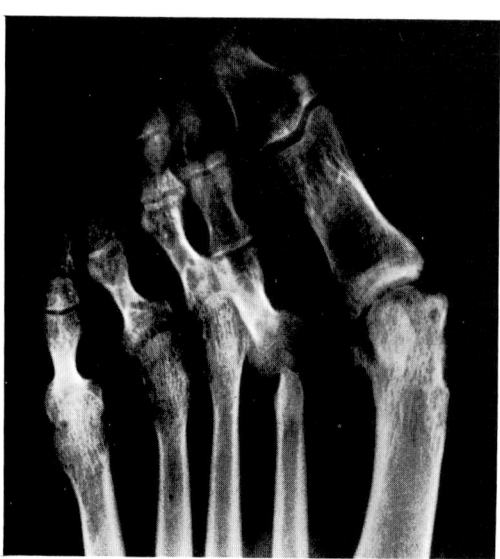

Fig. 5-10A. Pre-operative x-ray — see text.

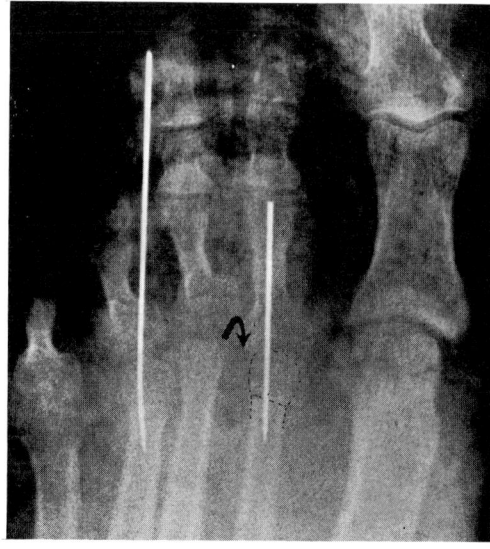

Fig. 5-10B. Post-operative x-ray — 3rd. metatarsal has been transferred to 2nd. metatarsal shaft. Note Reverdin Operation and Suppan Cap Technique on 4th.

PRINCIPLES OF BONE SURGERY

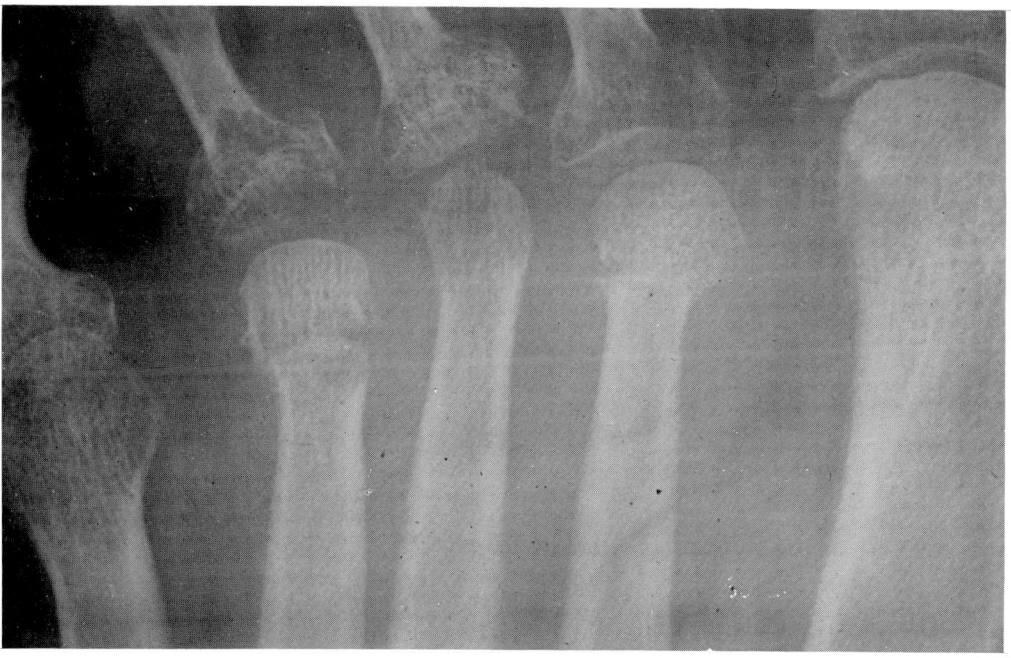

Fig. 5-10C. Three months after surgery — **Parabola** has been reestablished.

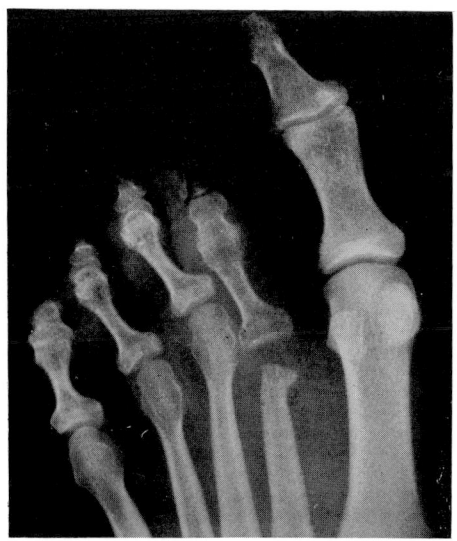

Fig. 5-11A. A total 2nd. metatarsal head resection has resulted in a transfer lesion under the 3rd.

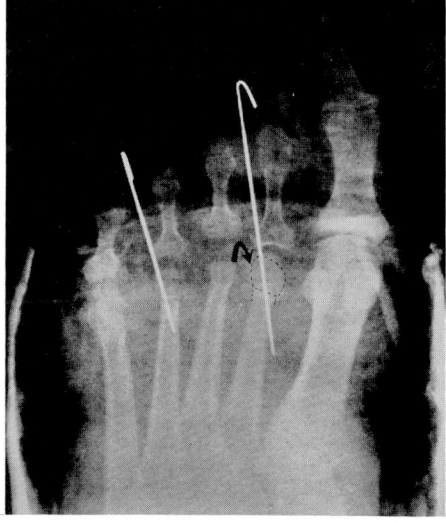

Fig. 5-11B. Post-operative x-ray — 3rd. metatarsal head has been transferred to the 2nd. shaft. Note Mercado-Smith osteotomy on 4th.

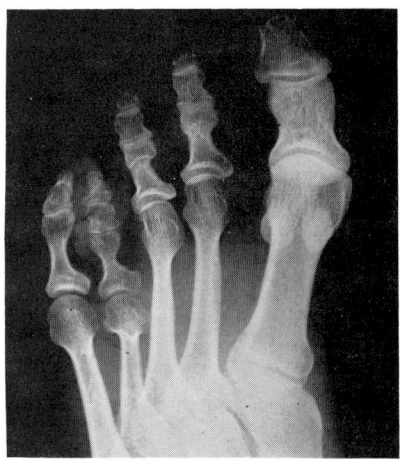

Fig. 5-12A. Pre-operative x-ray of patient with congenitally short 4th. metatarsal.

Creative Surgeries can be safely performed utilizing the principles outlined in this chapter. As an example, figure 5-12A is that of a patient with a congenitally short 4th. metatarsal which caused an overlapping 4th. toe. We decided to transfer the 5th. metatarsal head, which was normal, to the 4th. and the 4th. to the 5th.

Figure 5-12B shows the patient immediately after surgery; then 5th. metatarsal head is seen resting on the 4th. metatarsal shaft; and the stunted 4th. metatarsal head is on the 5th. metatarsal shaft.

One year later, the heads are **viable** and the overlapping toe has come down to a normal level (Fig. 5-12C).

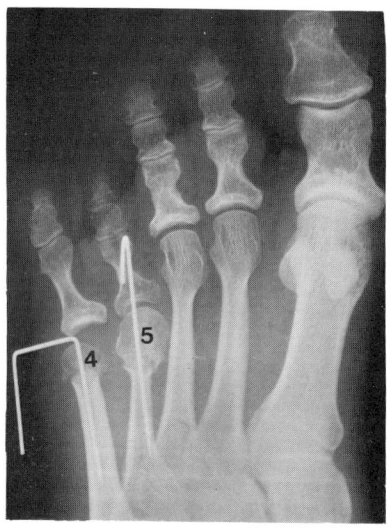 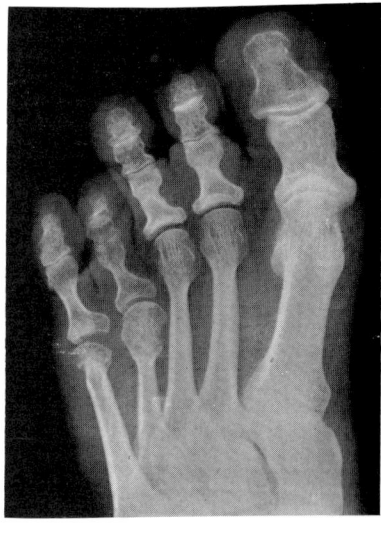

Fig. 5-12B. Post-operative x-ray — see text. *Fig. 5-12C.* One year after surgery — see text.

Dropped Metatarsal Head

In spite of the great care that we take during our metatarsal head transfer operations, I must admit that in the back of my mind I had always been worried about accidentally dropping a metatarsal head. One day, while performing a Suppan Cap Technique, the metatarsal head slipped from my hands and to the floor.

I had our circulating nurse **flash** the bone in the autoclave; the sterilized metatarsal head was returned to us a few minutes later and we continued with our surgery just as we would have done otherwise.

Figure 5-13A, shows the pre-operative view of the patient — she had an elongated 2nd. and 3rd. metatarsal shafts. Three weeks after the surgery the 2nd. metatarsal is completely healed; the 3rd. metatarsal, the one we dropped, has not healed as quickly but it is still viable (Fig. 5-13B).

Six months after the surgery, the 3rd. metatarsal has **healed** and the parabola has been reestablished (Fig. 5-13C).

This case serves very well to illustrate the fantastic healing faculties of bone. In fact it is this versatility that makes it such a wonderful biomaterial.

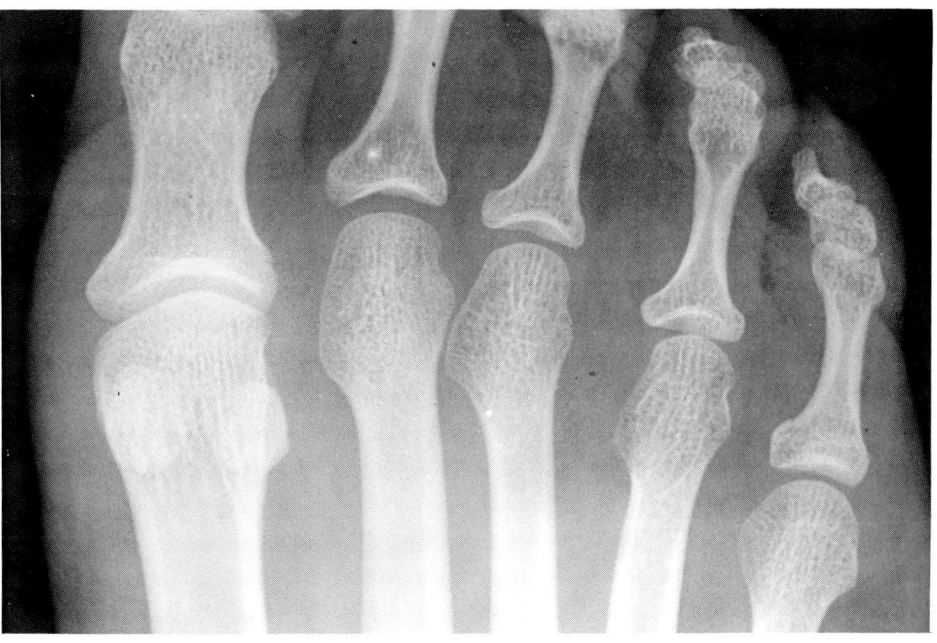

Fig. 5-13A. Pre-operative x-ray. Note elongated 2nd. and 3rd. metatarsal shafts.

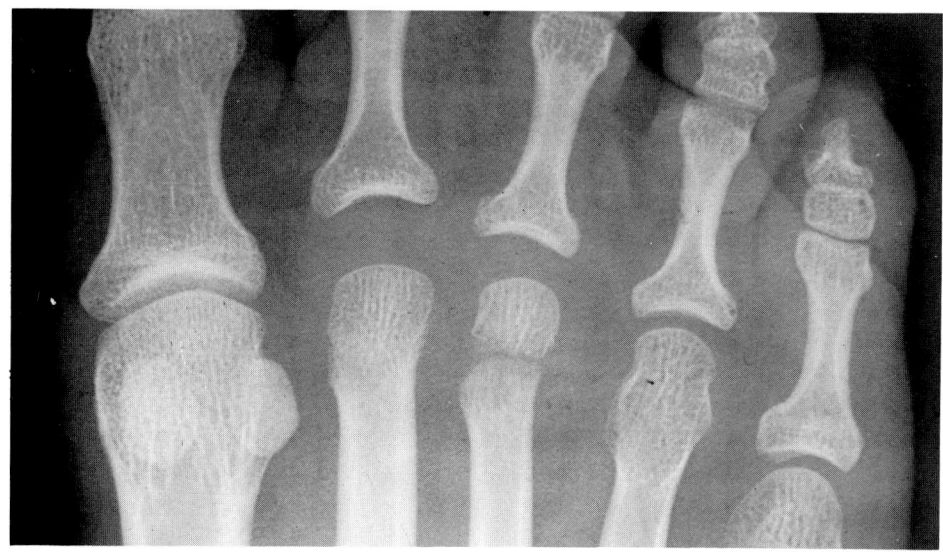

Fig. 5-13B. Post-operative x-ray (three weeks). Note that 2nd. metatarsal head has healed. The 3rd. metatarsal head (the one that was dropped during surgery) is viable.

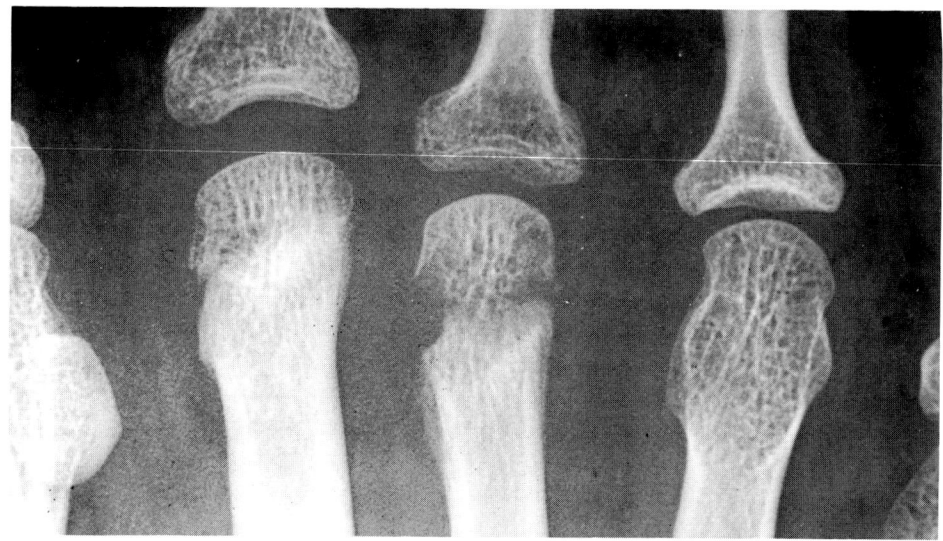

Fig. 5-13C. Six months after surgery. Parabola has been reestablished — compare this x-ray with Fig. 5-13A.

PRINCIPLES OF BONE SURGERY

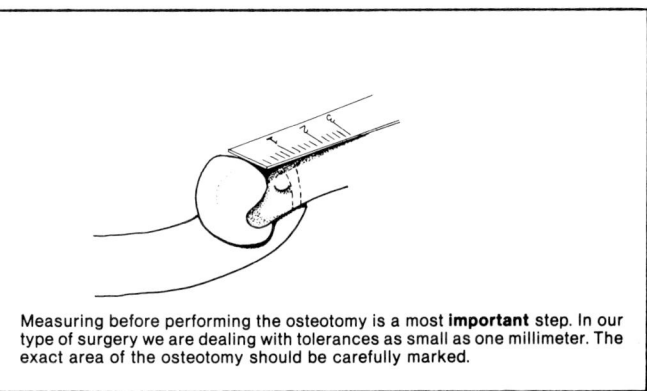

Measuring before performing the osteotomy is a most **important** step. In our type of surgery we are dealing with tolerances as small as one millimeter. The exact area of the osteotomy should be carefully marked.

Fig. 5-14

Performing the Osteotomy

Once the proper osteotomy site has been selected, the surgeon should keep the following points in mind to insure a problem free osteotomy. (Fig. 5-14)

1. Make sure that the osteotomy blade is **sharp.** Nothing will destroy a well planned and executed osteotomy as quickly as a **dull blade.** A dull blade cannot perform the nice clean cuts which are desirable in an osteotomy; a dull blade does not cut, it **tears.** Foot surgery calls for well executed osteotomies, within a tolerance of one to two millimeters; a dull blade **should not** be tolerated (Fig. 5-15).
2. Start the blade **moving** before it comes in contact with the bone. When the blade is rested against the bone and the saw is started, there will be an abrupt jump which will make starting an accurate cut difficult.
3. Don-t use a blade that's **too large.** Blades cut with an oscillating motion so that a blade has a cutting range **double** its width. A one centimeter blade will be adequate to perform all forefoot surgery (Fig. 5-16A-B).
4. Watch the **angle** of the osteotomy. Don't angulate the cuts unless they have to be angulated. Sometimes a surgeon will get so involved in the osteotomy that he will inadvertently drop his hand, thus causing an undesirable angle in the cut. It is a good idea to have your assistant's help in visualizing the proper cuts.
5. Take your time! I have seen surgeons hurrying and literally causing the bone to smoke — they are actually destroying the osteocytes.
6. Don't take a **big cut.** Its easy to take an extra piece of bone, if needed, but difficult to replace.

While the above rules may sound pedantic or even simplistic, we must remember that we are dealing with **living** bone not some innert material. Unlike a carpenter who doesn't have to worry about a piece of wood undergoing changes after he cuts it, the surgeon must **always** remember that the bone he cuts will undergo dynamic changes in the process of healing.

We are, for a fleeting moment, interlopers in Mother Nature's territory. Mother Nature will tolerate our trespass as long as we abide by her **rules**. She will even help by healing tissues that perhaps weren't cut or handled as gently as possible; but, break one of her rules and she will become treacherous and unforgiving.

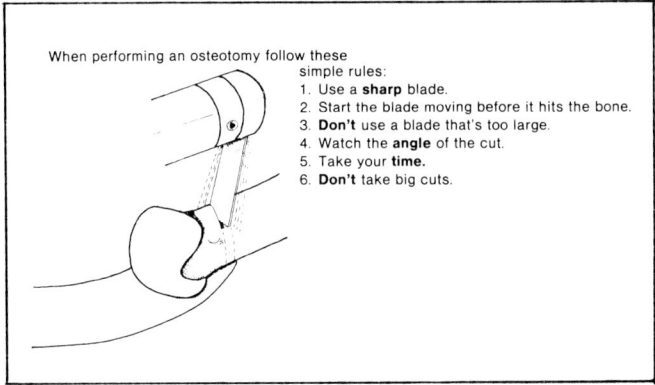

When performing an osteotomy follow these simple rules:
1. Use a **sharp** blade.
2. Start the blade moving before it hits the bone.
3. **Don't** use a blade that's too large.
4. Watch the **angle** of the cut.
5. Take your **time**.
6. **Don't** take big cuts.

Fig. 5-15

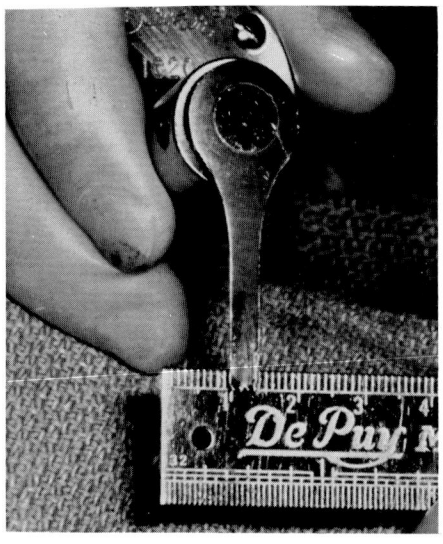

Fig. 5-16A. Blades cut with an **oscillating** motion ..

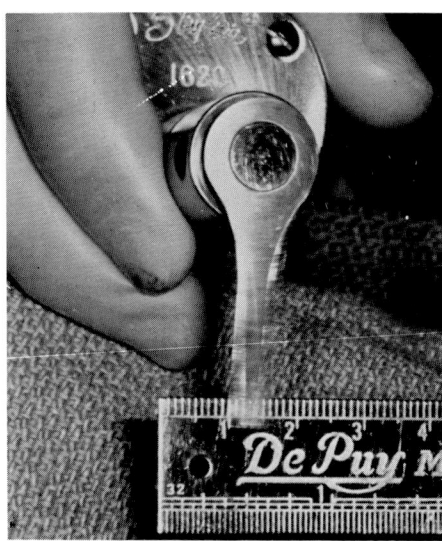

Fig. 5-16B. so that a blade has a cutting range double its width.

FIXATION OF BONE

Fixation of bone in an osteotomy is necessary to maintain correction while the bone heals. In foot surgery, there are essentially two methods of bone fixation:
  A. **External Fixation**
  B. **Internal Fixation**

External Fixation

External fixation calls for the fixation of bone with various size wires and pins which protrude outside the skin and are usually removed in three weeks, the time that it takes for cancellous bone to attain **clinical** healing.

The pullout wires that are used are called **Kirschner wires** (k-wire), they are available in three sizes; small (.035), medium (.045) and large (.062). The sizes given, incidentally, are measured in inches. The metric equivalent is as follows; small (0.85mm.), medium (1mm.) and large (1.5mm.).

As a rule, we use the **.035** k-wire for fixation of phalangeal and metatarsal-phalangeal-joint osteotomies. The **.045** k-wire is used for fixation of metatarsal base osteotomies (i.e. closing wedge, crescentic, Lapidus, etc.) and the **.062** k-wire is reserved for mid-tarsal and tarsal fusions.

The pins that can be used for external fixation are called **Steinman pins.** They are considerably larger to start with than the largest k-wire. There are seven sizes, beginning with the smallest, 5/64" (1.9mm.) and ending with the largest 3/16" (4.7mm.).

The use of Steinman pins in foot surgery should be **limited** to ankle fractures. It is **not necessary** to use anything larger than .062 k-wire to fixate the delicate bones of the foot. Good fixation of an osteotomy site is no secret. If the osteotomy is executed cleanly so that the bones meet at the proper angle, then fixation with low caliber k-wires is possible and desirable. (Fig. 5-17)

An improperly performed osteotomy will yield an **unstable** union that will resist proper fixation even with the largest Steinman pins. Somehow, it doesn't seem physiologically correct to fixate a delicate osteotomy with a large bore Steinman pin.

Another fixation pin which is available and very popular with hand surgeons is the **Riordan fixation pin** (see fig. 5-18). It is a pin which comes attached to a plastic luer-lock hub which can be loaded on a syringe. The pin is introduced and the hub is easily broken off. The Riordan pin is beneficial in office and emergency situations where the regular power equipment is not available.

Internal Fixation

Internal fixation calls for the fixation of bone with materials that are left inside the foot; or the shaping of bone in such a fashion as to form pegs, dowels and grafts.

The materials and methods that are usually used for internal fixation are the following:

A. Stainless Steel Materials
   1. wires
   2. staples
   3. screws
   4. bone plates
B. Bone
   1. pegs and dowlings
   2. ontogenous and exogenous pegs

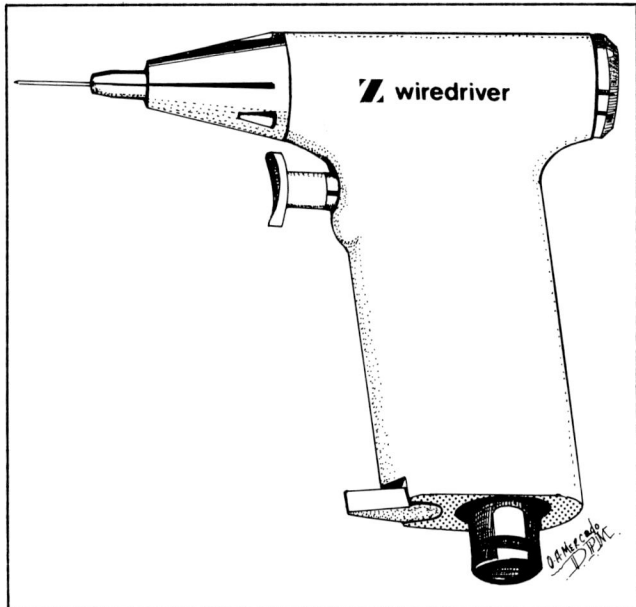

Fig. 5-17. Zimmer's new K-wire driver makes external fixation simple.

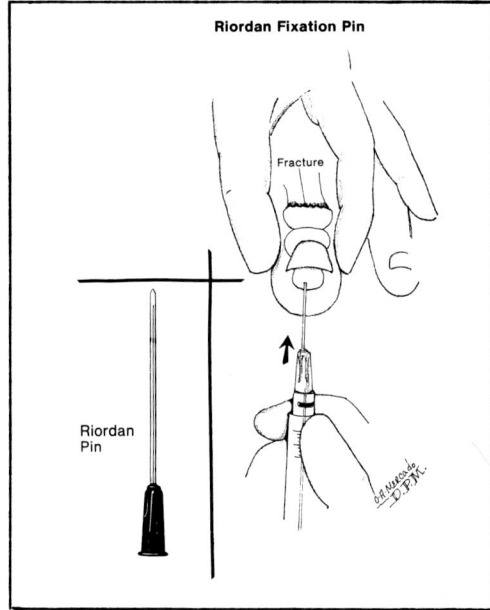

Fig. 5-18

Stainless Steel Wire

Internal fixation with stainless steel wire is common in foot surgery.. Stainless steel wire is available as a monofilament or braided; the most common sizes used are 35 gauge (approximately 5-0), 32 gauge (approximately 4-0) and 30 gauge (approximately 3-0). Most of the osteotomies performed in the foot can be fixated adequately with stainless steel wire.

Staples

Stapes are available in a wide variety of sizes and shapes (see fig. 5-19A). The most common staples are; the round staple, the barbed staple, the conventry staple, the osteoclasp and the Stone table staple. (Fig 5-19B) Staples can be used to approximate fractures or fixate osteotomy sites. The osteoclasp is an ingeniously shaped staple which actually creates compression on the osteotomy site thus enhancing healing.

PRINCIPLES OF BONE SURGERY

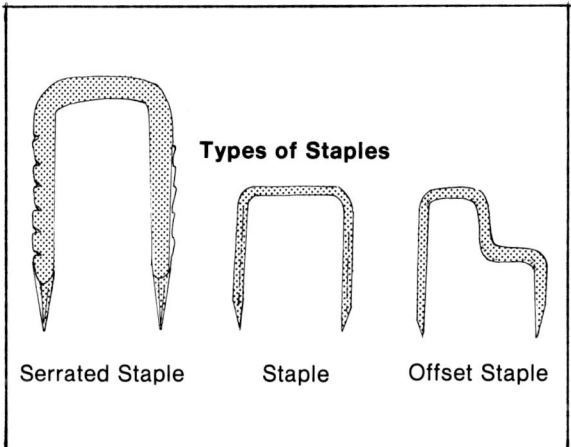

Fig. 5-19A

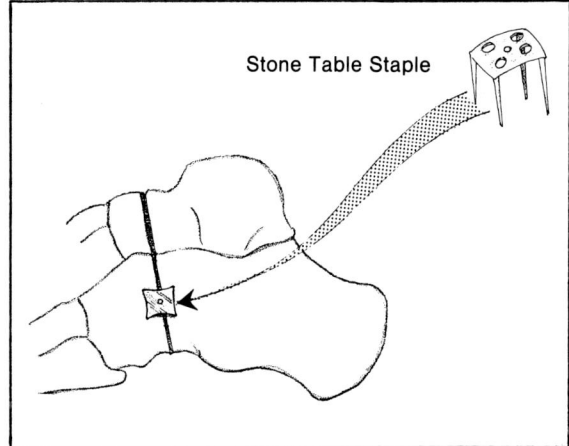

Fig. 5-19B

Screws

There is a great variety of sizes and shapes of bone screws, however, all screws fall into two general categories: 1. cortical bone screws and 2. cancellous bone screws (fig. 5-20A).

Cortical bone screws have small threads to better penetrate and fixate the bone. Cancellous bone screws have larger threads since they require more thread to bone contact for firm fixation.

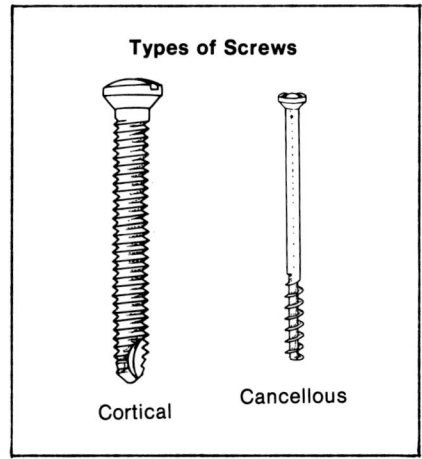

Fig. 5-20A

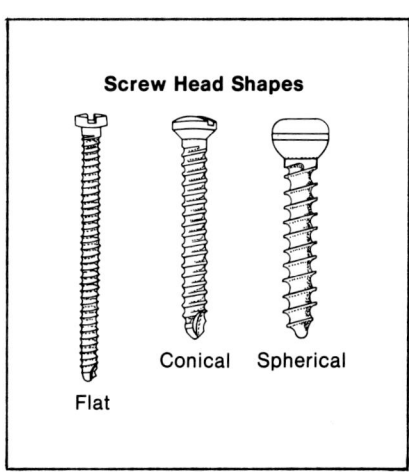

Fig. 5-20B

Bone screw heads may be classified as flat, conical or spherical. The shape refers to the undersurface of the screw. The flat head screw is used for fixation of short bones; the conical head screw is used to attach plates to bone; the spherical head screw can be used for the same purposes as the flat or conical heads except usually on larger bones (Fig. 5-20B).

The slot on the head of the screw can come in a variety of shapes, figure 5-20C illustrates some of these.

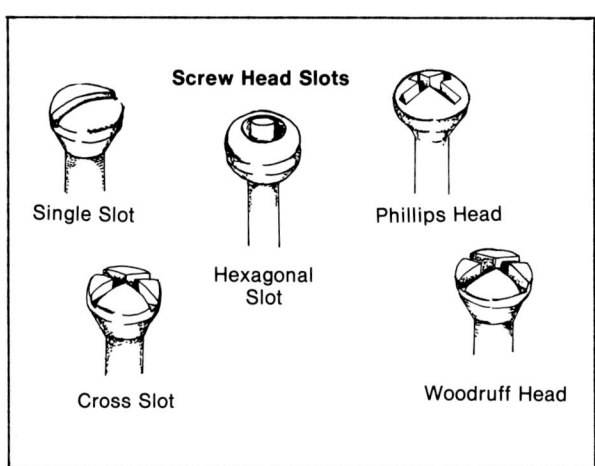

Fig. 5-20C

Bone plates

Bone plates come in a great variety of shapes and sizes. The student and surgeon alike will do well to spend sometime studying instrument catalogues and examining the plates available in the O.R. so that they can see what is available before they have to use them.

Incidentally two excellent orthopedic instrument catalogues are available from **Zimmer-Warsaw,** Indiana and **Richards Manufacturing Company,** 1450 Brooks Rd., Memphis, Tennessee.

As a rule, plates and screws are not used in forefoot surgery, they are mostly used for open reduction of ankle fractures.

Bone Pegs

Like any other building material, bone can be fashioned into a variety of shapes including pegs and dowlings. These pegs and dowlings can act as a **lattice framework** upon which the bone can grow; or they can be utilized for internal fixation, very much like a Kirschner wire.

PRINCIPLES OF BONE SURGERY

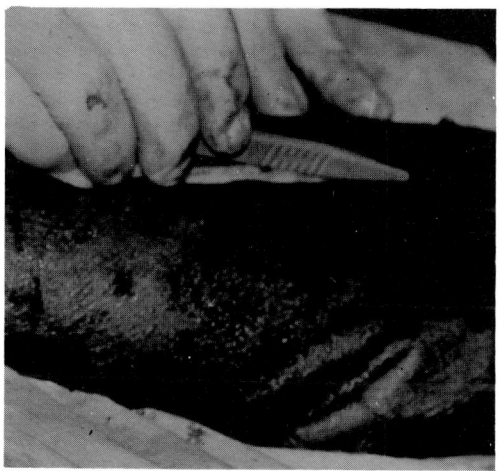
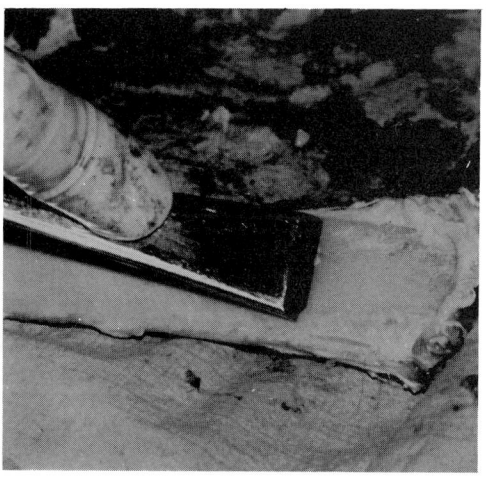

Fig. 5-21A. To start a bone bank, a freshly amputated leg is stripped of all muscles, tendons, fascia and periosteum.

Fig. 5-21B. The bone (usually the tibia) is then cut into large sections, sterilized and kept frozen until ready to use.

Starting a Bone Bank

Carrol Silver, has described a simple method for starting a bone bank which can easily be adopted by any surgeon or hospital.

He prepares his bone from a freshly amputated leg. All of the muscles, tendons, fascia and periosteum are stripped from the bone (Fig. 5-21 A-B). The bone, usually the tibia, is then cut into large sections; these sections are then sterilized and kept **frozen** inside a mason jar.

When the need for bone arises, all one has to do is to take a piece of bone from the freezer and cut the necessary size and use it — the unused portions can be re-sterilized a few more times.

At Franklin, we have been using our bone bank in this fashion for a number of years **without one** single incidence of rejection.

Before we had our bank, we would get our pegs from the shaft of the metatarsal — **ontogenous pegs** (fig. 5-22). Now, we cut our wedges from the preserved bone — **exogenous pegs.**

With the new power equipment we can fashion any size or shape of pegs that we will need (Fig. 5-23A-B). An assortment of sizes are kept available at all times and when the need arises they are ready for use.

In figure 5-24A, the x-rays reveal a deviated 5th. metatarsal ray. The surgery performed was a closing wedge which was fixated with an **intramedullary peg** (arrow — Fig. 5-24B).

The preoperative x-ray in figure 5-25A, reveals an Akin osteotomy three months after surgery. There is a non-healing osteotomy with a fractured lateral cortex which has resulted in a hallux varus.

A bone peg was used with excellent results to fixate the osteotomy and correct the hallux varus (Fig. 5-25B). In time, the intramedullary peg is absorbed by the bone.

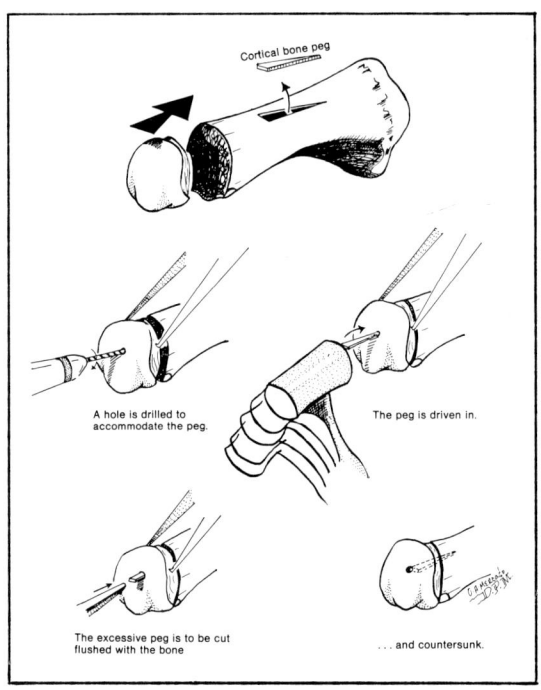

Fig. 5-22. Preparing ontogenous pegs.

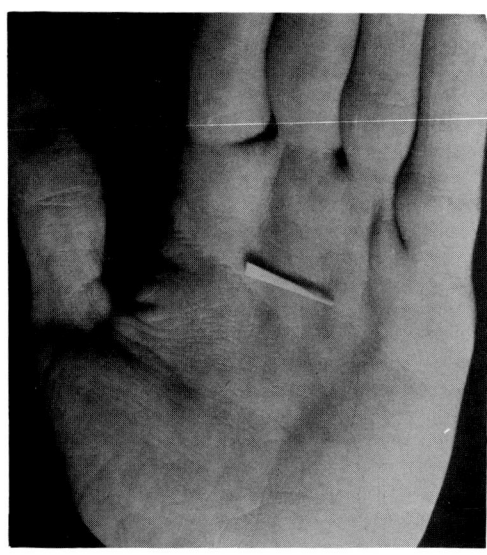

Fig. 5-23A. From the bone bank any size pegs can be prepared.

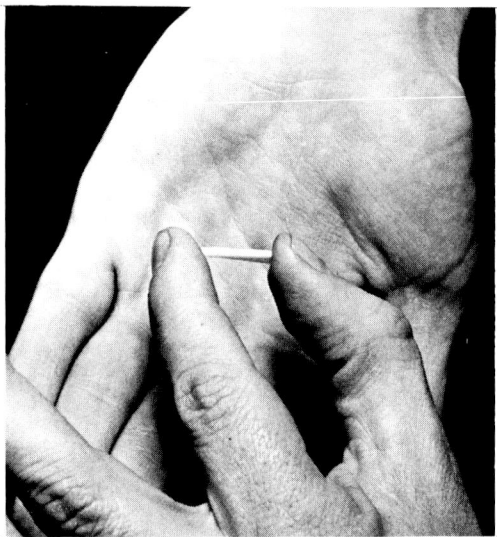

Fig. 5-23B. We keep an assortment of pegs available at all times.

PRINCIPLES OF BONE SURGERY

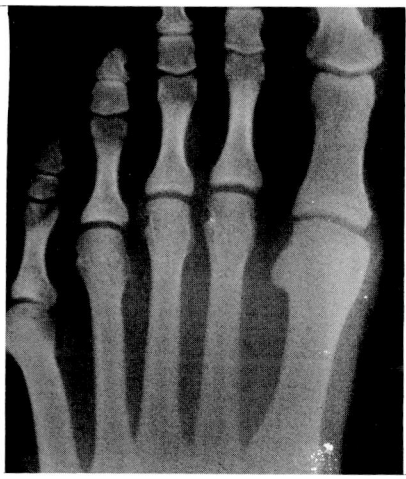

Fig. 5-24A. Pre-operative x-ray reveals deviated 5th. metatarsal shaft.

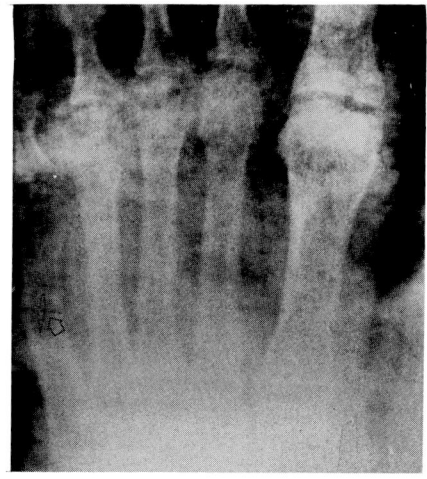

Fig. 5-24B. The osteotomy was fixated with an intramedullary peg (arrow).

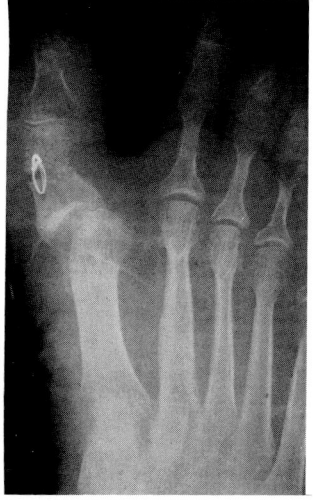

Fig. 5-25A. Pre-operative x-ray reveals a non-healing Akin osteotomy three months after surgery.

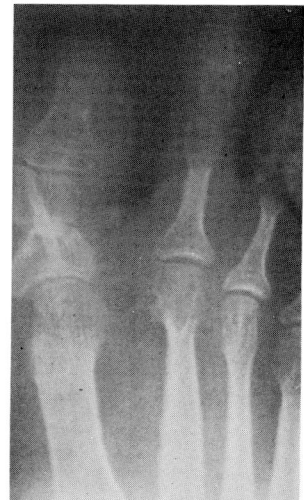

Fig. 5-25B. A bone peg was used to fixate the non-healing osteotomy.

Internal Fixation vs. External Fixation

The use of internal fixaton vs. external fixation is really one of taste among surgeons and training programs. At **Franklin** we lean more towards the use of Kirschner wire fixation because they are easy to use and painless to remove. In my personal experience with k-wire external fixation, I can think of only one malunion that has ever occured. Of course in the hands of someone capable and properly trained, I am sure that internal fixation will work just as well.

METATARSAL—PHALANGEAL JOINT SURGERY
CHAPTER 6

I. **M.P.J. Surgery**
   A. Historical Review
   B. Anatomy
   C. Etilogy
   D. Criteria

II. **Techniques for First Ray**
   A. Medial Sesamoidectomy
   B. Dorsi-Flectory Wedge Technique

III. **Techniques for Shortening the Metatarsal Ray**
   A. Partial and Complete Metatarsal Head Resectic
   B. Suppan Cap Technique
   C. Mercado-Smith Osteotomy
   D. McKeever Peg and Hole Technique
   E. Mercado Peg and Hole Technique

IV. **Techniques for Elevating the Metatarsal Ray**
   A. Osteoclasis
   B. V-Osteotomy
   C. Extensor Osteotomy (E.O.)
   D. Extensor Osteoarthrotomy (E.O.A.)

V. **Techniques for Fifth Ray**
   A. Ostectomy
   B. Partial Metatarsal Head Resection
   C. Reversed Reverdin
   D. Closing Wedge

VI. **Technique for Metatarsus Varus**
   A. Casting
   B. Heyman, Herdon, and Strong Release
   C. Base Crescentic Osteotomy

VII. **Techniques for Diseased Bone**
   A. Rheumatoid Arthritis
   B. Pan Metatarsectomy
   C. Freiberg's Infraction
   D. Bone Tumor

CHAPTER 6

METATARSAL PHALANGEAL JOINT SURGERY

Historical Review

The history of surgical procedures for the relief of plantar keratosis goes as far back as 1916, when **Meisenbach** (Fig. 6-1) suggested an osteotomy of the metatarsal shaft to elevate the metatarsal ray. This technique lay dormant in the literature until it was brought back into vogue during the late sixties.

In 1917, **George Davis** suggested the resection of the complete metatarsal head as his answer to the problem of plantar keratosis. This technique became the most commonly used procedure for the relief of intractable plantar keratosis in the fifties and sixties. Indeed, many metatarsal heads were taken out, only to have the plantar lesion reoccur under the adjacent metatarsal head as a **transfer lesion.**

In fact, the technique for metatarsal head transfer came about directly as the result of the need for a procedure which would allow the surgeon to re-establish weight-bearing patterns after the metatarsal parabola had been destroyed by ill-advised resection of metatarsal heads. Today, complete metatarsal head resections are only performed on diseased bone (i.e. Freiberg's Infraction, Rheumatoid Arthritis or in trauma where the bone cannot be repaired.)

Wedge ostectomy at the base of the metatarsal was described by **Mau** in 1940. Today, under the name of Extensor Osteotomy, it is used for the elevation of an elongated metatarsal ray. **Borggreve** in 1949 suggested a wedge ostectomy similar to Mau's, only it was performed at the site of the anatomical neck.

Dickson in 1948 described his pie-wedged resection of the total metatarsal phalangeal joint ray for the relief of all intractable plantar keratosis under the second metatarsal phalangeal joint. Unfortunately, some surgeons are still performing this crippling operation.

In 1952, **Duncan McKeever,** described his sub-capital peg and hole technique. This technique is still an excellent method of shortening a very long metatarsal ray while preserving the joint.

M.P.J. SURGERY

Plantar Condylectomies became very popular after **Henri DuVries** published his paper, "New Approach to Treatment of Intractable Verruca Plantaris (Plantar Warts)," in 1953. His technique called for the resection of the hypertrophic plantar condyles. In reality, the plantar condyles are seldom hypertrophic to the point of causing a plantar lesion. As a result, DuVries' plantar condylectomy gave a high incidence of poor results. Not because the technique was bad per se, but because it was overused and misapplied.

Giannestras described a method of shortening an elongated metatarsal ray. His technique, written in 1957, look deceptively easy in a drawing (see Fig. 6-1). In reality, it is a very difficult technique to execute and is seldom used.

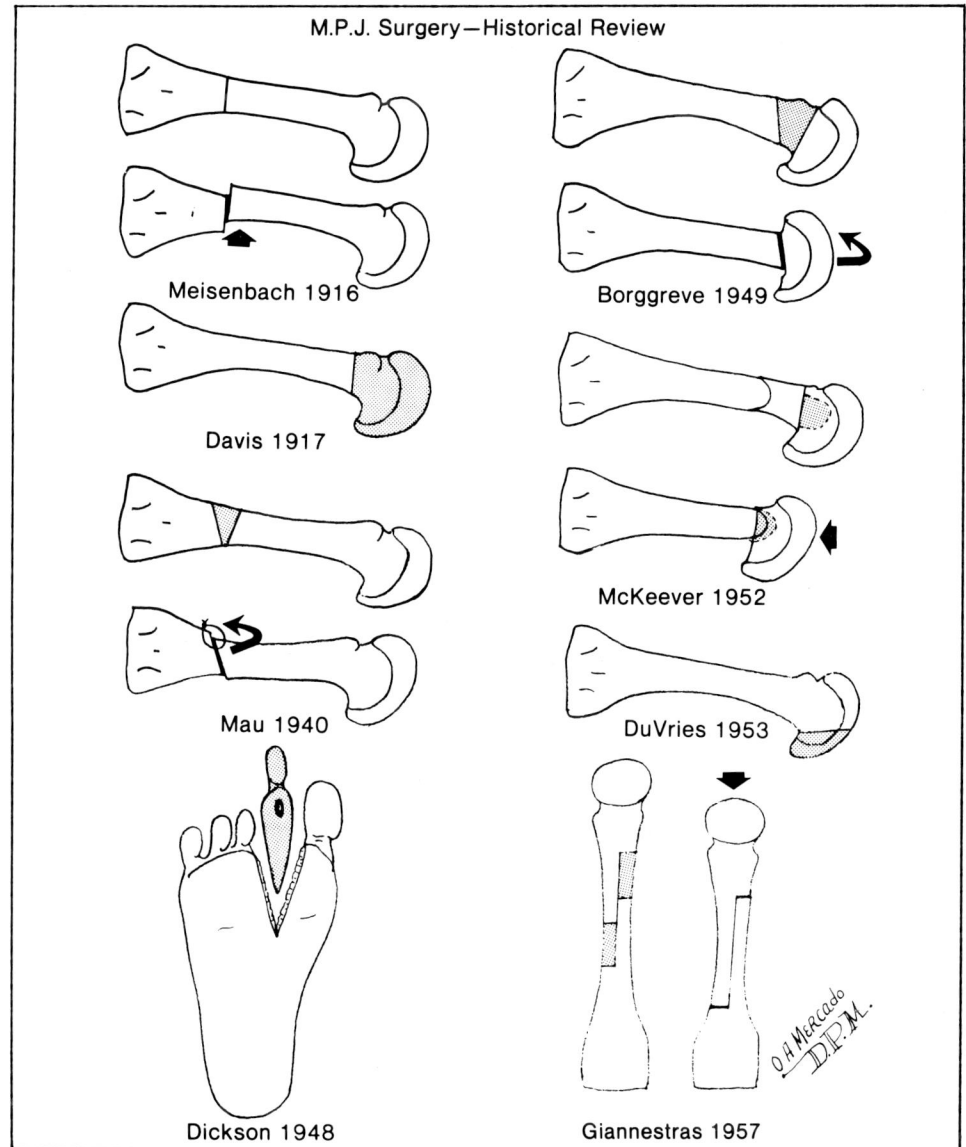

Fig. 6-1

In looking back at the history of metatarsal-phalangeal-joint surgery, it appears that surgeons have all been looking for the one technique which will correct all intractable plantar keratosis. Unfortunately, there is no panacea in surgery. The surgeon must evaluate each case individually, and choose, from the many techniques that are available, the one that will best correct the patient's problem. In the pages that follow, we hope to make the surgeon's task of choosing a technique a little easier.

Anatomy of the Metatarsal-Phalangeal-Joint

Before we can choose a technique, we must first understand what a complex mechanism the metatarsal-phalangeal-joint is.

Osteology

The metatarsal phalangeal joint is composed of the metatarsal head and the base of the proximal phalanx.

From a lateral perspective, the metatarsal head presents an articulate facet which extends more posteriorly on its plantar aspect than on its dorsal aspect. This plantar extension makes up the medial and plantar condyles. There is a groove in between these condyles for the passage of the flexor tendons. (see Fig. 6-2).

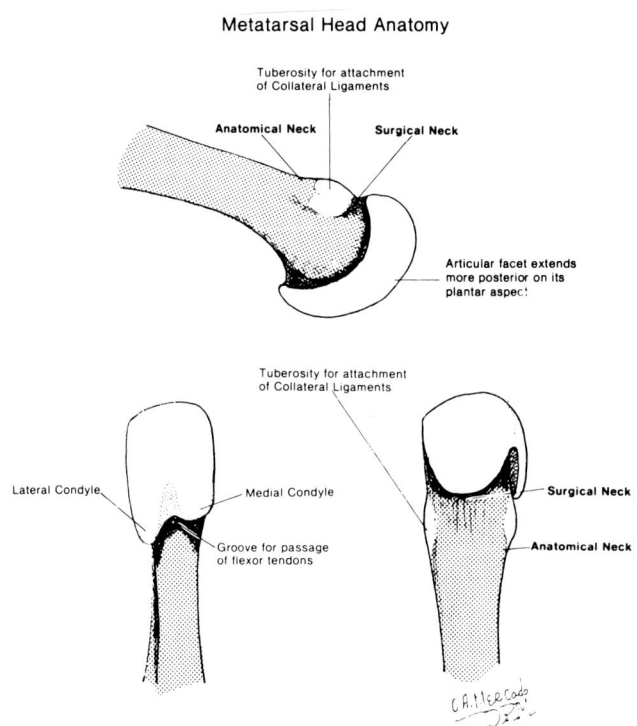

Fig. 6-2

The lateral condyle is larger than the medial condyle. There is a normal inward rotation of the metatarsal head on its axis, causing the lateral condyle to be more involved on weight bearing that the medial condyle.

On the dorsal aspect of the metatarsal, at the end of the shaft, are two tuberosities to either side of the shaft (medial and lateral) for the attachment of the collateral ligaments. The groove that is formed in between these tuberosities and the beginning of the articulate cartilage on the dorsal aspect is known as the **surgical neck.** The area immediately proximal to the tuberosities (the end of the shaft) is known as the **anatomical neck.**

The base of the proximal phalanx is approximately three times thicker than its head. On its lateral and medial aspects it presents a facet for the attachment of the collateral ligaments. On the plantar aspect it has two eminences separated by a groove (or tunnel) for the pasage of the flexor tendons.

Collateral Ligaments

The metatarsal phalangeal joint is held together first by a strong cord like collateral ligament which extends from the metatarsal tuberosities to the facets on the base of the proximal phalanx. This collateral ligament is quite unique. Most collateral ligaments go from side to side, as do the interphalangeal ligaments or even the metacarpal-phalangeal collateral ligaments in the hand. The metatarsal phalangeal joint collateral ligament crosses the joint line at approximately 45°, also, it is inside the capsular ligament. In the hand the collateral ligament is outside the capsule (see Fig. 6-3).

Capsular Ligament

The next component of the metatarsal phalangeal joint is the capsular ligament, this too is quite unique because the capsule is thin on the dorsal aspect but on the plantar aspect it is reinforced by the **transverse metatarsal ligament.**

Muscles and Tendons

There are a number of muscles and tendons around the metatarsal phalangeal joint. First we have the **extensor tendons.** There are two, the extensor digitorum longus, the most superificial and extensor digitorum brevis. On the plantar aspect we have the **flexor tendons.** There are also two, but while on the dorsum of the foot the longus tendon is the most superficial, on the plantar aspect the flexor digitorum brevis is the most superficial tendon and the longus is the deeper tendon. This creates a problem for mother nature, since the brevis tendon has to become the deepest tendon in the digital area so as to be able to insert into the base of the proximal phalanx.

Mother nature resolves the problem admirably, by having the brevis tendon bifurcate to allow the flexor digitorum longus to pass to its attachment into the base of the distal phalanx, and join again to insert as a single tendon into the base of the middle phalanx.

The other muscles around the metatarsal phalangeal joint are the **Lumbricales.** These arise from within the tendons of flexor digitorum longus, passing forward and dorsally to insert into the expanse of extensor digitorum longus. There are two lumbricales around the metatarsal phalangeal joint, one to either side.

The **interosseous muscles** arise from in between the metatarsal shaft and insert into the base at either side of the proximal phalanx. There are two interossei muscles around the metatarsal phalangeal joint.

Plantar Fascia

The plantar fascia sends down fibers to make up the tendon sheaths of the flexor tendons and at the same time to surround fatty tissue into a sort of **fat pad.**

Components of the Metatarsal Phalangeal Joint

You must marvel and respect the complexity of the metatarsal-phalangeal-joint when you think that there are fifteen individual anatomical components around this small but important joint.

The anatomical components are: two collateral ligaments, the transverse metatarsal ligament, the capsular ligament, extensor digitorum longus, extensor digitorum brevis, two interossei muscles, two lumbricales, flexor digitorum brevis, flexor digitorum longus, tendon sheath fibers from the plantar fascia, the fat pad, and the plantar fascia.

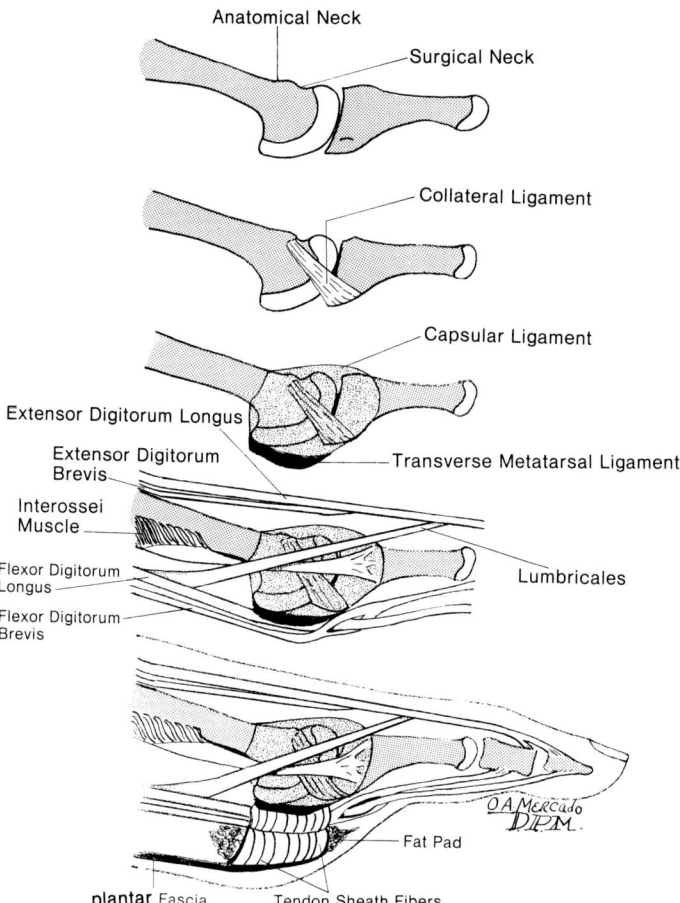

Fig. 6-3

M.P.J. SURGERY

Etiology of Intractable Plantar Keratosis (I.P.K.)

There have been many theories about the causation of intractable plantar keratosis. **DuVries** advanced the idea that the reason for the formation of the keratosis is a hypertrophic plantar condyle, usually the lateral condyle. To prove his point, he shows an illustration of a metatarsal very similar to that shown in Fig. 6-4A, where the plantar condyle appears very prominent. This is supposed to cause irritation to the plantar skin, which in turn will result in the formation of a keratosis.

While the illustration would seem very convincing, we must remember that the metatarsal shaft does not lie parallel to the plantar of the foot but descends at an angle of 30°-40°. Because of this angle of **declination,** even if the condyles were hypertrophic they would be rotated out of the way (see Fig. 6-4A1). Weight bearing occurs on the anterior one-third of the metatarsal head.

There are number of etiological factors involved in the formation of a plantar keratosis which becomes intractable and requires surgical treatment. One of these factors is the anterior displacement of the fat pad (see Fig. 6-4B). Under the normally functioning M.P.J., there is a fat pad. Sometimes, due to contraction of the digit, this pad is anteriorly displaced. Since there is no protective padding under the metatarsal head a pressure keratosis forms.

Another factor causing a plantar keratosis is a planti-flexed metatarsal ray (see Fig. 6-4C). This entity is quite simple to diagnose. In a dorsal-plantar weight bearing x-ray, the metatarsal parabola (metatarsal length pattern) appears normal. On examination, a normal metatarsal head will dorsi-flex readily when plantar pressure is applied; puckering will occur when the head is pushed with the thumb (see Fig. 6-5A).

A **planti-flexed** ray will cause elevation of the plantar skin, in relationship to the other metatarsals. When pressure is applied, puckering will not readily occur. Also, when the adjacent heads are pressed, they will dorsi-flex to a higher level than the involved metatarsal ray (see Fig. 6-5B).

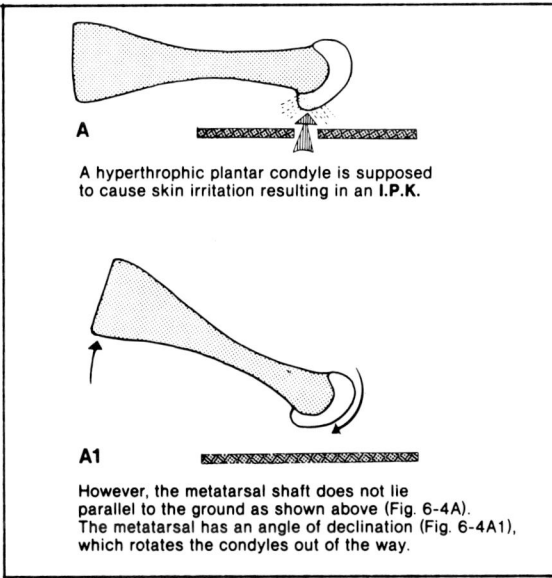

A. A hyperthrophic plantar condyle is supposed to cause skin irritation resulting in an **I.P.K.**

A1. However, the metatarsal shaft does not lie parallel to the ground as shown above (Fig. 6-4A). The metatarsal has an angle of declination (Fig. 6-4A1), which rotates the condyles out of the way.

Fig. 6-4A

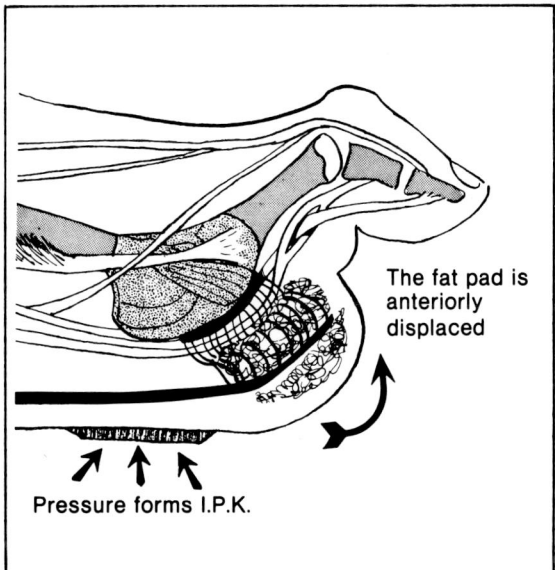

The fat pad is anteriorly displaced

Pressure forms I.P.K.

Fig. 6-4B

The metatarsal heads must dorsi-flex easily as on weight bearing, they have to adjust to the walking surface in such a manner as to distribute the weight evenly. When a metatarsal ray is planti-flexed, it carries the brunt of the body weight, resulting in the formation of a plantar keratosis. In order to distribute the weight more evenly, the surgeon has to elevate the involved metatarsal head so that on weight bearing, it will be at the same level as the other metatarsal heads.

An **elongated metatarsal** ray is a common factor causing a plantar keratosis (see Fig. 6-4D). The surgery to correct this problem calls for the shortening of the metatarsal to a level where a normal **parabola** will be created.

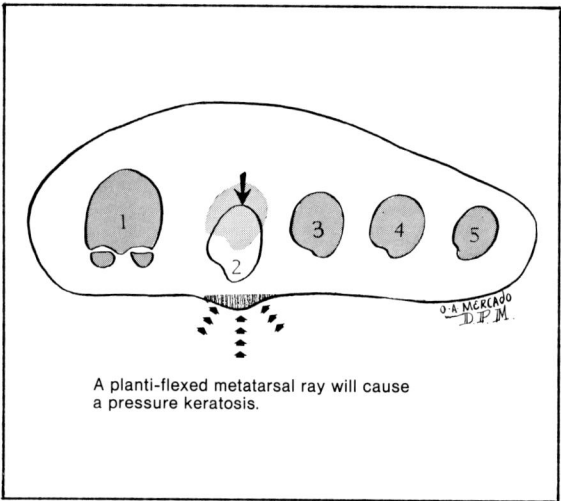

A planti-flexed metatarsal ray will cause a pressure keratosis.

Fig. 6-4C

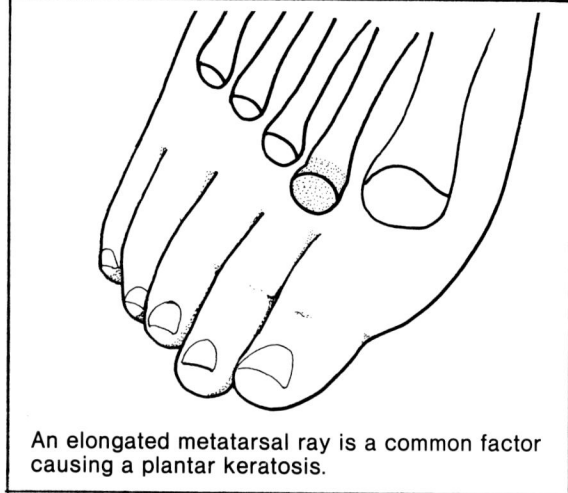

An elongated metatarsal ray is a common factor causing a plantar keratosis.

Fig. 6-4D

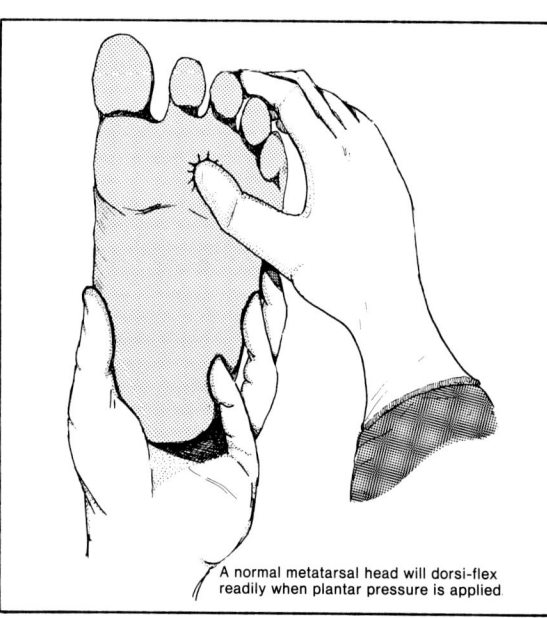

A normal metatarsal head will dorsi-flex readily when plantar pressure is applied.

Fig. 6-5A

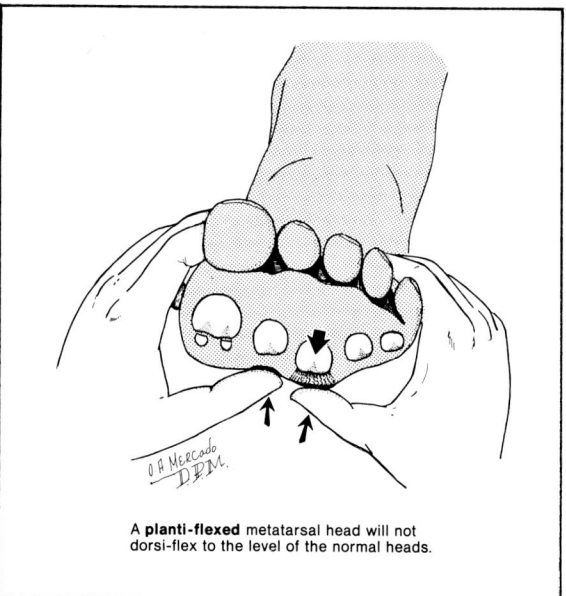

A **planti-flexed** metatarsal head will not dorsi-flex to the level of the normal heads.

Fig. 6-5B

Metatarsal-Phalangeal-Joint Surgery Criteria

For the last few years, we have been using a simple surgical criteria at Franklin Boulevard Commuity Hospital, which has served us well. Obviously, no criteria will work 100% of the time, but if the surgeon is imaginative and flexible, the results will be consistently good (see Fig. 6-6).

First Metatarsal Ray

The procedure to use for relief of a plantar keratosis under the first, will depend on whether the lesion is caused by a hyperthrophic medial sesamoid or a planti-flexed ray.

For a hypertrophic sesamoid a medial sesamoidectomy is performed.

For a planti-flexed ray a dorsi-flectory wedge is performed.

Fifth Metatarsal Ray

Hyperostosis on lateral aspect (Tailor's bunion) — use simple ostectomy.

Intractable Plantar Keratosis under the 5th metatarsal head — use partial metatarsectomy

Medially displaced articular facet - use Reversed Reverdin

Deviated metatarsal shaft — use closing wedge

Elongated Metatarsal Ray

The metatarsal should be shorten so as to create a normal **parabola.**

If ray has to be shortened .5cm. or less— 1. Suppan cap
    2. Mercado-Smith osteotomy

If ray has to be shortened .5cm. or more— 1. McKeever peg and hole
    2. Mercado peg and hole

Planti-Flexed Metatarsal Ray

Surgery aims at elevating the involved metatarsal (or metatarsals) to an even level, so that all of the metatarsals are meeting the ground together.

For single planti-flexed ray   — 1. Osteoclasis
    2. Extensor osteotomy (E.O.)

For single planti-flexed ray   — 1. Extensor osteoarthrotomy (E.O.A.)
with unstable metatarsal base
join

For multiple planti-flexed ray — 1. Osteoclasis
(not more than three)

M.P.J. Surgery Criteria

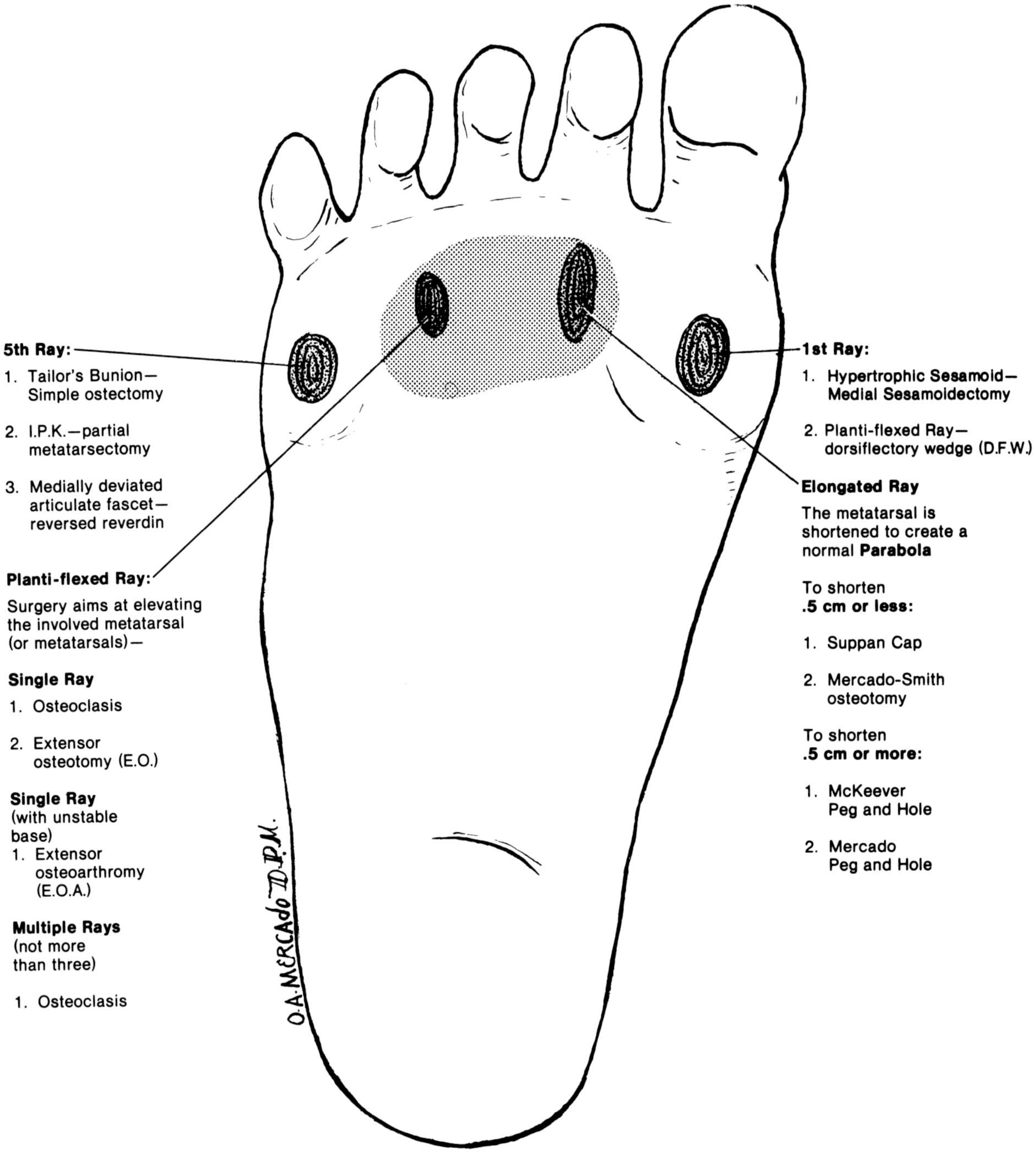

5th Ray:

1. Tailor's Bunion—
   Simple ostectomy

2. I.P.K.—partial metatarsectomy

3. Medially deviated articulate fascet—reversed reverdin

Planti-flexed Ray:

Surgery aims at elevating the involved metatarsal (or metatarsals)—

Single Ray

1. Osteoclasis

2. Extensor osteotomy (E.O.)

Single Ray (with unstable base)

1. Extensor osteoarthromy (E.O.A.)

Multiple Rays (not more than three)

1. Osteoclasis

1st Ray:

1. Hypertrophic Sesamoid—
   Medial Sesamoidectomy

2. Planti-flexed Ray—
   dorsiflectory wedge (D.F.W.)

Elongated Ray

The metatarsal is shortened to create a normal **Parabola**

To shorten **.5 cm or less:**

1. Suppan Cap

2. Mercado-Smith osteotomy

To shorten **.5 cm or more:**

1. McKeever Peg and Hole

2. Mercado Peg and Hole

Fig. 6-6

TECHNIQUES FOR FIRST RAY

Medial Sesamoidectomy

The procedure for resection of the medial sesamoid is indicated whenever there is an intractable plantar keratosis on the first metatarsal-phalangeal-joint, with an associated **hyperthrophic** medial sesamoid. It is important to first ascertain that the first metatarsal ray is not **planti-flexed**. If the ray is planti-flexed, then the medial sesamoidectomy procedure **will not** work — the technique of choice would then be a dorsi-flectory wedge.

Differential Diagnosis

The most important points in the differential diagnosis between an intractable plantar keratosis caused by a hypertrophic medial sesamoid and one caused by a planti-flexed ray are: (1) In a **dorsal-plantar x-ray view,** the medial sesamoid will be much larger than the lateral sesamoid; in a planti-flexed ray, the sesamoids appear normal. (2) In a **sesamoidal view x-ray,** (the beam of the x-ray tube is aimed just behind the sesamoids when the patient is weight bearing and the heel is raised) the medial sesamoid will be larger and not infrequently somewhat (plantarly) pointed; on a planti-flexed ray, the sesamoids will appear normal. (3) On a **lateral x-ray view,** the first ray will have a normal angle of declination; a planti-flexed first will have an acute angle of declination. (4) On **palpation,** when the foot is loaded and the intractable plantar keratosis is pressed, the first metatarsal head will move to the level of the adjacent heads; on the planti-flexed ray, the first metatarsal head will remain lower (more plantarwards) than the adjacent heads. (5) **Statistically,** hypertrophic medial sesamoids are more common than the planti-flexed first ray.

Techiques

A lineal incision 5-6 cm. long is made on the medial-plantar aspect of the first metatarsal-phalangeal-joint. The incision is deepened and the superficial bleeders are ligated. The incision is underscored so as to expose the capsular ligament of the first metatarsal-phalangeal-joint.

The plantar aspect of the wound is carefully explored and if a bursal sac (sometimes a fibroma or infrequently a neuroma) is found, it is resected in toto. The bursa, incidentally, will be inferior to the sesamoids and will extend across the total metatarsal-phalangeal-joint (Figure 6-7A).

The hallux is then vigorously flexed dorsally and plantarly; this is done so that the medial sesamoid can be felt. **Remember,** the medial sesamoid is attached to the medial head of flexor hallucis brevis, so that when the hallux is flexed, it will glide on the articulate facet of the metatarsal head (Figure 6-7A-B). In fact, the purpose of any sesamoid (the patella included) is to allow the tendon to glide smoothly over a joint without irritation or likelihood of getting inpinged when the joint is flexed.

Once the moving sesamoid is felt, it is quite simple to make an incision right at the point where the sesamoid articulates with the head (Figure 6-7B). A small stab incision can be made first, if you are not sure of the articulation, and then elongated distally and proximally to expose the sesamoid.

The capsule is then carefully retracted medially and plantarly to expose the sesamoid. Incidentally the capsule at this level is reinforced by the aponeurotic tendon fibers of abductor hallucis (Figure 6-7C).

The sesamoid is then grasped with a thumb and finger forceps and literally peeled from the tendon (medial head) of flexor hallucis brevis. The sesamoid has a strong inter-sesamoidal ligament which must be carefully cut in order to free it from the adjoining lateral sesamoid. Extreme care must be exercised during this maneuver as the tendon of flexor hallucis longus lies immediately below (Figure 6-7A). The capsule is then carefully closed as are the deep, superficial tissues and skin with the suture material of choice.

Medial Sesamoidectomy

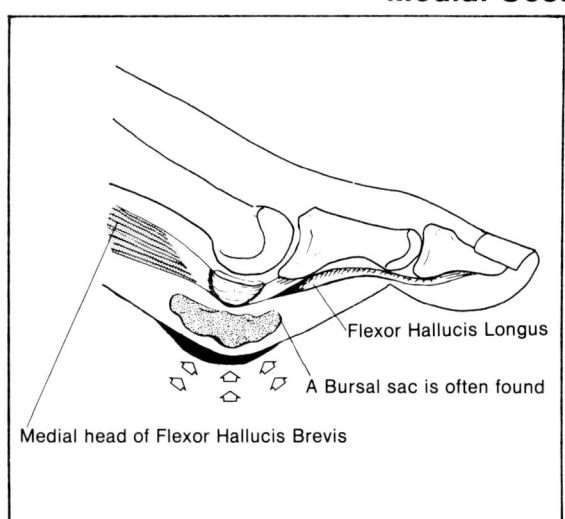

Fig. 6-7A

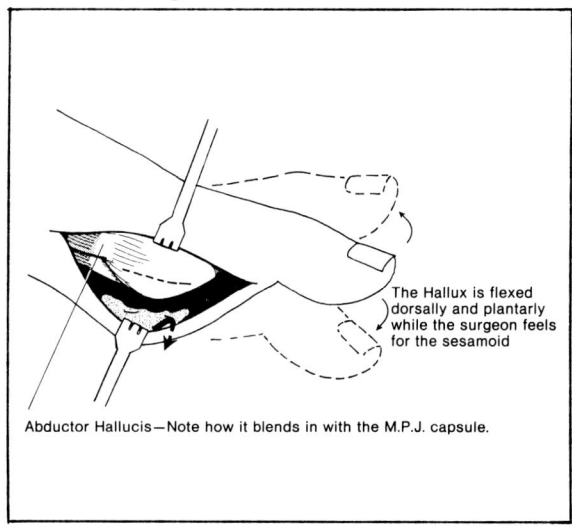

Fig. 6-7B

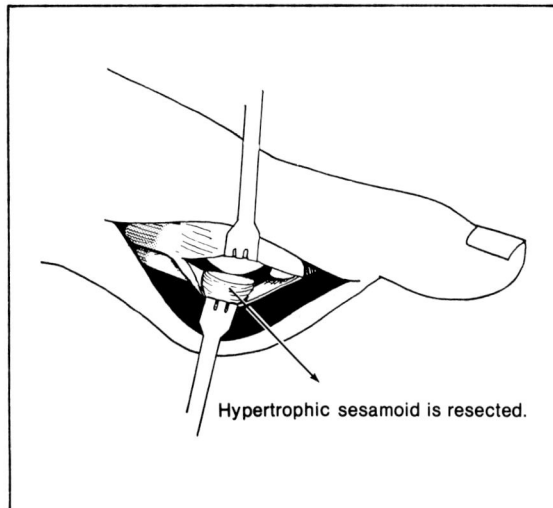

Fig. 6-7C

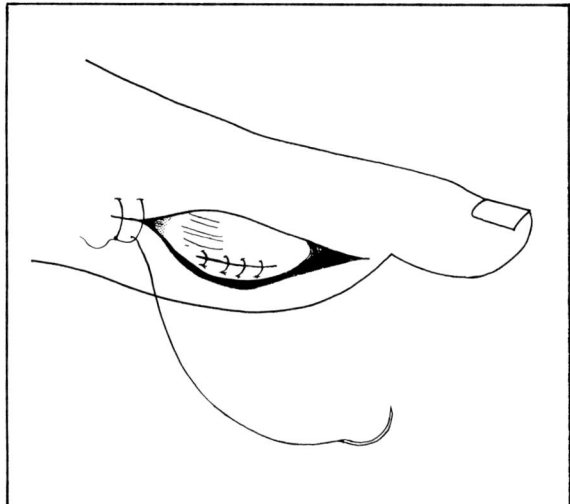

Fig. 6-7D

There is a **variation** of this procedure which was brought to my attention by **Dr. William Carpino,** of Pittsburg, Kansas. Instead of removing the hypertrophic sesamoid, he performs a medial-plantar condylectomy (Figure 6-7E-F), this allows the sesamoid to ride deeper (more dorsally), thus relieving the pressure on the first metatarsal-phalangeal-joint plantar aspect. As of this writing, I do not have enough experience with this modification to make a judgement on its efficacy.

Variation of Medial Sesamoidectomy

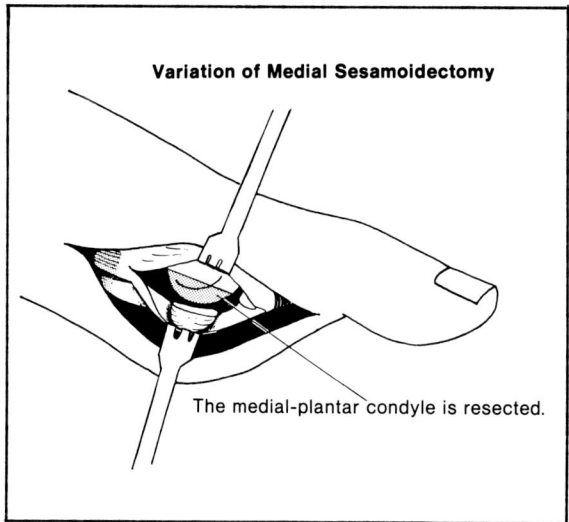

Variation of Medial Sesamoidectomy

The medial-plantar condyle is resected.

Fig. 6-7E

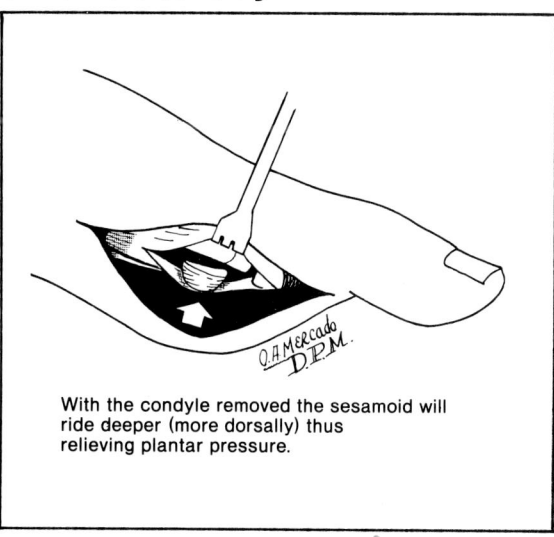

With the condyle removed the sesamoid will ride deeper (more dorsally) thus relieving plantar pressure.

Fig. 6-7F

Precautions
1. Make certain that the cause of the plantar keratosis is indeed a hypertrophic medial sesamoid and not a planti-flexed ray.
2. The skin incision should be made medial-plantar and long enough to insure adequate exposure.
3. Flex the hallux dorsally and plantarly a number of times to feel the sesamoid (remember, the sesamoid moves, but the head is still). Make the incision just in between the sesamoid and the articular facet of the metatarsal head (Figure 6-7B).
4. Underscore the sesamoid carefully to **preserve** the capsule and tendon (medial head) of flexor hallucis brevis.
5. Take care when cutting the intersesamoidal ligament not to stray too far plantarly with the blade as the tendon of flexor hallucis longus could be cut.
6. Close the capsule carefully to preserve the integrity of the joint.

Conclusion

I sometimes tell my students the story about my aunt who was one of my first surgery patients when I started practice well over a decade ago. I performed a medial sesamoidectomy on her to relieve a painful keratosis which to this day has **never** bothered her again. More important, a hallux valgus **did not** form as a result of the procedure.

I do believe that when a medical sesamoidectomy procedure is performed using the same indications, precautions, meticulous dissection and closure as described here, the chances of a hallux valgus forming as a result of the procedure, would be **rare.** In fact, I have not seen one single case of post surgical hallux valgus that could be attributed to this technique.

Medial sesamoidectomy, when performed properly, will yield consistently good results.

Dorsi-Flectory Wedge Technique

The dorsi-flectory wedge technique is indicated for the relieve of an intractable plantar keratosis under the first metatarsal-phalangeal-joint when it is caused by a **planti-flexed** first ray. This procedure **is not** indicated when the underlying problem is a hypertrophic medial sesamoid (for differential diagnosis see medial sesamoidectomy procedure, this chapter).

Technique

A lineal incision approximately 4 cm. long is made over the base of the first metatarsal extending proximally past the first metatarsal-cuneiform-joint (Figure 6-8A).

The incision is carefully deepened and retracted. You will immediately notice a large vein running across the incision, this vein is part of the **irregular dorsal venous network** and drains into the medial marginal vein (Figure 6-8B). The tendon of extensor hallucis longus runs immediately below this vein.

Sometimes, a small (and more superficial) vein is found in this area, in addition to the large vein mentioned above. The small vein can be ligated, but the large vein is preserved.

The large vein is carefully underscored and retracted with a small Penrose drain (Figure 6-8C). Incidentally, veins and arteries are quite elastic and are easily retracted.

The tendon of extensor hallucis longus is carefully retracted. Care is taken when retracting as the neurovascular bundle lies immediately below the tendon in this area. The **dorsalis pedis** gives off its two final branches, the first dorsal metatarsal artery and the deep plantar artery (Figure 6-8C).

A lineal incision is then made into the capsule and periosteum of the metatarsal base extending past the proximal joint line (Figure 6-8D). The capsule and periosteum are underscored, first with a number fifteen blade and then with a sharp periosteal elevator. The idea is to literally peel the periosteum and capsule from the bone so as to expose the dorsal, medial and lateral aspect of the base. By staying inside the capsule and periosteum, the fragile **deep plantar artery** will not be damaged. The blunt ends of a Senn retractor are used to retract the capsule and periosteum. A measurement is then taken on the dorsal aspect from the cuneiform-metatarsal-joint line distally to the base. This distance should be **at least 1 cm.** This will ensure the positioning of the osteotomy right on cancellous bone (see Chapter Five — Principles of Bone Surgery).

The proximal osteotomy line is marked lightly with an osteotome (Figure 6-8D). The second (or distal) osteotomy line is marked just distal to the first. The amount of wedge to be taken depends **entirely** on the clinical judgement of the surgeon. We have tried measuring angles and dangles and we usually (quite honestly) rely on our judgement as to how much we should raise the ray.

The idea is to raise the ray so that on loading the foot (or on weight bearing) all of the metatarsal heads meet the ground at the same level. Always start by removing the **smallest** possible amount of bone, if after the wedge is removed, the elevation of the ray is not adequate, more bone can be removed.

The proximal cut is made first, this is a straight cut from dorsal to plantar. The cut **does not** go all the way through the plantar cortex as we want to create a **hinge.** The second (distal) cut is angulated somewhat from dorsal to plantar so as to create a wedge; this cut meets the plantar end of the first cut. Again, the plantar cortex is left intact (Figure 6-8D).

The wedge thus formed is then resected and the plantar cortex (hinge) is thinned out to allow the distal end of the metatarsal to dorsi-flex, thus joining the raw bone surfaces of the osteotomy tightly together. Remember that you want a tight fit with compression as this will enhance the healing of cancellous bone (Figure 6-8E).

The **importance** of the plantar cortical hinge cannot be over-emphasized. The hinge will allow plantar to dorsal movement and at the same time prevent medial or lateral shifting of the shaft on the base. Also, it will ensure a good tight fit between the raw bone surfaces.

Fixation of the osteotomy can be accomplished internally with stainless steel or with an osteoclasp; or externally with a Kirschner wire. My personal preference is by external Kirschner wire fixation. (Figure 6-8 F). The Kirschner wire can be easily pulled out in the office without anesthesia at the time the cast is removed.

After the bone is fixated, the capsule and periosteum are carefully closed as are the deep and superficial structures and skin, utilizing the suture materials of choice. A short cast (above the ankle) is applied. The cast is removed in three weeks as are all sutures and Kirschner wire. Healing usually is uneventful.

Precautions

1. Make certain that the first ray is indeed planti-flexed.
2. Meticulous dissection should preserve the large dorsal vein as well as the deep plantar artery.
3. Make your wedge in cancellous bone at least **1 cm.** from the joint line.
4. **Do not** cut all the way through the bone when cutting the wedge. Make sure that a plantar cortical hinge is left.
5. Fixate the osteotomy line securely. My preference is external fixation with Kirschner wire.
6. Apply a short cast (above the ankle) for three weeks.

Conclusion

The dorsi-flectory technique, when performed as described here will give consistently good results.

Dorsi-Flectory Wedge Technique

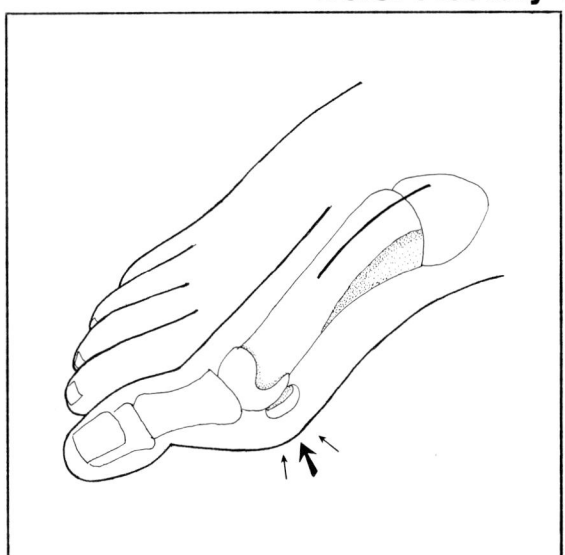

Fig. 6-8A

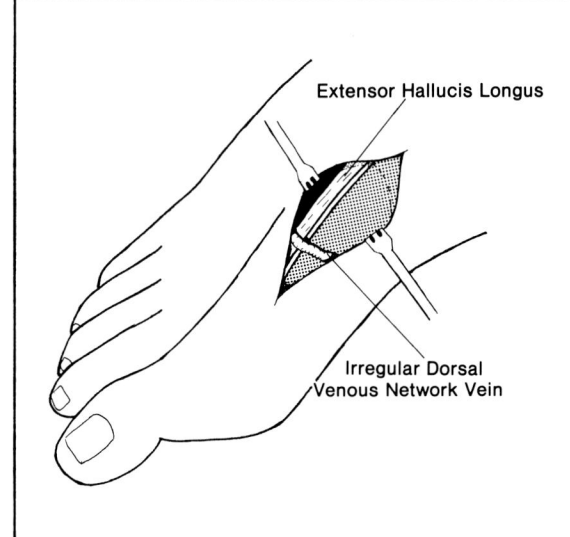

Fig. 6-8B

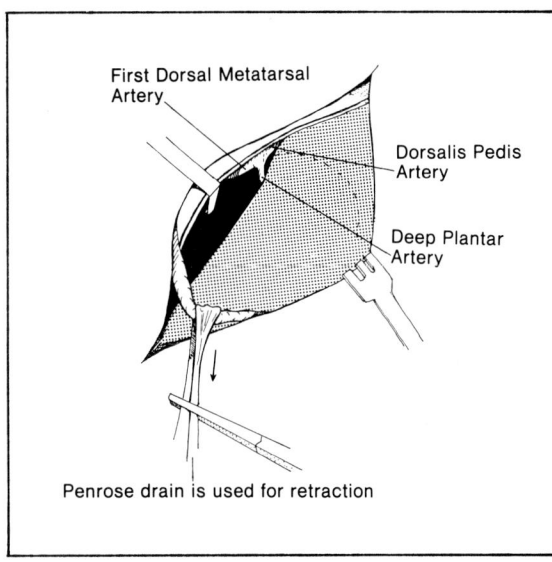

Fig. 6-8C

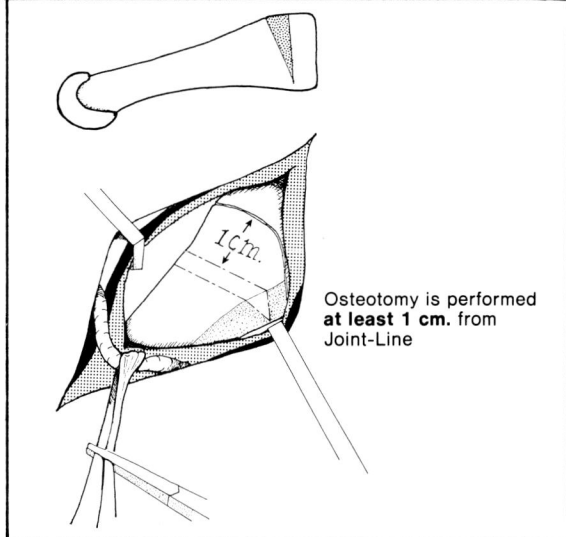

Fig. 6-8D

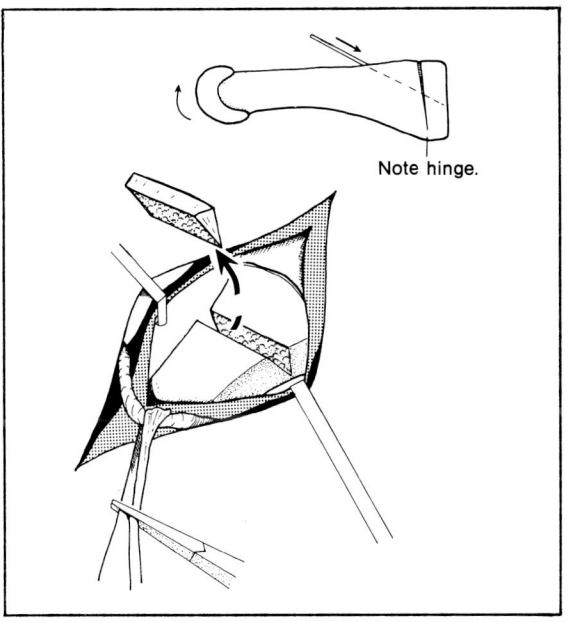

Fig. 6-8E

Note hinge.

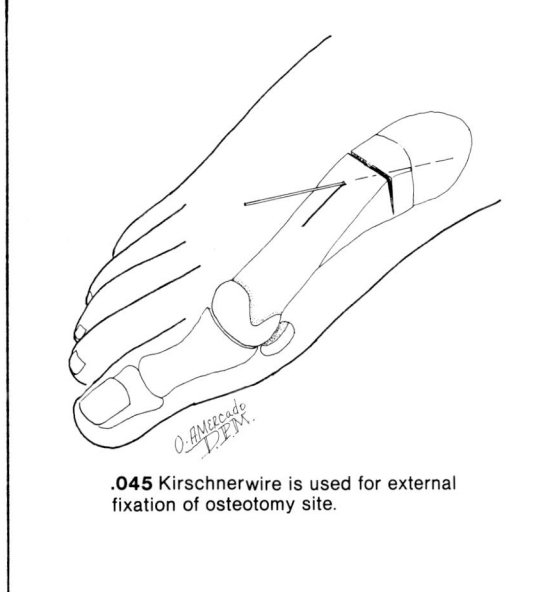

.045 Kirschnerwire is used for external fixation of osteotomy site.

Fig. 6-8F

Techniques for Shortening the Metatarsal Ray

The most obvious way of shortening a metatarsal ray is to remove, partially or completely, the metatarsal head. While this method is direct, we have found through hard experience that it is not the best technique.

For over a decade, from the mid-fifties through the late sixties, metatarsal head resection for the relief of plantar keratosis became the most widely used surgical technique for metatarsal-phalangeal-joint surgery. While some patients achieved some measure of good results, the vast majority developed **transfer lesions** on the adjacent metatarsal heads which were just as bad if not worse than the original problem. In time, most podiatric surgeons began performing partial metatarsal head resections and their results improved somewhat, but not to the point of being predictably good.

The underlying problem, of course, was not the technique, but the misapplication of the technique. Today, we use partial or complete metatarsal head resections for the removal of diseased bone (I.E. Freiberg's Infraction, Rheumatoid Arthritis); in trauma where the bone cannot be repaired; and for the relief of an intractable plantar keratosis under a straight fifth metatarsal ray (we use a partial metatarsectomy).

Incidentally, the difference between a partial and complete metatarsal head resection is as follows. In a partial metatarsal head resection, the head is resected at the surgical neck and then the condyles are resected. In a complete metatarsal head resection, the head is completely resected at the anatomical neck (see Figure 6-9).

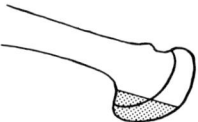

Plantar Condylectomy

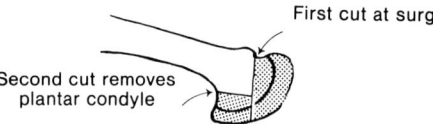

Partial Metatarsal Head Resection

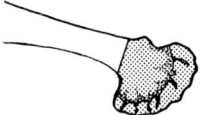

Complete Metatarsal Head Resection
Fig. 6-9

Partial Metatarsal Head Resection

A partial metatarsal head resection is a method of shortening a metatarsal ray. Today it is only used for diseased bone or for the relief of a plantar keratosis under a fifth metatarsal head that has an essentially straight shaft.

Technique

The classic incision is shown in Figure 6-10 A, extending from the shaft distally into the dorsal aspect of the toe. This incision is seldom used because there is a tendency for fibrosis to form around the extensor tendon sheath, resulting in a contraction of the digit on the metatarsal.

The incision of choice, is the one recommended by **Henri DuVries.** His incision starts on the dorsal aspect of the metatarsal shaft, and glides just into the innerspace (Figure 6-12 A). This incision avoids placing the scar over the tendon sheath and healing occurs without digital contraction.

Once the incision is deepened, the dorsal tendons are carefully retracted so as to expose the metatarsal-phalangeal-joint capsular ligament (Figure 6-10 B-C). A lineal incision is made into the capsular ligament and the capsule is carefully retracted.

The collateral ligaments lie immediately under the capsule — they stabilize the proximal phalangeal base on the metatarsal head. A number 15 blade is used to cut the ligaments (see Figure 6-10 D). Once the ligaments are cut a **Seeburger** retractor is slipped under the metatarsal head and the head is delivered (Figure 6-10 E).

Using bone forceps, the metatarsal head is cut at the level of the surgical neck. This cut must be made at 90° to the shaft so as to avoid beveling of the bone. Once the head is resected, what remains of the plantar condyles is easily removed (Figure 6-10 E). It is important to cut the condyles even with the metatarsal shaft to avoid forming any sharp points.

The bone is then rasped smooth. The capsule is carefully closed with 4-0 Dexon. The deep and superficial fascia are closed in layers. The skin is closed with the suture material of choice. Healing is usually uneventful.

M.P.J. SURGERY

Conclusion

1. The partial metatarsectomy technique has a very limited use in modern foot surgery.
2. The technique fell into disrepute not because it was a bad technique per se, but because it was overused and misapplied.
3. Partial metatarsectomies are only useful for **diseased bone;** in **trauma** where the head cannot be repaired; and for the relief of a plantar keratosis under a fifth metatarsal head with an essentially straight shaft.

If used for the proper indications and as described here, the technique will yield consistently good results.

Partial Metatarsal Head Resection

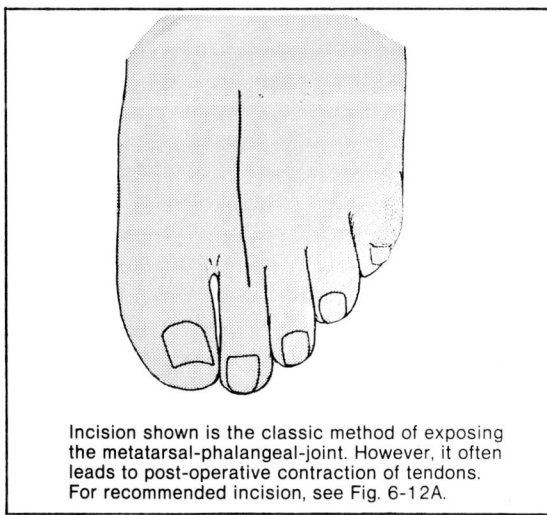

Incision shown is the classic method of exposing the metatarsal-phalangeal-joint. However, it often leads to post-operative contraction of tendons. For recommended incision, see Fig. 6-12A.

Fig. 6-10A

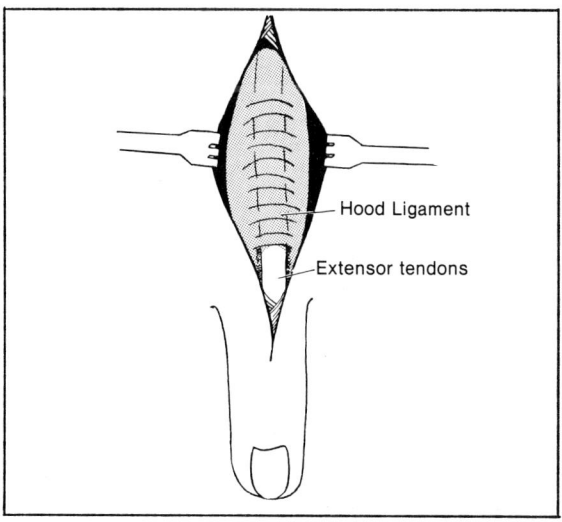

Fig. 6-10B

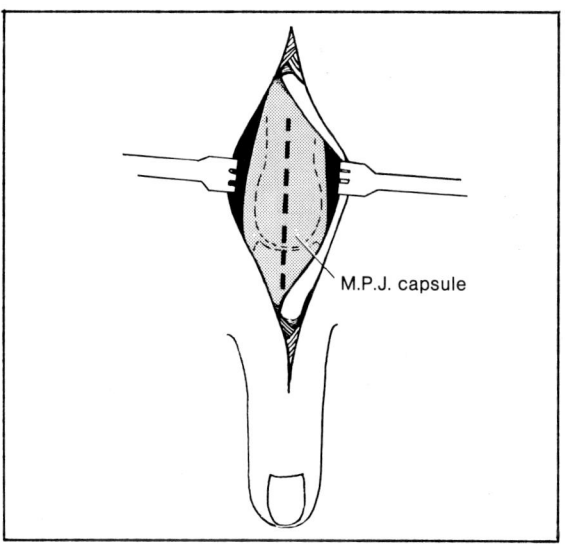

Fig. 6-10C

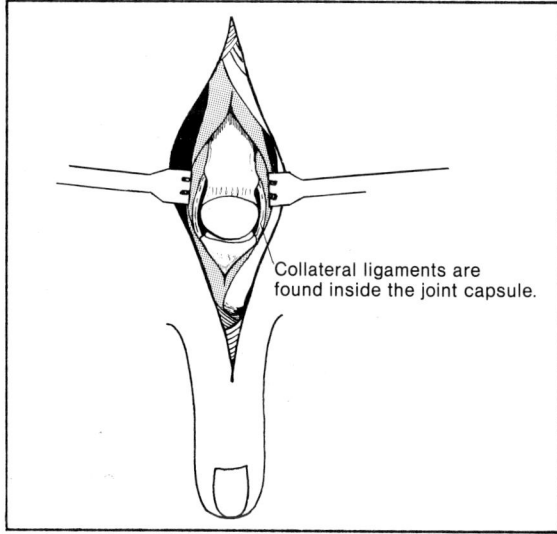

Fig. 6-10D

139

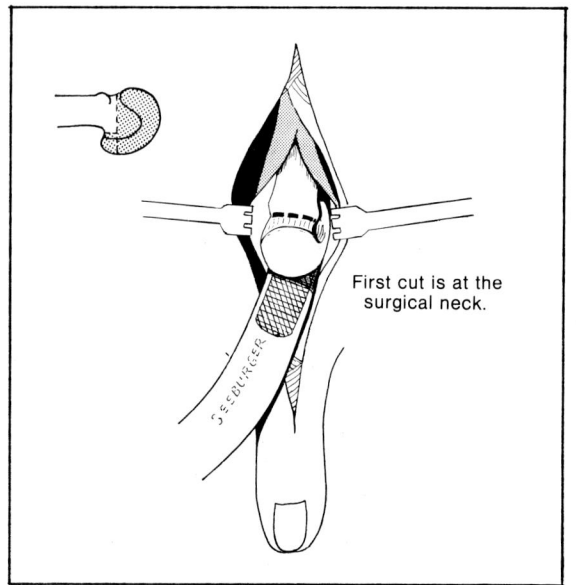
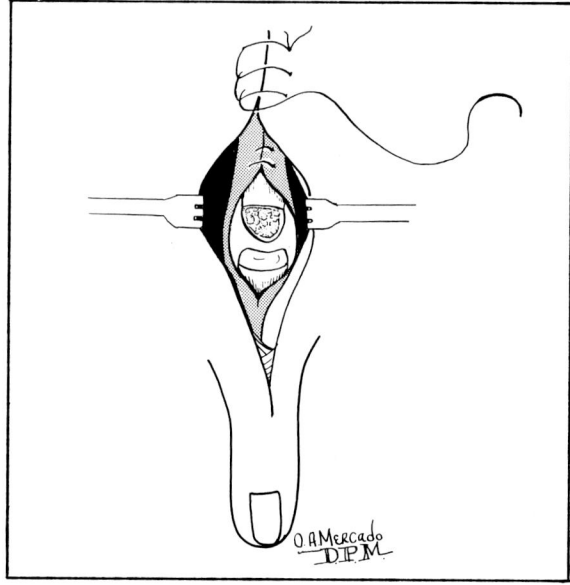

Fig. 6-10E *Fig. 6-10F*

The Suppan Cap Technique

The Suppan cap technique is a method of shortening the metatarsal ray while preserving the integrity of the articular facet. This technique was devised by **Dr. Raymond J. Suppan** and it is used whenever the metatarsal ray must be shortened, **0.5 cm.** or less.

Technique

An incision approximately 4.5 cm. long is made over the metatarsal shaft extending into the interdigital space. The incision is deepened and retracted and the superficial vessels are ligated. The dorsal tendons are underscored and retracted.

A lineal incision is made into the metatarsal-phalangeal-joint capsular ligament and the ligament is carefully retracted. The collateral ligaments can be seen immediately under the capsular ligament to either side of the joint. With a number 15 blade, the collateral ligaments are cut (from distal to proximal) and the metatarsal head thus freed, is retracted out of the wound using a Seeburger retractor (Figure 6-11A).

Next, the metatarsal head is cut, using power equipment, at the level of the surgical neck (the groove just proximal to the articular facet). It is important to cut the head at this level as this will not only preserve all of the dorsal articulate facet, but the cap thus formed will be thick enough to ensure adequate blood supply and **viability.** In fact, some of the original problems that were inherent to this procedure (mostly aseptic necrosis of the cap) were due to cutting the cap too thin (Figure 6-11B). The articular cap is then placed in saline solution and we move to the next step of the operation, the shortening of the metatarsal ray.

M.P.J. SURGERY

The amount that the metatarsal is to be shortened will depend on how much longer the metatarsal is than the adjacent heads. The exact length is determined by drawing the outline of the metatarsal heads (from a dorsal-plantar x-ray view) onto a piece of paper. The metatarsals are then cut out (much like making a paper doll) and the elongated metatarsal is cut until the **desirable parabola** is formed. The amount that is necessary to shorten the metatarsal paper cut-out to create an ideal parabola, will be the amount of bone that must be resected. It should be noted here that if that amount of bone is more than 0.5 cm., then a McKeever peg and hole technique should be considered.

Once we have established the amount of shortening necessary, we measure the correct amount (usually 2-4 mm.) on the dorsal aspect of the bone and mark the area with an osteotome (by striking it with a mallet). The correct amount of bone is then resected taking care that the power blade is held at exactly the same angle as in the first cut. This will ensure a perfect fit between the cap and the shaft. The plantar condyles are then cut even with the shaft (Figure 6-11C).

The cap is then taken out of the saline solution and carefully dried. At this time the condyles of the cap are removed using a bone forceps (Figure 6-11 C). It is important not to make the cap too small so that it will fit snugly against the shaft.

The cap is then held, with thumb and finger forceps, tightly against the shaft. A Kirschner wire is then used to fixate the osteotomy. The Kirschner wire is inserted obliquely on the dorsal aspect of the articular facet into the metatarsal shaft and cortex (Figure 6-11 D).

The periosteum, capsule, deep and superficial tissues and the skin are closed using the suture materials of choice. A short (above the ankle) cast is applied. The cast is removed in three weeks as are the sutures and Kirschner wire. Healing is usually uneventful.

The Suppan Cap Technique

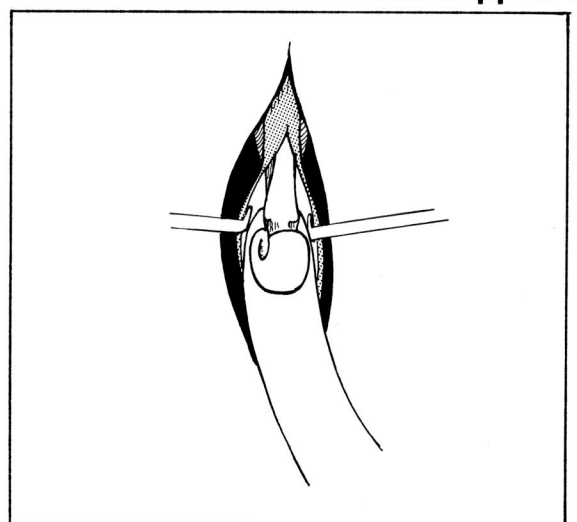

Fig. 6-11A

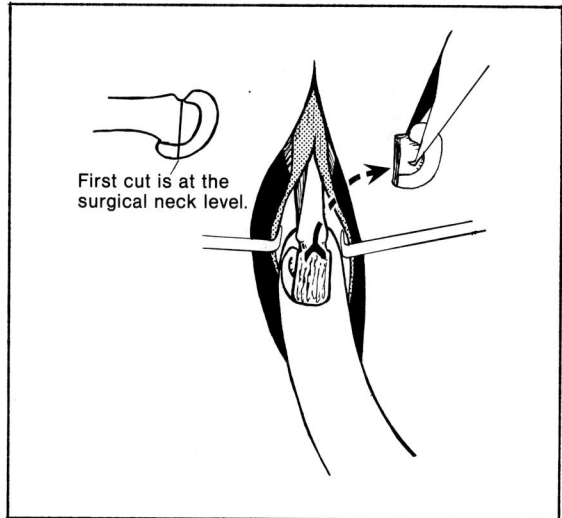

First cut is at the surgical neck level.

Fig. 6-11B

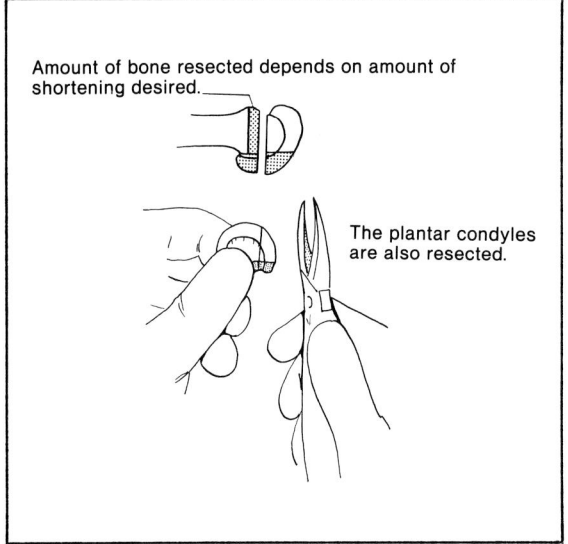

Fig. 6-11C

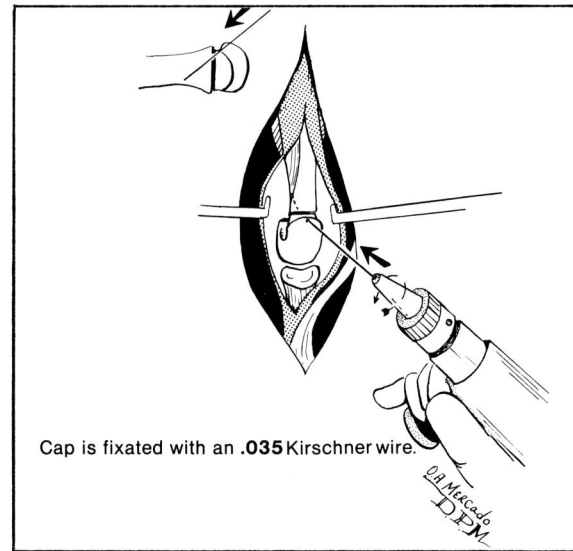

Fig. 6-11D

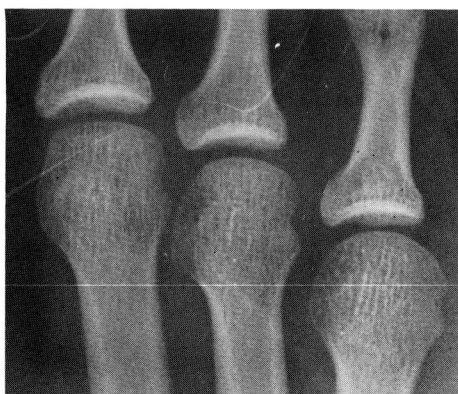

Fig. 6-11E. Pre-operative x-ray reveals elongated 2nd. metatarsal ray.

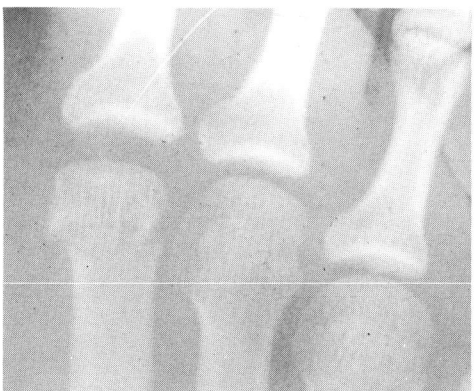

Fig. 6-11F. Three weeks after surgery. The 2nd. metatarsal has been shorten by a Suppan Cap Technique.

Precautions

1. Make sure that the cap is thick enough to ensure adequate blood supply and viability.
2. If the metatarsal ray must be shortened more than 0.5 cm. then a McKeever peg and hole technique should be considered.
3. The cap should be fixated with a Kirschner wire and the foot casted for three weeks.
4. The procedure will work well on the second, third or fourth metatarsals. However, when more than one metatarsal head is shortened at one time, fixation becomes difficult.

Conclusion

The Suppan cap procedure will work well when used for the proper indications with the proper precautions.

The Mercado-Smith Osteotomy—
Shortening Osteoclasis

The Mercado-Smith osteotomy technique is utilized whenever it is necessary to shorten the metatarsal ray by **0.5 cm.** or less. The technique is usually used on the second, third or fourth metatarsal head.

Technique

An incision approximately 4.5 cm. long is made on the intermetatarsal space extending somewhat into the interdigital space. The second intermetatarsal space is used to expose the second and/or third metatarsal head. The third intermetatarsal space is used to expose the third and/or fourth metatarsal head. As a rule, we avoid going into the first intermetatarsal area to expose the second metatarsal head as this area is highly vascular and contains the deep peroneal nerve.

The incision is carefully retracted. The superficial vessels crossing the incision are ligated. The hood ligament of the extensor tendons is incised and the tendons are retracted (Figure 6-12 A).

A lineal incision is made into the capsular ligament extending from proximal to the joint line to the shaft of the metatarsal (it is not necessary to expose the whole joint). The anatomical neck of the metatarsal shaft is identified. Care is taken, by exploring underneath the shaft with a curved hemostat, that the osteotomy line falls behind (proximal to) the end of the condyles.

The distal osteotomy line is carefully marked by striking the bone with an osteotome. The location of this line is exceedingly important as we have seen in Chapter Five. The closer we can come to the **cancellous bone** of the metatarsal head, the better the healing of the osteotomy will be. If, however, we place our osteotomy line too far distally, we run the very real danger of placing our cut into the condyles.

After the distal osteotomy line is marked, we carefully measure the amount of the bone that is to be resected. The amount of bone resected will depend on **how much** the metatarsal ray has to be shortened to establish a more normal metatarsal parabola (Figure 6-12B). With a power saw we carefully cut down on the distal osteotomy line. Care is taken to hold the blade at ninety degrees to the horizontal axis of the shaft, both on the dorsal to plantar plane and the medial to lateral plane. The second (proximal) cut is then made, making certain that the blade is kept at the same angle as the first cut. The section of bone that is thus cut is then resected (Figure 6-12C).

Once this section of bone is resected, the head will easily move back (proximally) into its new shortened position. At this time the **most important** step of the operation is performed; the head is held tightly against the shaft of the metatarsal, at the same time, the forefoot is loaded and the surgeon carefully feels the metatarsal heads to make certain that they will be striking the ground at the same level. Usually, it is only necessary to hold the metatarsal head down against the shaft. Sometimes, however, it will be necessary to also elevate the metatarsal head ever so slightly to ascertain that it will not be planti-flexed in relation to the other metatarsal heads.

Once the **proper level** of the metatarsal head is ascertained, the head is held tightly with a large thumb and finger forceps and a small Kirschner wire is inserted (Figure 6-12D). If at all possible, the wire is inserted just proximal to the articular facet. The wire will go in easier if it is inserted somewhat obliquely to the longitudinal axis of the metatarsal shaft.

The capsule is carefully sutured with 3-0 Dexon. The deep and superficial fascia are closed with 4-0 Dexon. The skin is approximated with a suture material of choice. The Kirschner wire is carefully bent proximally, and the wound is dressed with Vaseline gauze, sterile gauze and Kling. A boot cast (above the ankle) is then applied.

The boot cast is removed in three weeks. The sutures and K-wire are removed at this time. The patient is encouraged to commence weight bearing and ambulate to tolerance soon after. Healing of this procedure is usually uneventful.

Precautions

1. This technique is **contra-indicated** in osteoporosis, rheumatoid arthritis and when the underlying cause of a plantar lesion is a plantiflexed metatarsal ray.
2. It is **important** that the osteotomy cuts be made at the same angle so that the head can meet the shaft properly when the bone is resected.
3. Adequate fixation (with Kirschner wire) is important so that healing can occur.
4. Make the osteotomy cuts as close as possible to the metatarsal head **(cancellous bone)** but avoid cutting into the plantar condyles.
5. The osteotomy site needs **immobilization** with plaster of paris to ensure proper alignment and healing.

The Mercado-Smith Osteotomy

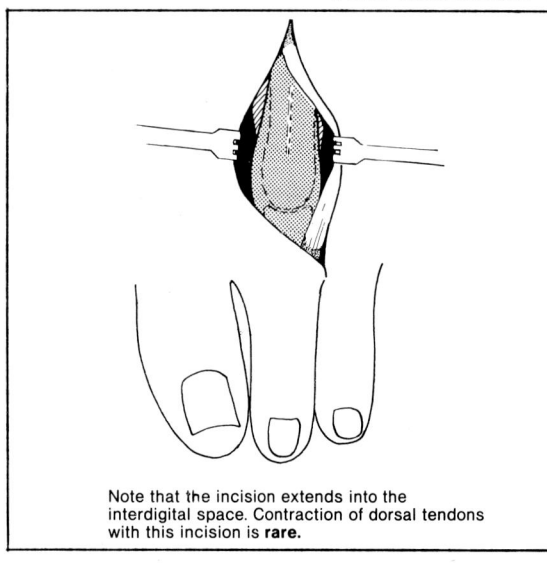

Note that the incision extends into the interdigital space. Contraction of dorsal tendons with this incision is **rare**.

Fig. 6-12A

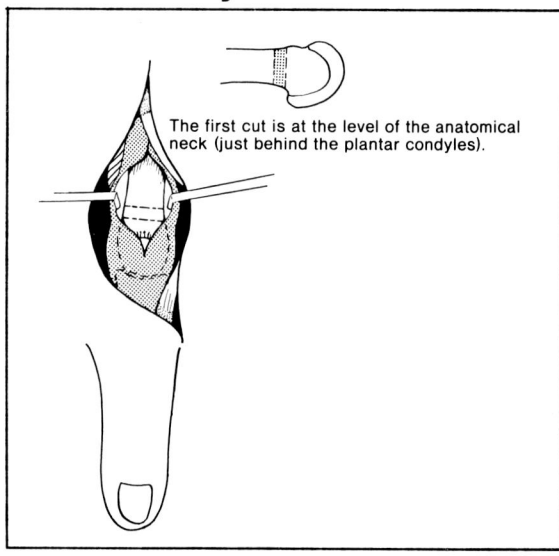

The first cut is at the level of the anatomical neck (just behind the plantar condyles).

Fig. 6-12B

M.P.J. SURGERY

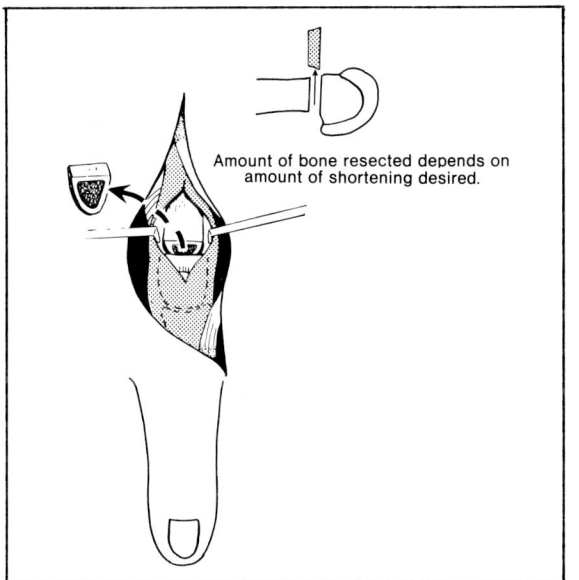

Fig. 6-12C

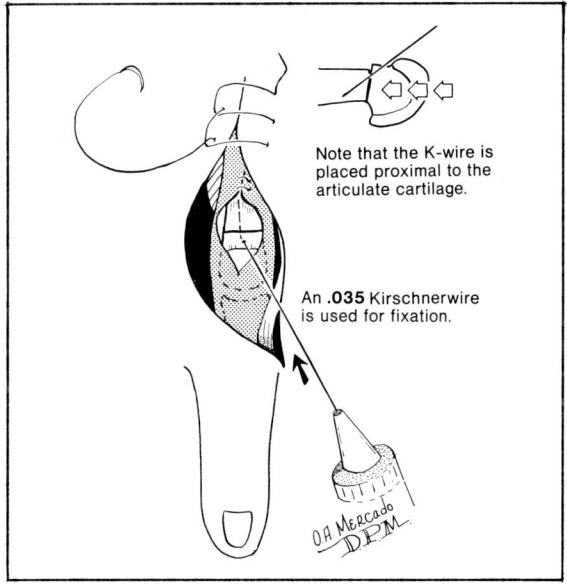

Fig. 6-12D

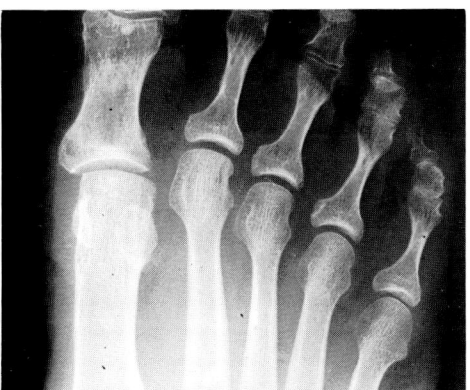

Fig. 6-12E. Pre-operative x-rays reveal elongated 2nd. metatarsal shaft.

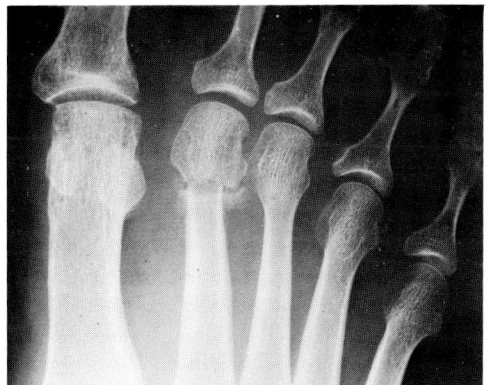

Fig. 6-12F. Three weeks after the surgery. The 2nd. metatarsal has been shortened by a Mercado-Smith Osteotomy.

Conclusion

The Mercado-Smith osteotomy technique is used to shorten the metatarsal up to 0.5 cm. It can be performed on one or two metatarsals. As a rule, if there is an intractable plantar keratosis underneath the second, third and fourth metatarsals, and the corresponding metatarsal rays appear long, it is best to perform a triple osteoclasis to elevate all three metatarsals.

In all of the cases we have performed to date, there has not been one single incident of mal-union of the bone. Healing has been uneventful and the results have been consistently good.

As with any technique, it is important that it be utilized for the proper reason (i.e. shortening of the metatarsal ray).

The McKeever Peg and Hole Technique

Duncan McKeever, first described his operation in 1952. The technique is used to shorten elongated lesser metatarsal rays, and it is ideally suited for **Morton's** type syndrome, where the elongated second metatarsal ray has caused an intractable plantar keratosis (I.P.K.). In years past, the most common operation used to shorten metatarsal rays was a metatarsal head resection. This often led to an unstable metatarsal-phalangeal-joint and frequent transfer lesions to the adjacent metatarsal heads.

The McKeever operation, when performed properly, will shorten the metatarsal ray, restore the metatarsal parabola and have much less tendency to create transfer lesions (Figure 6-13).

Technique

An incision approximately 4.5 cm. long is made over the metatarsal shaft, extending somewhat into the interdigital space. The incision is deepened, the superficial veins in the line of the incision are ligated. The wound is carefully underscored and the dorsal tendons are retracted so as to expose the capsular ligaments (Figure 6-14 B).

A lineal incision is made, the capsule is retracted, the collateral ligaments are cut and the metatarsal head is exposed out of the wound utilizing a **Seeburger** retractor. Using power equipment, the metatarsal head is cut just proximal to the anatomical neck (Figure 6-14 C). The head is then retracted outside the wound and placed in saline solution (Figure 6-14). The shaft of the metatarsal is underscored and with a bone forceps and drill, the shaft is fashioned into a peg (Figure 6-14 E).

The metatarsal head is removed from the saline solution and carefully dried. The surgeon then, being careful to rest his hand on the table so as not to drop the metatarsal head, **reams out** the metatarsal head. It is important that the hole shelled out of the metatarsal head is of sufficient caliber to accomodate the truncated metatarsal shaft snuggly (Figure 6-13 A-D and 6-14 F-G).

Sometimes it is necessary to try the metatarsal head on the peg several times until it fits just right. Once the metatarsal head is fitted on the metatarsal head to the surgeons' satisfaction, the back of a blade handle is used to further **compress** the head on the shaft (Figure 6-14 H-I). While doing this, it is important to hold the head steady with large thumb and finger forceps so as to prevent accidental dropping of the head.

In all of the years that we have been performing this procedure we have **never** dropped a metatarsal head. We have, once by accident, dropped a head while performing a Suppan cap procedure. The head was immediately "flashed" in the autoclave and the operation continued as planned. The healing was slow, but uneventful. (X-rays of this particular case can be seen in Chapter Five).

The capsule, subcutaneous tissues and wound are then closed and dressed in the usual manner. A short (above the ankle) walking foot cast is applied for three weeks. Healing is usually uneventful.

McKeever Peg and Hole Technique

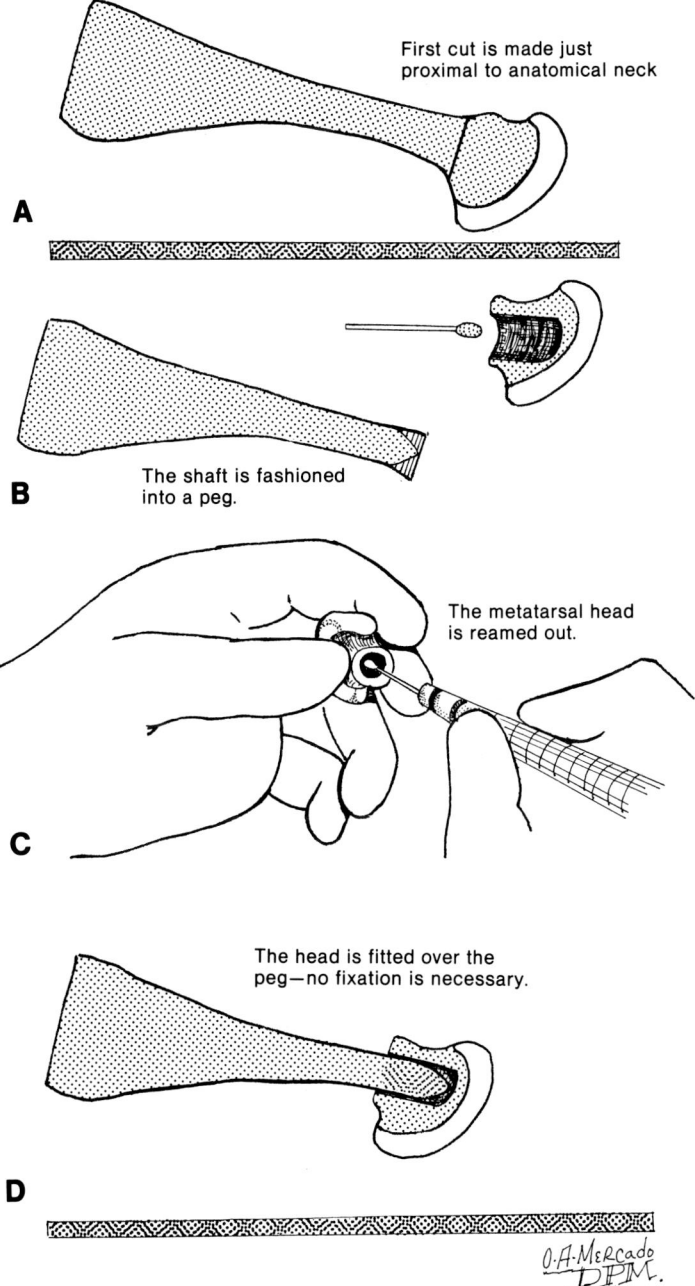

Fig. 6-13

Precautions

1. The McKeever operation is used only to shorten an elongated metatarsal ray. A planti-flexed metatarsal ray requires elevation, not shortening (i.e., E.O.A., E.O., osteoclasis, etc.).
2. The metatarsal ray must be shortened **at least** 0.5 cm. in order to obtain an adequate peg on the shaft and enough depth in the metatarsal head to ascertain a solid fixation.
3. Extreme care is needed in the handling of the metatarsal head while it is being drilled to avoid accidental dropping.
4. The head must fit snuggly on the metatarsal shaft since wire fixation is not used with this technique.
5. This technique is usually used to shorten one single metatarsal (as in Morton's type syndrome).

Conclusion

While it requires a high degree of surgical dexterity and patience, the McKeever peg and hole technique is an excellent method of **shortening** an elongated metatarsal ray. Patients who have had this technique performed, retain an almost full range of motion of the metatarsal phalangeal joint, with no contraction of the digit on the metatarsal head. When performed for the proper indication, it will yield consistently good results.

The McKeever Peg and Hole Technique

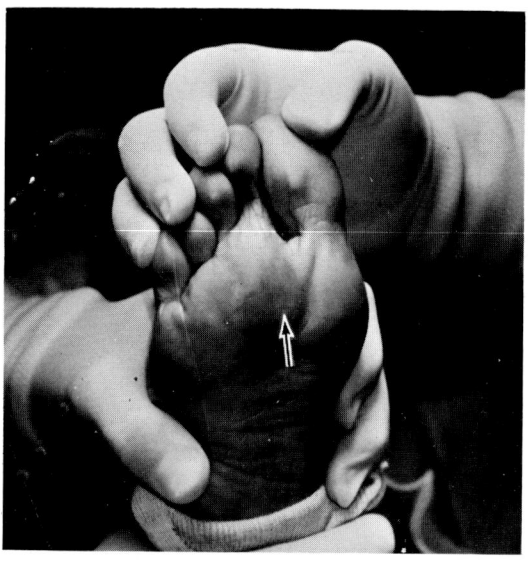
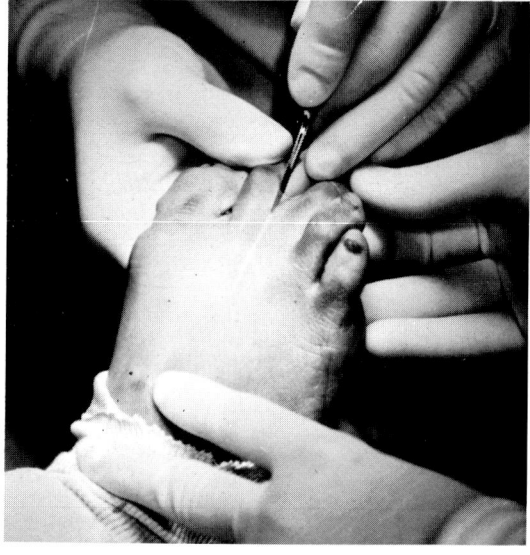

Fig. 6-14A. Arrow points to painful I.P.K. caused by elongated 2nd. metatarsal ray.

Fig. 6-14B. Incision is made over metatarsal shaft, extending somewhat into the interdigital space.

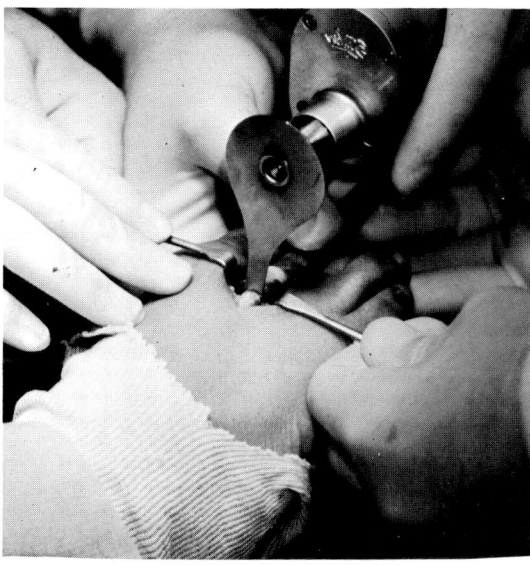

Fig. 6-14C. The metatarsal head is cut proximal to the **anatomical neck.**

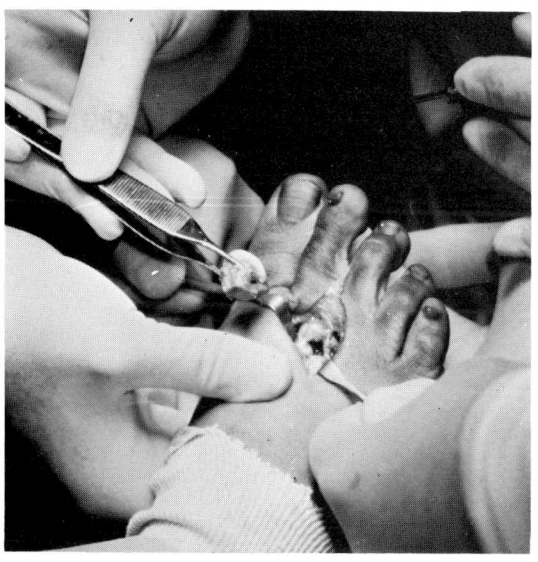

Fig. 6-14D. The head is retracted outside the wound and placed in saline solution.

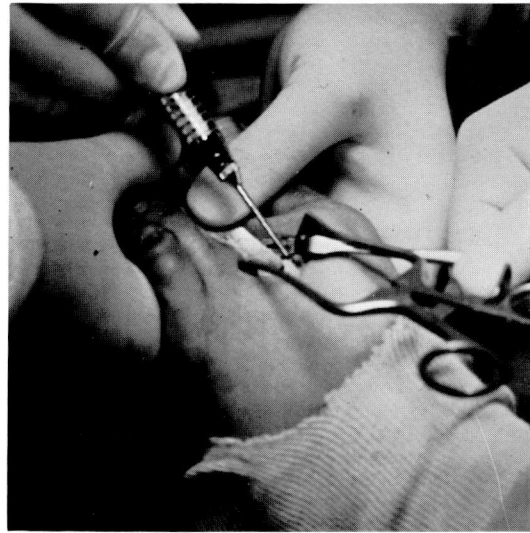

Fig. 6-14E. The metatarsal shaft is then fashioned into a **peg.**

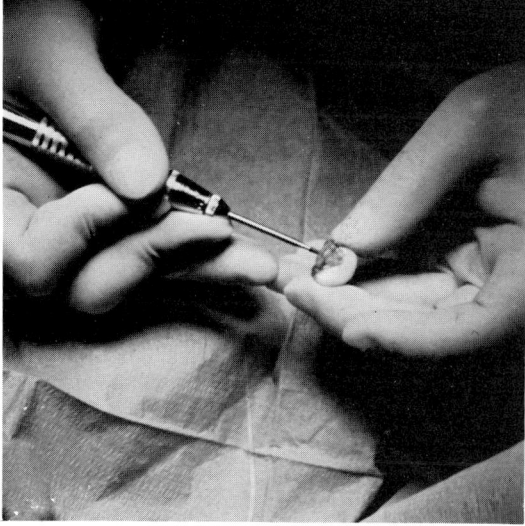

Fig. 6-14F. The metatarsal head is reamed out to accomodate the peg.

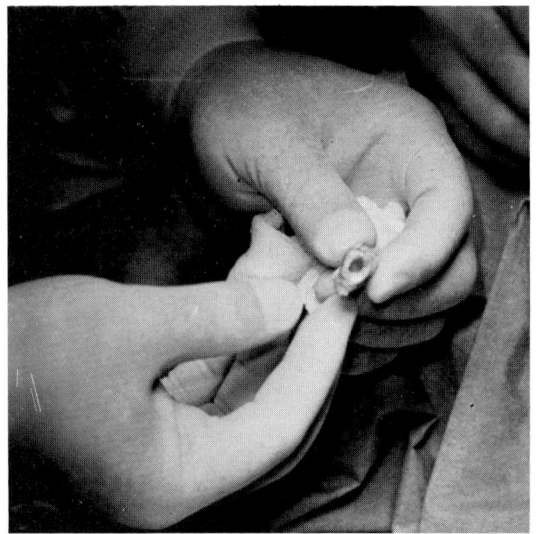

Fig. 6-14G. The shelled-out hole of the metatarsal head must accomodate the peg snuggly.

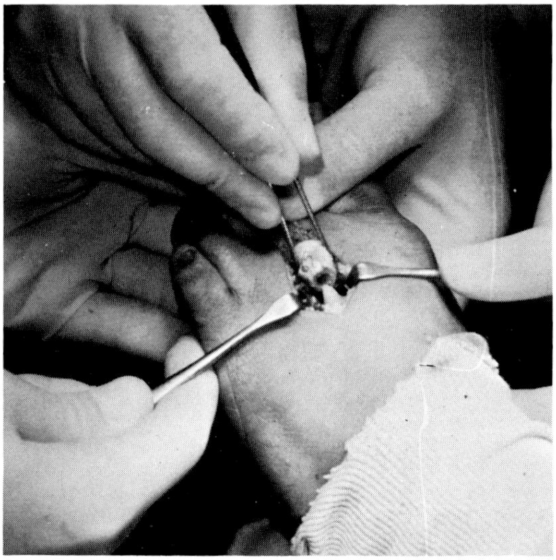

Fig. 6-14H. The metatarsal head is fitted over the peg.

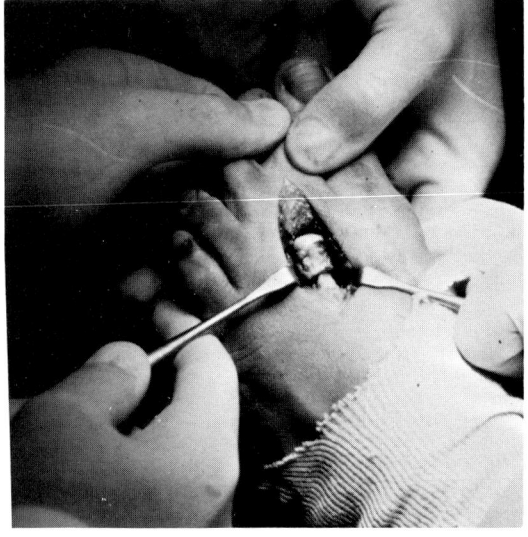

Fig. 6-14I. The head is **compressed** over the peg...no other fixation is necessary.

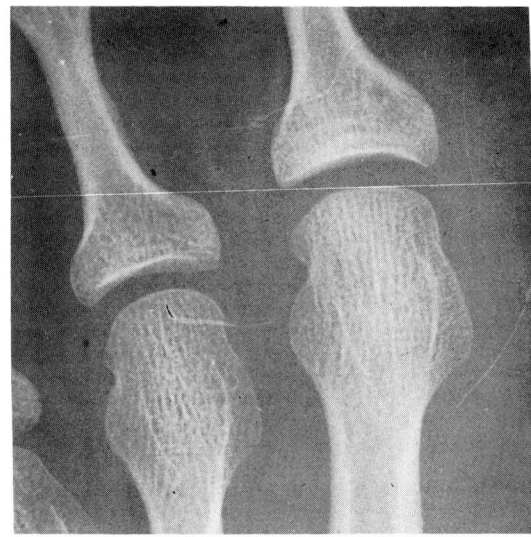

Fig. 6-14J. Pre-operative x-ray of elongated 2nd. metatarsal ray.

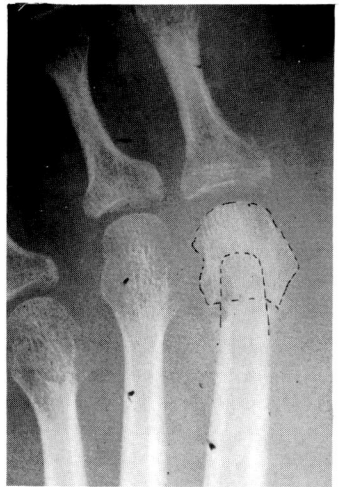 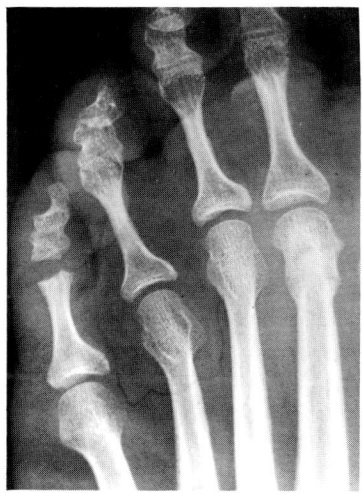

Fig. 6-14K. Three weeks after the surgery. The dotted-lines show the way the head of the metatarsal fits over the metatarsal ray.

Fig. 6-14L. Six months after the McKeever Peg and Hole technique the bone has healed.

The Mercado Peg and Hole Technique

The Mercado peg and hole technique is an operation which we devised to shorten the metatarsal ray and at the same time create a certain amount of elevation. The procedure is used for the relief of an intractable plantar keratosis when examination and x-rays reveal a need for shortening the corresponding metatarsal ray.

Technique

A lineal incision approximately 4.5 cm. is made over the corresponding metatarsal shaft and carried somewhat into the intermetatarsal space (Figure 6-15A). The incision is deepened and the exposed dorsal tendons are retracted. The metatarsal shaft is exposed and the periosteum is incised and freed from the bone (Figure 6-1 5B and 6-15C).

The metatarsal is cut transversely, using power equipment, at the junction of the middle and distal one-third of the shaft (Figure 6-15C).

The distal end of the shaft is retracted dorsally out of the wound and a peg is fashioned from the shaft (Figure 6-15D). The size of the peg will depend on the amount of shortening desired. The peg is readily fashioned with bone forceps and a power drill.

Once the Peg is fashioned, the medullary canal of the proximal shaft is reamed out to allow for the insertion of the peg. Incidentally, reaming out of the canal is not difficult since the tissues are spongy and yielding (Figure 6-15 E).

The peg is inserted into the canal, and the periosteum is sutured around the bone (Figure 6-15 F). The fibers of the interossei muscles, which are found to either side of the shaft, are sometimes sutured around the shaft to maintain the position of the osteotomy line and the peg. The subcutaneous tissues and the wound are closed in the usual manner and a short (above the ankle) walking cast is applied for three weeks.

Healing of the Osteotomy

Our osteotomy site is on **cortical** (compact) bone. Cortical bone, which is found along the shafts of any long bone, heals quite different from cancellous bone which is contained on the bases and heads of long bones. While cancellous bone heals very fast with little proliferation, cortical bone heals more slowly, with a great amount of periosteal proliferation and callus formation. This bone callus, however, is absorbed in time and remodeling of the metatarsal shaft occurs (see Chapter Five).

Precautions

1. the technique is used where shortening with some elevation of the metatarsal ray is needed.
2. When cutting the peg, make the peg long enough so that it will fit into the reamed-out medullary canal snuggly. A good fit will prevent medial or lateral shifting of the metatarsal shaft.
3. The metatarsal shaft needs to be shortened **at least** 0.5 cm. so that an adequate peg can be obtained.
4. The patient should be warned that after the surgery, there will be **enduration** of the osteotomy site for months after the surgery (because of the callus formation). However, this enduration will subside in time.
5. This technique is usually used to shorten a single metatarsal ray.

Conclusion

The peg and hole technique was devised at Franklin Boulevard Community Hospital a number of years ago to provide shortening of the metatarsal ray with some elevation.

When used for the proper indications, the results will be consistently good.

The Mercado Peg and Hole Technique

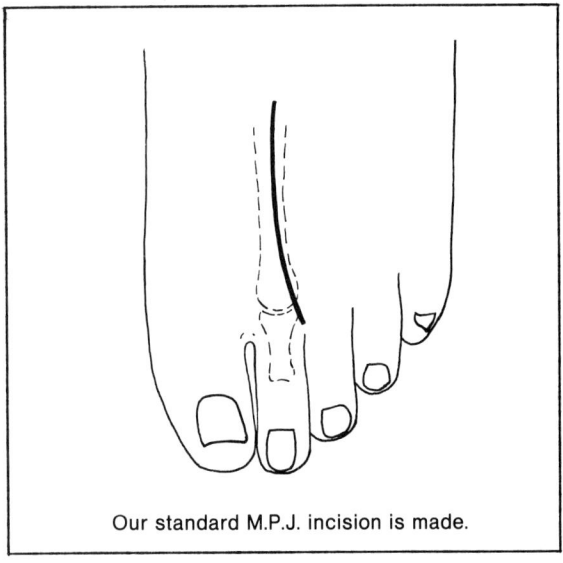

Our standard M.P.J. incision is made.

Fig. 6-15A

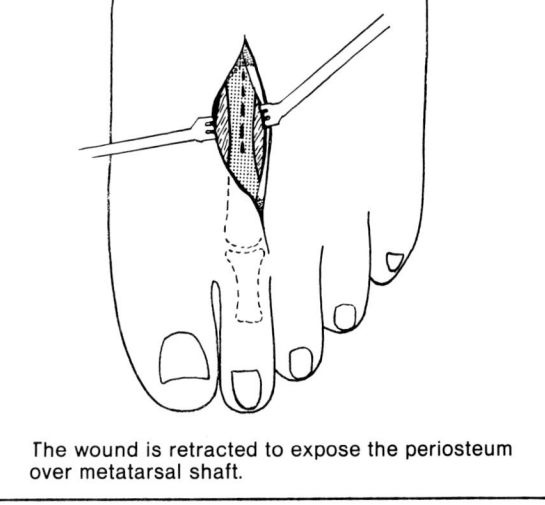

The wound is retracted to expose the periosteum over metatarsal shaft.

Fig. 6-15B

M.P.J. SURGERY

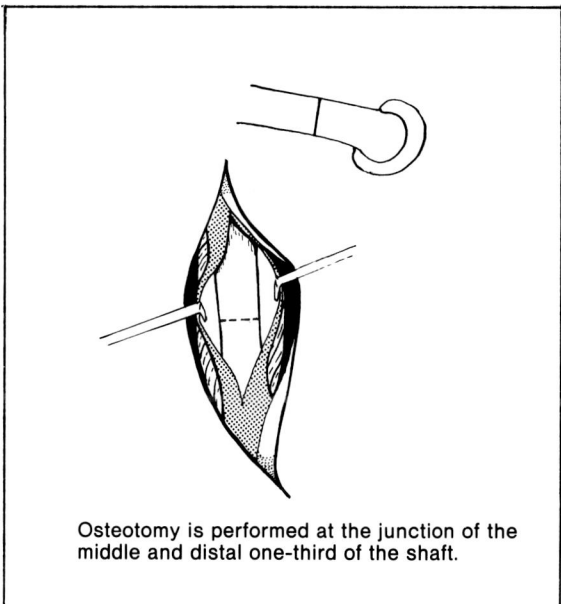

Osteotomy is performed at the junction of the middle and distal one-third of the shaft.

Fig. 6-15C

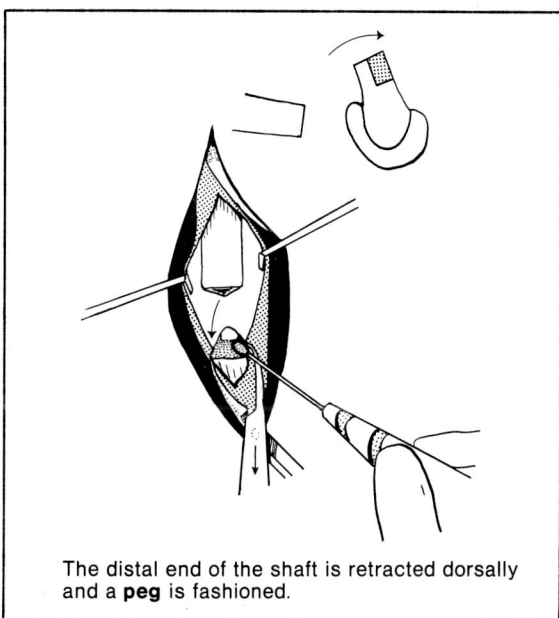

The distal end of the shaft is retracted dorsally and a **peg** is fashioned.

Fig. 6-15D

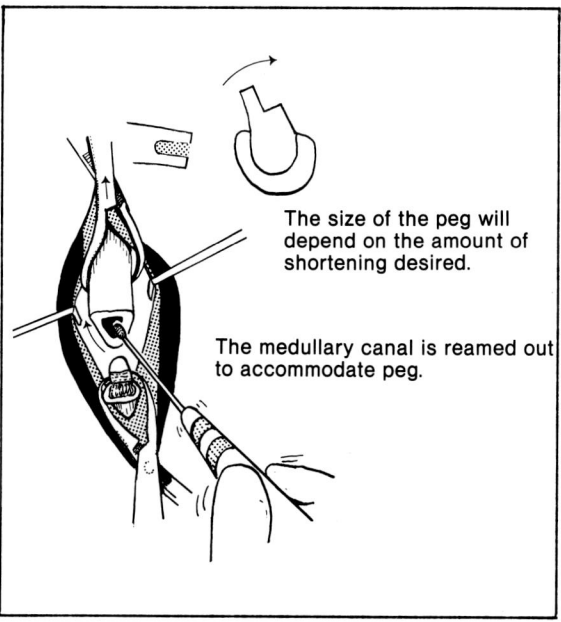

The size of the peg will depend on the amount of shortening desired.

The medullary canal is reamed out to accommodate peg.

Fig. 6-15E

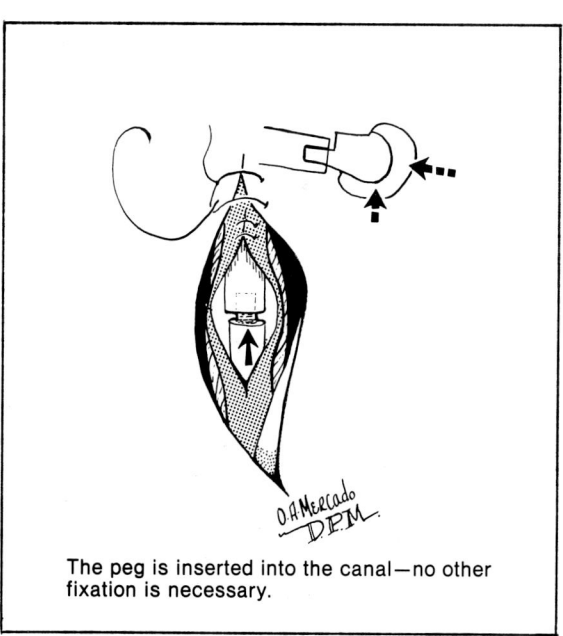

The peg is inserted into the canal—no other fixation is necessary.

Fig. 6-15F

Osteoclasis

The osteoclasis technique is an operation performed to elevate one or more planti-flexed metatarsal heads to relieve an underlying plantar keratosis. The foundation of this technique lies back with the writing of **R.O. Meisenbach,** who in 1916 devised an osteotomy of the metatarsal shaft to raise the head to a higher plane.

Because the technique is quite simple to execute, it is probably the most **commonly used** and, unfortunately, **misused** technique performed for the relief of plantar keratosis today.

Many surgeons are under the **false** impression that all one needs do to relieve a plantar keratosis is to cut (fracture) the metatarsal and allow the head to **"seek its own level".** Never mind the instrument used for the osteotomy (rasp, drill, osteotome, bone forceps, rongeur, or power equipment) nor the location of the osteotomy (base, low-shaft, mid-shaft, high-shaft, neck, or head). It is no small wonder that there is such a high incidence of transfer lesion with this procedure.

To begin with, Meisenbach's idea to elevate the metatarsal head to relieve the underlying plantar keratosis is **correct,** but **only** if the metatarsal shaft is indeed planti-flexed. If the metatarsal shaft is too long, then an osteoclasis **WILL NOT WORK.**

Secondly, the location of the osteotomy site is of **utmost importance** in this (and for that matter, any) procedure. Since we know that compact bone heals with marked proliferation and callus formation, it makes sense to place the osteotomy site in cancellous bone.

An osteotomy on the base of the metatarsal would not work as it could raise the head too much and be prone to medial or lateral shifting.

The **ideal site** for the osteotomy is right at the anatomical neck. As close to the head as possible, but being careful that the cut is placed just proximal to the plantar condyles (see Figure 6-16 A).

To avoid medial or lateral shifting of the head, the collateral ligaments are left intact — this is possible since the collateral ligaments lie inside and are independent of the capsular ligament.

Finally, the instrument used for the osteotomy is a power saw. It will give a controlled even cut which will allow the smooth gliding and positioning of the head on the shaft.

Technique

An incision approximately 4.5 cm. long is made on the metatarsal shaft extending into the interdigital space. The wound is underscored and the superficial vessels are ligated. The dorsal tendons are underscored and retracted.

An incison is made on the capsule just proximal to the joint line. The capsule and periosteum are carefully underscored and retracted taking care to leave the collateral ligaments intact (Figure 6-16 A).

A curved hemostat is used to feel underneath the metatarsal shaft to ascertain that the osteotomy will be located proximal to the plantar condyles. The osteotomy site is carefully marked with an osteotome — by striking it with a mallet.

Using a power saw, the bone is cut transversely from dorsal to plantar. As with any osteotomy, the operator will find that the power saw will work best if the oscillation of the blade is started prior to coming in contact with the bone and continued in one straight cut until the osteotomy is completely performed. One frequent mistake is to stop the blade just prior to cutting through the plantar cortex; this usually will cause a small fracture at this site which **will not** allow the head to glide smoothly on the shaft. Time is then wasted trying to remove the spicule left behind.

Once the osteotomy is performed, the toe is pulled distally to separate the osteotomized bone. The foot is loaded and the metatarsal head is carefully elevated so that all of the heads are on an even level and are able to meet the ground evenly (Figure 6-16 B).

Surprisingly, **very little** elevation (one to three millimeters) is needed to correct the problem. In the cases where we did get a transfer lesion with this procedure, it was due to **too much** elevation of the metatarsal head.

Once the proper (elevated) position is ascertained, the head is held carefully with a large thumb and finger forceps and a Kirschner wire is used to fixate the osteotomy site. The Kirschner wire is placed just proximal to the articulate facet and runs obliquely into the cortex of the shaft. You will notice that there will be a puckering visible on the plantar aspect since the head is now in a corrected position and is no longer planti-flexed (Figure 6-16 D).

The periosteum, capsule, deep and superficial tissues as well as the skin are closed with suture material of choice. A short (above the ankle) cast is applied for three weeks. The patient is encouraged to ambulate to tolerance soon thereafter. The recovery is usually uneventful.

Precautions

1. Make sure that the osteotomy is performed **without** fragmentation of the plantar cortex, so as to allow for a smooth positioning of the metatarsal on the shaft.
2. **Do not** cut the collateral ligaments. It is not necessary (as in the Suppan cap and McKeever procedures) to retract the head out of the wound.
3. Load the foot and elevate the metatarsal head so that it is on an even plane with the other metatarsal heads. **Do not over correct.**
4. Once the head is placed at the proper level, fixated with a Kirschner wire. The metatarsal left alone (without fixation) **will not** seek it's own level.
5. A cast must be applied to maintain the correction and ensure proper healing.
6. This technique **will not** work on long metatarsal shafts unless all three shafts are osteotomized (triple osteoclasis).

Conclusion

The osteoclasis technique performed as outlined here will yield consistently good results with a low incidence of transfer lesion.

Osteoclasis

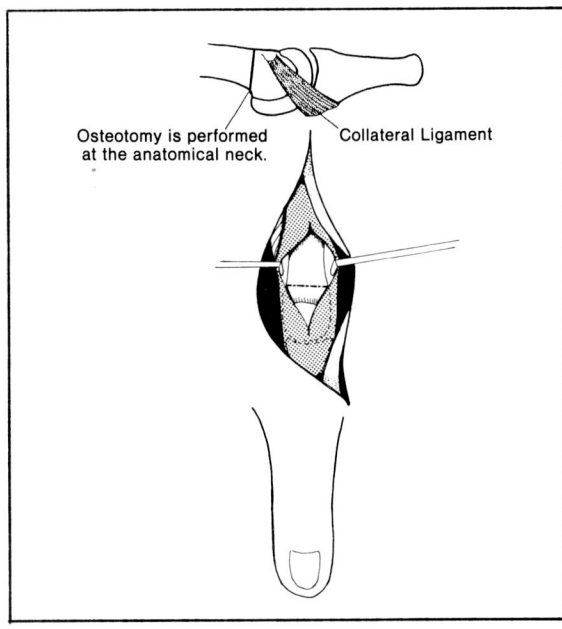

Fig. 6-16A

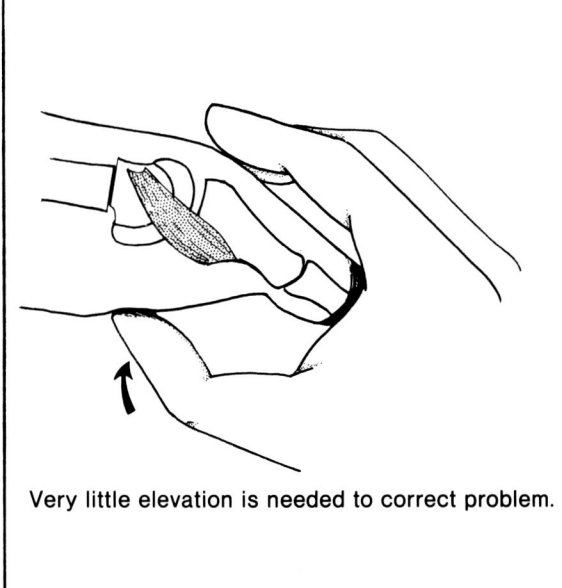

Very little elevation is needed to correct problem.

Fig. 6-16B

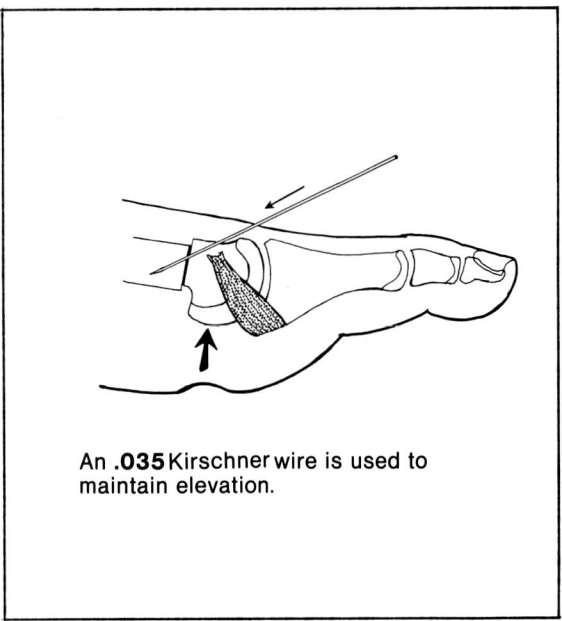

An .035 Kirschner wire is used to maintain elevation.

Fig. 6-16C

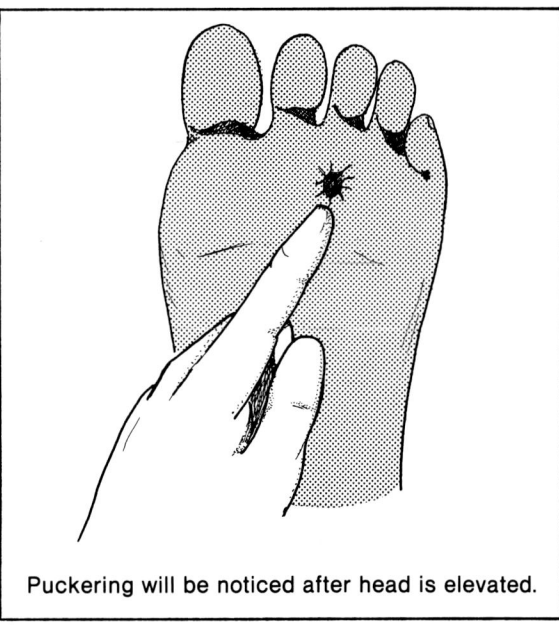

Puckering will be noticed after head is elevated.

Fig. 6-16D

M.P.J. SURGERY

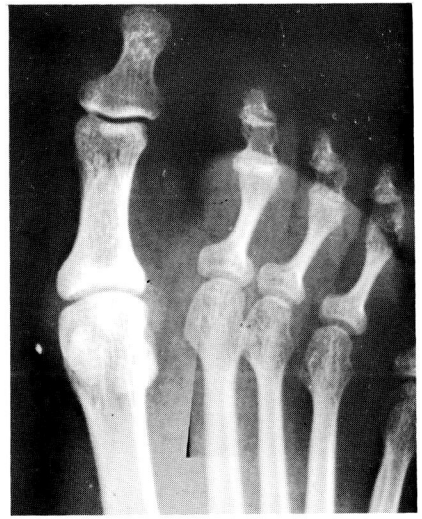

Fig. 6-16E. Pre-operative x-ray. Patient has painful I.P.K. Under second metatarsal head.

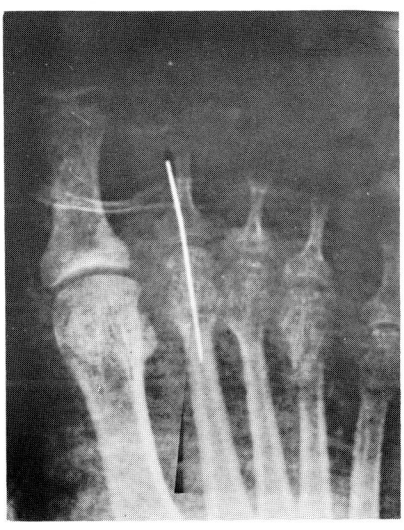

Fig. 6-16F. Post-operative x-ray shows Kirschner wire fixation.

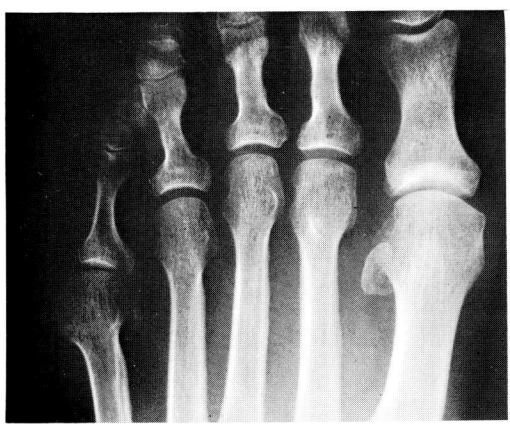

Fig. 6-16G. Pre-operative x-ray. Patient has planti-flexed second metatarsal ray. Osteoclasis, to elevate metatarsal head, is indicated.

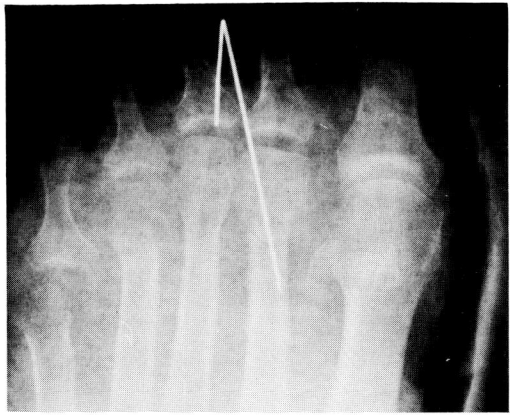

Fig. 6-16H. Post-operative x-ray shows Kirschner wire fixation of osteoclasis.

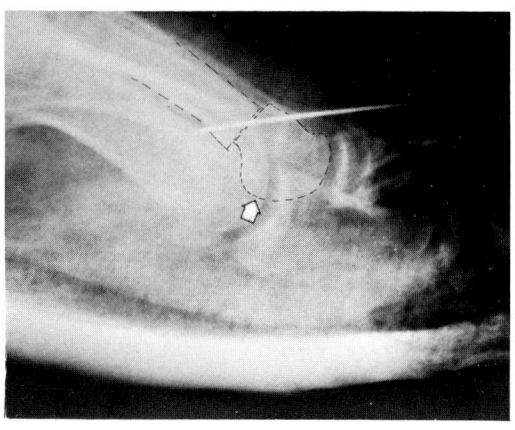 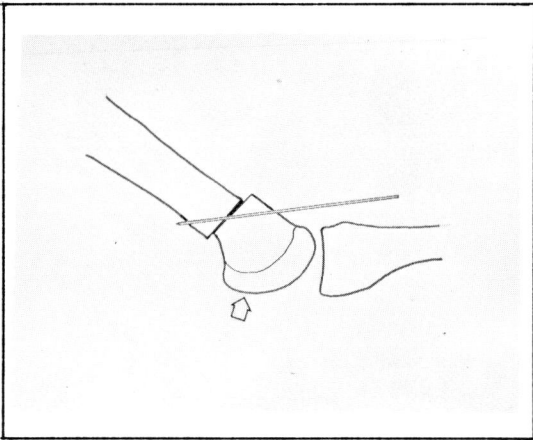

Fig. 6-16I. Lateral view of post-operative x-ray. Dotted line shows metatarsal head elevated and fixation with Kirschner wire.

Fig. 6-16J. Outline of x-ray on left.

V-Osteotomy

The V or Chevron osteotomy for the elevation and fixation of planti-flexed metatarsal head came about because of the problem that existed with medial or lateral deviation of a metatarsal head and shaft following osteoclasis. The reason that a displacement occurred was due to the osteoclasis being performed (1) at the level of the shaft and (2) the lack of fixation and casting postoperatively. When an osteoclasis is performed as described elsewhere in this chapter, displacement or shifting of the head does not occur. This is not to say, however, that the V-Osteotomy is not a useful technique. Quite the contrary, V-Osteotomy when performed for the proper indications (i.e. planti-flexion of the metatarsal ray) will yield as good a result as an osteoclasis.

Technique

A lineal incision approximately 4.5 cm. long is made extending from the metatarsal shaft into the interdigital space. The incision is deepened and the dorsal tendons are retracted. A lineal incision is made into the capsule extending distally to the middle of the metatarsal shaft just proximal to the joint line (Figure 6-17 A).

The capsule and periosteum are carefully peeled from the metatarsal shaft using a periosteal elevator. The blunt ends of Senn retractors are used to retract the capsule. Using a small blade on the power saw, two cuts are made extending from just behind the surgical neck proximal to the medial and lateral borders of the shaft, forming a V-shaped osteotomy (Figure 6-17 B). The V-shaped osteotomy can also be placed so that the apex lies proximally.

Incidentally, **Dr. William Goldfarb**, has devised an extremely useful V-shaped osteotome (available from G·H·G Products, Inc. 417-419 Mill St., Bristol, Pa. 19007) which makes placement of the V-Osteotomy accurate and simple.

M.P.J. SURGERY

Once the cuts are made, the toe is pulled distally to separate the bone. Then, the foot is loaded and the metatarsal head is elevated to the level of the adjacent members. The head is then **pushed hard** against the shaft of the metatarsal. The compression of the head against the shaft will accomplish two things. First, fixation of the metatarsal and secondly prevent excessive periosteal proliferation since cortical bone will not proliferate as readily when covered by cancellous bone (Figure 6-17 C-D).

The capsule, deep and superficial fascia as well as the wound are then sutured with the material of choice. An above the ankle cast is applied for three weeks. Healing is usually uneventful.

Precautions

1. The V-Osteotomy is used for the **same** indications as an osteoclasis.
2. It does not require Kirschner wire fixation.
3. It can be used to shorten the metatarsal rays but not more than 0.5 cm. This is accomplished by cutting a double V-Osteotomy. However, this is quite difficult to perform. Consequently, it is best to use V-Osteotomy for **elevation only.**
4. The patient should be casted for three weeks.

Conclusion

The V-Osteotomy can be performed for the same indications as an osteoclasis. The only real advantage that it has over the osteoclasis is that it **does not** require Kirschner wire fixation. The main disadvantage is the difficulty encountered in performing the V cuts.

V-Osteotomy

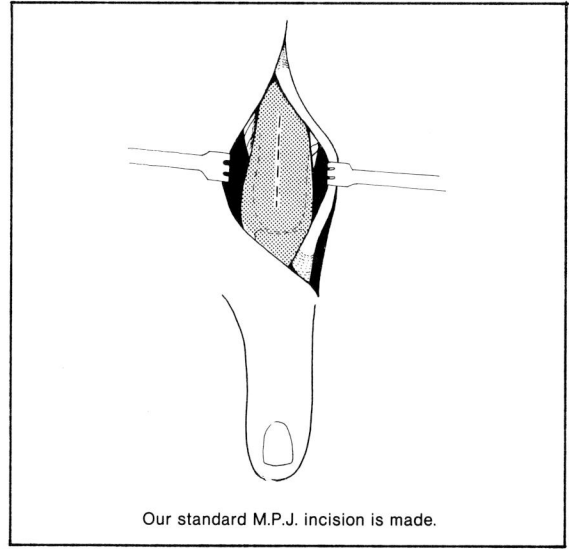

Our standard M.P.J. incision is made.

Fig. 6-17A

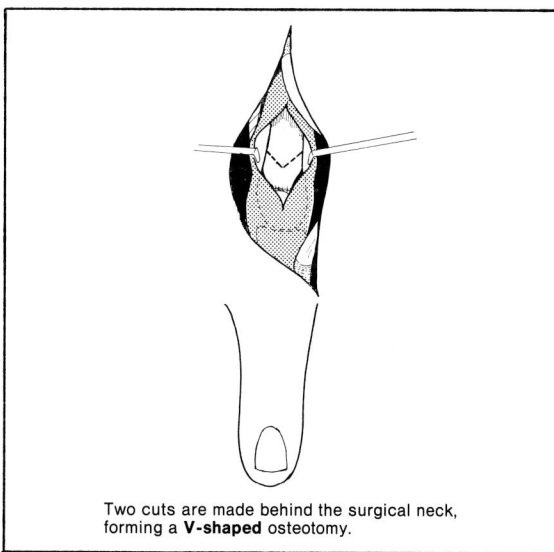

Two cuts are made behind the surgical neck, forming a **V-shaped** osteotomy.

Fig. 6-17B

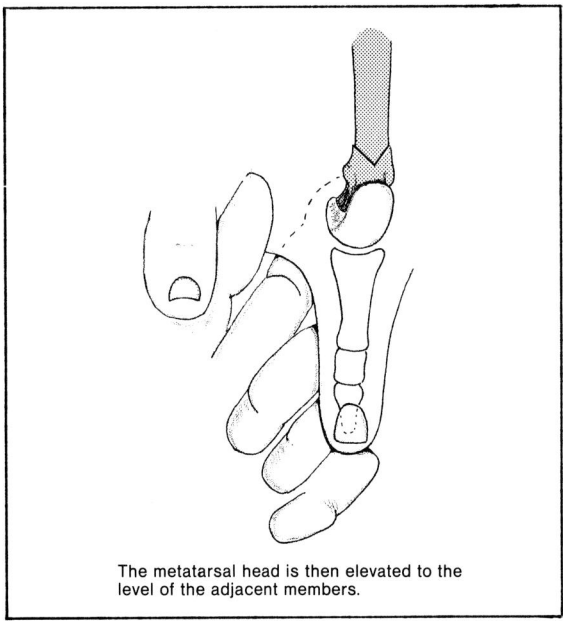

The metatarsal head is then elevated to the level of the adjacent members.

Fig. 6-17C

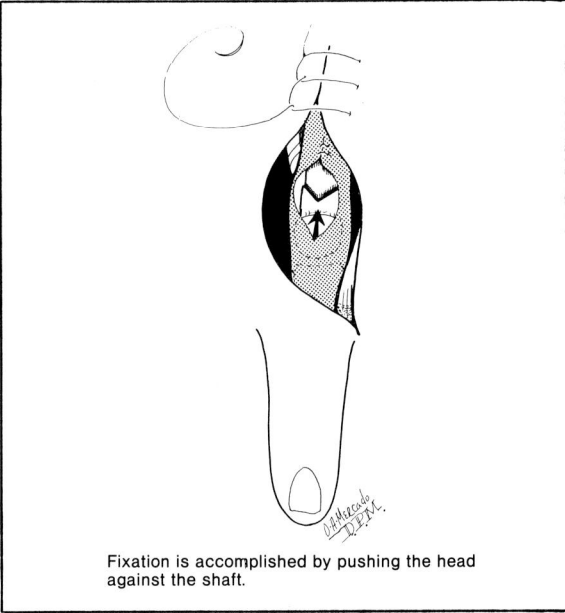

Fixation is accomplished by pushing the head against the shaft.

Fig. 6-17D

Extensor Osteotomy (E.O.)

Extensor osteotomy is a technique used for the elevation of a planti-flexed metatarsal ray. As with the other techniques in metatarsal-phalangeal-joint surgery, it is important to evaluate the patient and x-rays thoroughly before deciding on which procedure to use.

The indications for the technique are the same as for an osteoclasis (i.e. elevation of metatarsal ray). It is used less frequently than an osteoclasis because it is more difficult to perform.

Techniques

Making an incision for an extensor osteotomy can be confusing, since it is sometimes difficult to locate the individual metatarsal bases. Figure 6-18 A, demonstrates the approaches to the metatarsal bases. As a rule of thumb, the metatarsal base for the first toe can be found by drawing an imaginary line proximally from the waist of the foot to the second toe. Similarly, the base of the second metatarsal lies straight back from the third toe; the base of the third metatarsal lies straight back from the fourth toe; the base of the fourth metatarsal straight back from the fifth toe. The fifth metatarsal base is easy to find since its tuberosity can be palpated.

Once the proper metatarsal base is identified, a lineal incision approximately 4.0 cm. long is made. The incision is deepened and the dorsal tendons are retracted (Figure 6-18B). A lineal incision is made on the capsule extending from just proximal to the metatarsal-cuneiform-joint line distally to the shaft. The capsule and periosteum are carefully underscored (peeled) from the metatarsal shaft and base. Care is taken to make the dissection intra-capsularly so as to avoid cutting the **posterior perforating arteries** which descend in-between the metatarsal bases. Should a perforating artery be inadvertently cut, the circulation in this area is so abundant that it should not present a healing problem.

A measurement is taken from the joint line extending at least **1.0 cm.** distally to the base of the metatarsal. This area is carefully marked with an osteotome and will be the site of the proximal osteotomy line. It is important to go at least 1.0 cm. from the joint line as this will place the osteotomy well into cancellous bone (Figure 6-18C).

The second osteotomy line is marked with an osteotome just in front of the first line. The distance in-between the two lines will determine the size of the wedge to be taken and hence the amount of elevation that will be obtained. There is no method available at this time which will give the exact amount of elevation needed to bring the planti-fixed ray to a level with its adjacent members. The amount of wedge taken will depend entirely on the **clinical judgement** of the surgeon. As a rule, it is best to resect a small amount of bone first, then, if more elevation is needed, more bone can be resected.

The **proximal cut** is made first. A small power saw blade is used to make the transverse cut. The osteotomy **does not** go all the way through the plantar aspect of the bone. The second (distal) cut is made. This cut is **angulated** somewhat from dorsal to plantar to create a wedge shaped osteotomy. The second cut meets the plantar aspect of the first ostetomy and the wedge of bone thus formed is resected.

After the wedge of bone is resected, there will remain a plantar cortical HINGE. This hinge will prevent medial or lateral displacement but will allow plantar to dorsal movement. (Figure 6-18 D).

The metatarsal ray is then pushed from the plantar aspect to elevate the ray, thus closing the wedge and coaptating the osteotomized bone. If the metatarsal ray does not move readily, the cortical hinge is thinned out with a power saw blade.

If the wedge is inadvertently made **too big** (wide), trying to close it will cause excessive elevation of the shaft. It is best not to close the wedge all the way. Bone chips from the resected bone can be used to pack the osteotomy site to fill in the gaping space.

The metatarsal ray is elevated and the osteotomy line is fixated by inserting a small Kirschner wire (Figure 6-18 D). The capsule, deep and superficial fascia as well as the wound are closed with the suture materials of choice. An above the ankle cast is applied for three weeks at which time the sutures and the Kirschner wire are removed. Healing is usually uneventful.

Precautions

1. Be sure that the metatarsal ray **needs** elevation and not shortening.
2. Make your wedge in cancellous bone at least **1.0 cm.** from the joint line.
3. It is not necessary to resect a **great deal** of bone to obtain the desired elevation.
4. Leave a plantar cortical **hinge** when cutting the wedge.
5. Fixate the osteotomy line securely. My preference is external fixation with Kirschner wire.
6. **Immobilize** the osteotomy with an above the ankle cast for three weeks.

Conclusions

The extensor osteotomy procedure is another method of elevating the metatarsal ray. It has the same indications as an osteoclasis technique, but is a bit more difficult to perform.

Extensor Osteotomy (E.O.)

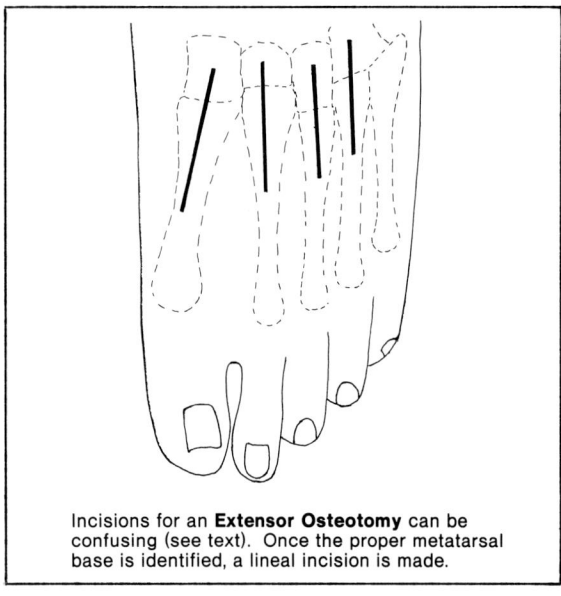

Fig. 6-18A

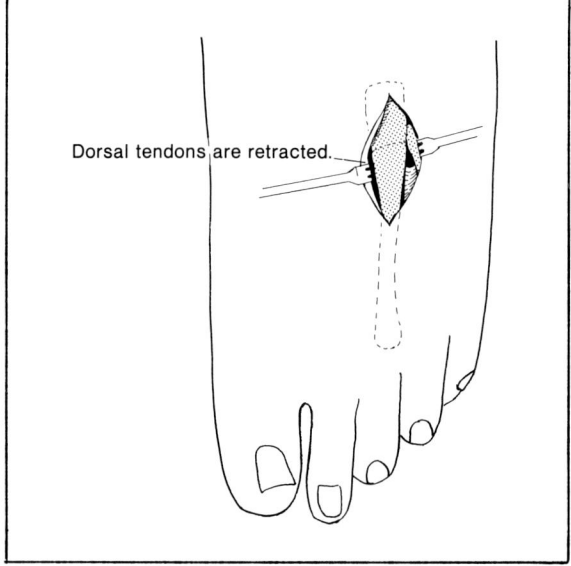

Fig. 6-18B

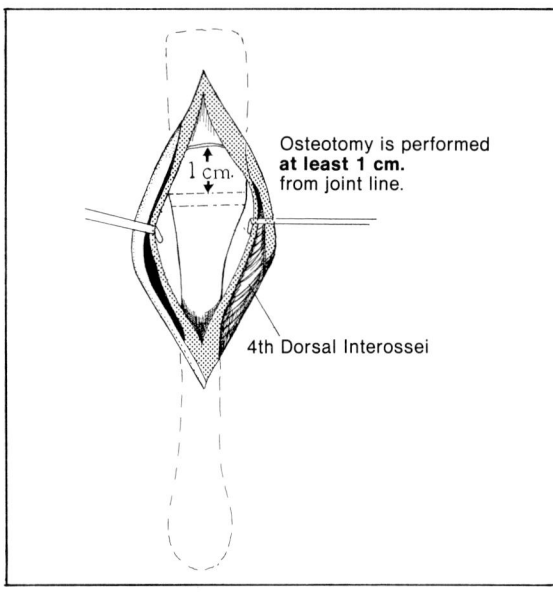

Fig. 6-18C

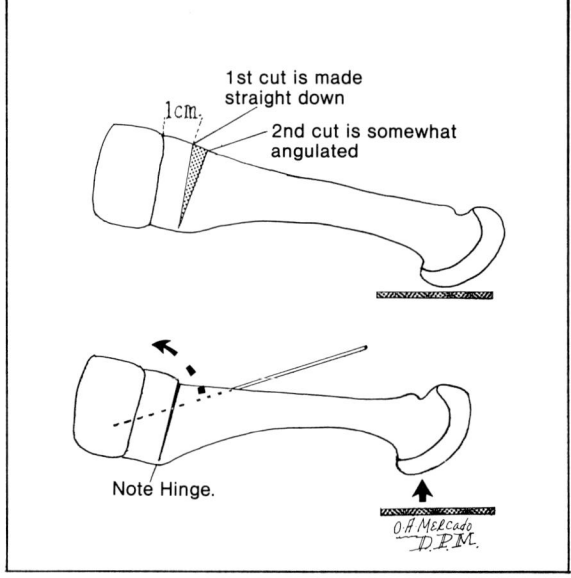

Fig. 6-18D

Extensor Osteoarthrotomy (E.O.A.)

Extensor osteoarthrotomy (E.O.A) is a technique used essentially for the same indications as the extensor osteotomy, except that it is used when stabilization of the metatarsal base joint is desirable.

The technique will work for any of the inner metatarsals. It is usually performed to relieve an isolated intractable plantar keratosis.

Technique

A lineal incision is made immediately over the corresponding metatarsal-cuneiform-joint (or metatarsal-cuboidal-joint in the case of the 4th metatarsal). The metatarsal base joint line can be found by tracing an imaginary line from the toe lateral to the involved metatarsal head, back to the waist of the foot (I.E., the base of the 2nd metatarsal will be found by tracing an imaginary line from the 3rd toe back to the waist of the foot, see Figure 6-18 A).

The incision is deepened and the dorsal tendons are retracted, so as to expose the metatarsal base joint capsule. The involved metatarsal head is then grasped and pulled vigorously back and forth a number of times to fascilitate locating the metatarsal base joint line. As the metatarsal is pulled, the joint capsule is stretched and a **puckering** of the tissues will occur at the joint line.

A lineal incision is made directly over the joint line, extending into the base of the metatarsal. The capsule and periosteum are carefully retracted (peeled) from the bone and the joint line is exposed.

Two cuts are carefully marked with an osteotome. The first is proximal to the joint line. The second is distal to the joint line (Figure 6-19 A). As in the extensor osteotomy procedure, it **is not** necessary to resect a great deal of bone. A minimal amount of bone removed will raise the metatarsal head the required amount as it is only necessary to elevate the ray a few millimeters.

Utilizing the power saw, the first (proximal) cut is made parallel to the joint line. The second (distal) cut is angulated from dorsal to plantar to form a slight wedge with its apex directed plantarwards (Figure 6-19 B). The wedge of bone thus formed will contain the metatarsal-cunneiform (or metatarsal-cuboidal) joint. The joint is removed in-toto. No plantar hinge is left in this procedure.

The foot is loaded and the involved metatarsal ray is elevated to the desired plane (even with the adjacent metatarsal heads) and a Kirschner wire is used to externally fixate the osteotomy line. The wound is closed in the ususal manner. An above the ankle cast is applied for three weeks at which time the cast, Kirschner wire, and sutures are removed. Healing is usually uneventful.

Precautions

1. This technique is used when a single ray needs **elevation** and **stabilization.**
2. It is not necessary to remove a great deal of bone to obtain the desired elevation.
3. If too much bone is accidentally resected, do not try to close the osteotomy all the way as this will result in over correction. Bone chips obtained from the wedge can be used to pack in between the osteotomy until the proper elevation is obtained.
4. In essence, this technique will **fuse** the metatarsal-cuneiform (or metatarsal-cuboidal) joint. Remember that the movement of the inner metatarsal base joints is limited to one plane (dorsal-plantar). In reality, the planti-flexed ray is already in a rigid state, so that by fusing the joint, the surgeon is merely stabilizing the ray at a more functionable plane.

    In my experience, not only with the E.O.A. technique but with the Lapidus procedure (which calls for the fusion of the 1st metatarsal-cuneiform joint), I have not seen any deleterious sequela after the fusion of the metatarsal base joints. This is not to say that injudicious fusion of these or any other joint should be advocated, but rather, that the fusion of a joint sometimes is necessary to stabilize and enhance function.

Conclusion

The E.O.A. technique is useful whenever a ray needs elevation along with stabilization of the metatarsal base joint. When performed as indicated here, it will yield consistently good results.

Extensor Osteoarthrotomy (E.O.A.)

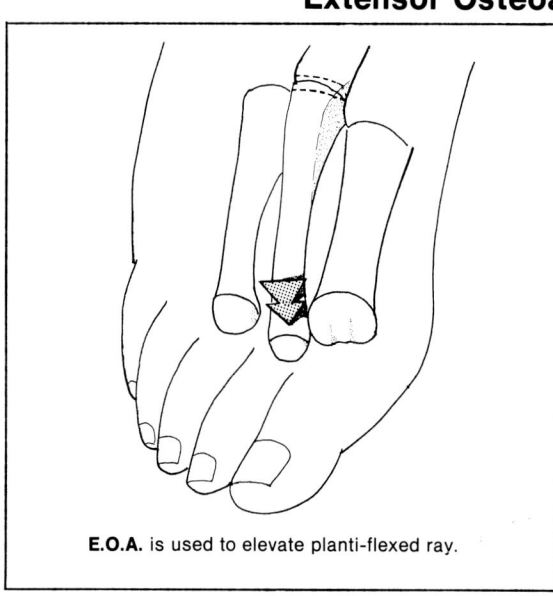

Fig. 6-19A

E.O.A. is used to elevate planti-flexed ray.

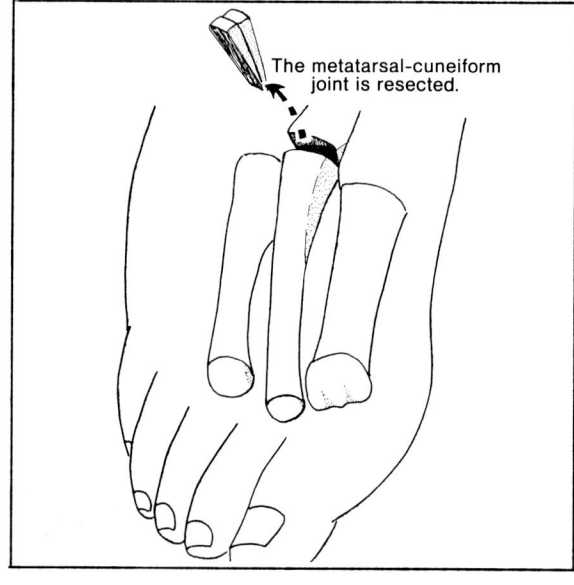

Fig. 6-19B

The metatarsal-cuneiform joint is resected.

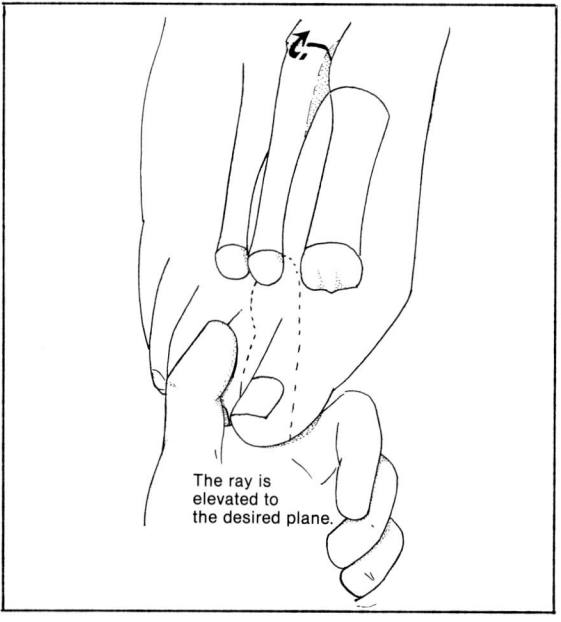

Fig. 6-19C

The ray is elevated to the desired plane.

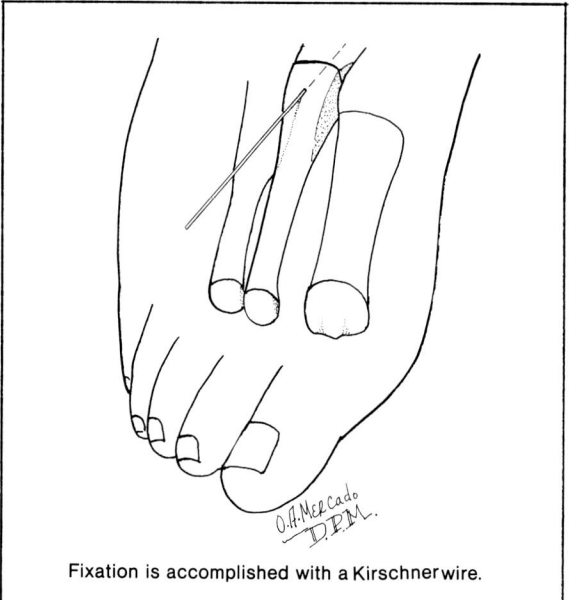

Fig. 6-19D

Fixation is accomplished with a Kirschner wire.

Techniques for the Fifth Metatarsal Ray

Problems affecting the fifth metatarsal ray can be usually classified as follows:
1. A hyperostosis on the lateral aspect of the fifth metatarsal head (a tailor's bunion).
2. An I.P.K. under the fifth metatarsal head.
3. A medially displaced articular facet (causing **retrograde** pressure on the head.)
4. A laterally deviated metatarsal shaft.

Tailor's Bunion (Figure 6-20) is nothing more than a hyperostosis on the lateral aspect of the fifth metatarsal head. If the shaft is straight, and the metatarsal-phalangeal-joint is congruous, then a simple ostectomy is performed.

Technique

A lineal incision approximately 5 cm. long is made on the lateral aspect of the metatarsal-phalangeal-joint. The wound is deepened and the superficial bleeders are ligated. The wound is underscored and the joint capsule is exposed. A lineal incision is made into the joint capsule. The capsule and periosteum are carefully retracted; the collateral ligaments are cut and the metatarsal head is delivered.

The hyperostosis on the lateral aspect of head is then resected flush with the metatarsal shaft. The bone is rasped smooth. The capsule, deep and superficial fascia as well as the skin are sutured with the material of choice.

I.P.K. under Metatarsal Head (Figure 6-20)

An I.P.K. under the fifth metatarsal head will respond to a partial metatarsal head resection as long as the shaft is not deviated. Partial metatarsal head resections, as we have mentioned before, are only used for diseased bone (I.E. Freiberg's and R.A.), and for fifth metatarsal head I.P.K.'s.

In my lectures to different groups in various parts of the country, when I ask if they agree with a partial metatarsectomy for an I.P.K. under the essentially straight shaft, the answer is overwhelmingly "yes".

Medially Displaced Articular Facet (Figure 6-20)

A medially displaced articular facet occurs somewhat **infrequently** on the fifth metatarsal head. When it is present, the base of the fifth proximal phalanx will cause retrograde pressure causing lateral displacement of the head, resulting in symptoms very similar to a tailor's bunion.

The surgery performed is a sub-capital osteotomy, actually a **reversed Reverdin,** to realign the articular facet. There is also a small amount of shortening occurring with this technique, which will in turn increase the joint space.

Lateral Deviated Metatarsal Shaft (Figure 6-20)

When the shaft is laterally deviated, a closing wedge is used to correct the deviation.

Techniques for the Fifth Metatarsal Ray

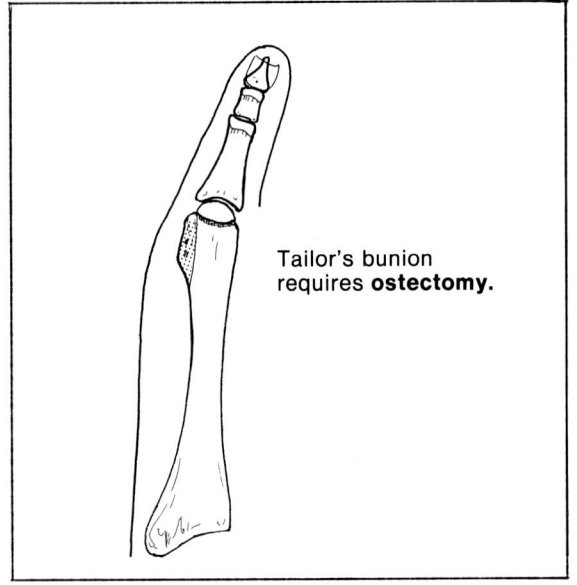

Tailor's bunion requires **ostectomy**.

Fig. 6-20A

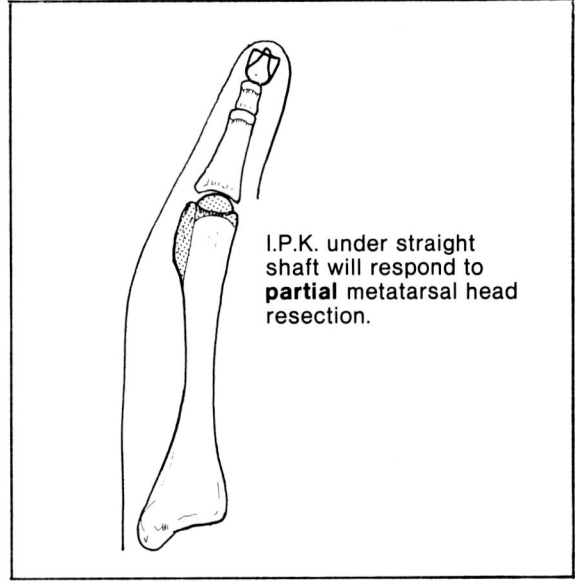

I.P.K. under straight shaft will respond to **partial** metatarsal head resection.

Fig. 6-20B

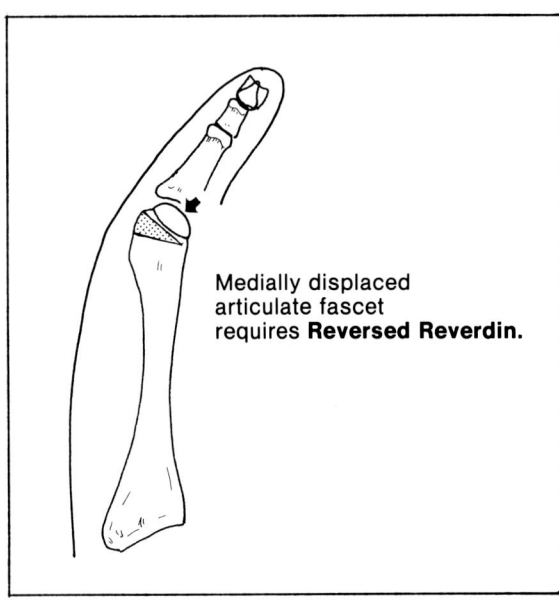

Medially displaced articulate fascet requires **Reversed Reverdin**.

Fig. 6-20C

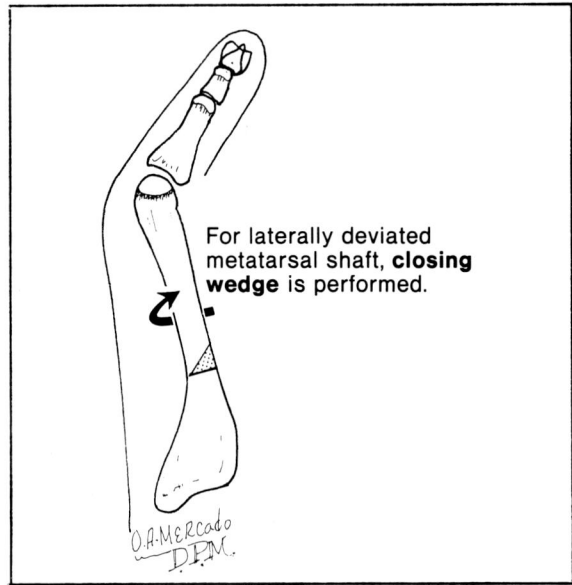

For laterally deviated metatarsal shaft, **closing wedge** is performed.

Fig. 6-20D

Closing Wedge Osteotomy for Deviated Fifth Metatarsal Shaft

A closing wedge osteotomy is indicated for the correction of a deviated fifth metatarsal shaft.

Technique

An incision approximately 5 cm. long is made immediately over the metatarsal shaft. The incision is deepened and the superficial bleeders are ligated (Figure 6-21 A).

The metatarsal shaft is exposed and an incision is made into the periosteum. Using a periosteal elevator the periosteum is carefully underscored and the metatarsal shaft is exposed (Figure 6-21 B-C).

The **site** of the osteotomy is determined by the x-ray. It is usually at the point where the greatest deviation of the shaft occurs. This point will vary from patient to patient so that the osteotomy will be located distally sometimes and other times it will be proximal.

Once the location is determined, the osteotomy is marked with an osteotome. The first cut is parallel with the articular facet of the metatarsal base. The second cut is distal to the first and it is angulated from lateral to medial to form a **pie shaped** wedge. Note that the cuts do not go through the lateral cortex, but a hinge is left. This hinge is extremely important as it will only allow movement from lateral to medial, it **will not** allow dorsal or plantar movement (Figure 6-21 C-D).

Sometimes, a bit of dorsal movement is desirable particularly in the case where there is an intractable plantar keratosis under the fifth metatarsal head along with the deviation of the shaft. In such cases **Gerbert, Sgarlato,** and **Subotnick** advocate a bi-plane osteotomy. Simply stated it requires nothing more than angulating the distal cut not only from lateral to medial, but from dorsal to plantar. In this manner when the osteotomy is closed, movement will occur not only on a lateral to medial plane, but a plantar to dorsal plane as well.

Once the osteotomy site is closed, it is fixated with a small Kirschner wire. The periosteum, sub-dermal tissues and skin are closed with the suture materials of choice. An above the ankle cast is applied for three weeks. Healing is usually uneventful.

Conclusion

1. The closing wedge technique will work well when the correction of a deviated metatarsal shaft is desired.
2. **Do not** take too much bone out or an over correction will occur.
3. Fixation of the osteotomy site can be also accomplished with an intermedullary cortical bone peg graft (see Chapter 5 — Principles of Bone Surgery).

Closing Wedge Osteotomy for Deviated Fifth Metatarsal Shaft

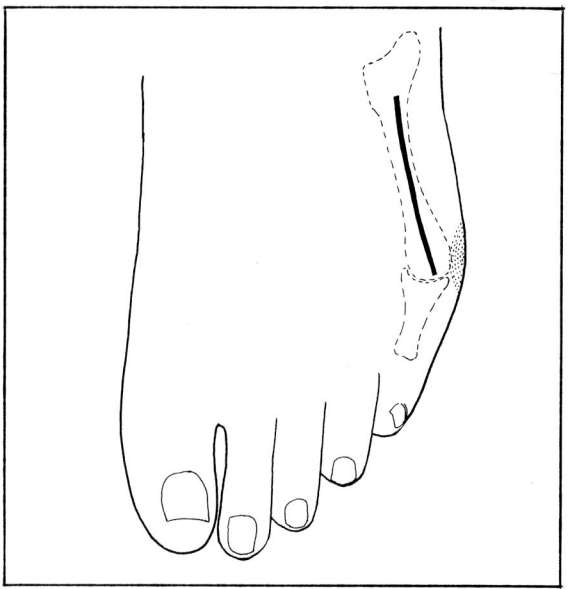

Fig. 6-21A

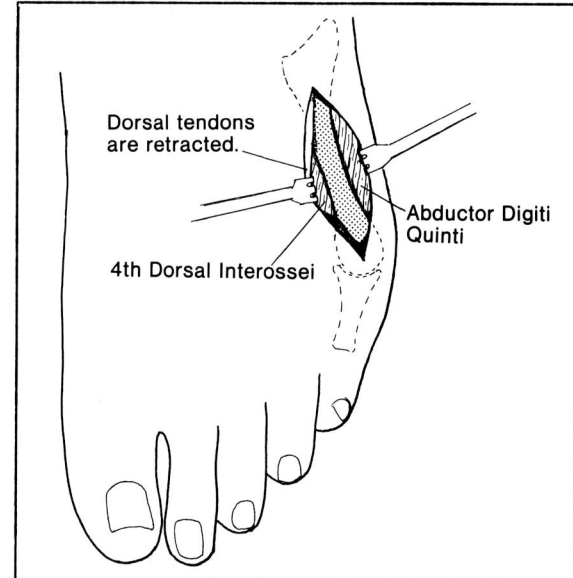

Fig. 6-21B

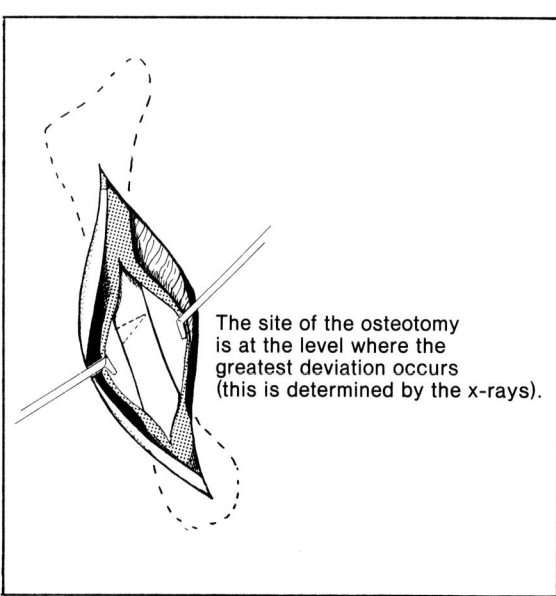

Fig. 6-21C

The site of the osteotomy is at the level where the greatest deviation occurs (this is determined by the x-rays).

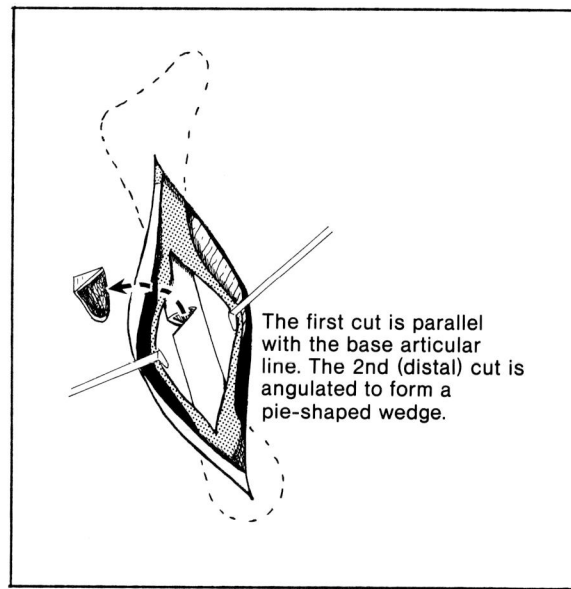

Fig. 6-21D

The first cut is parallel with the base articular line. The 2nd (distal) cut is angulated to form a pie-shaped wedge.

M.P.J. SURGERY

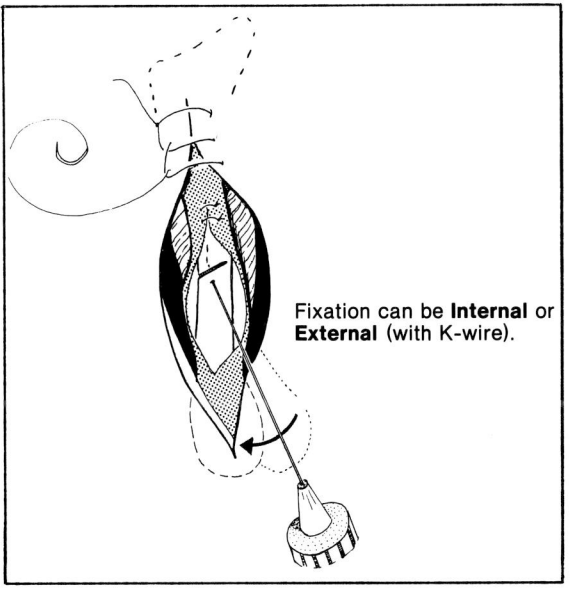

Fig. 6-21E

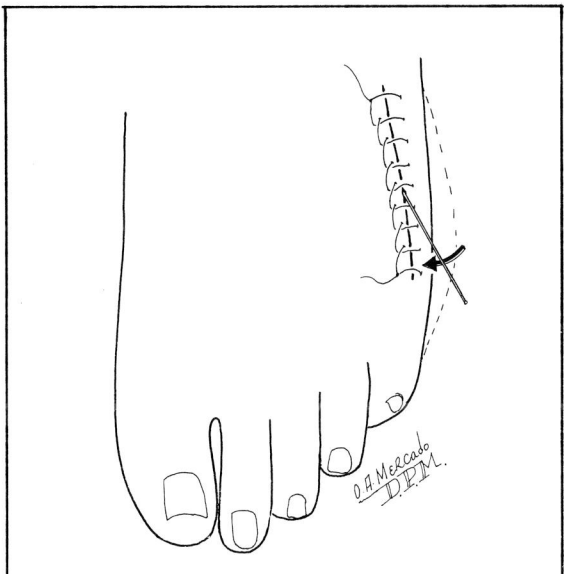

Fig. 6-21F

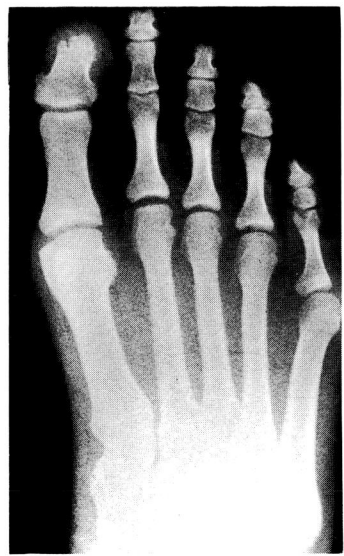

Fig. 6-21G. Pre-operative x-ray reveals **deviated** 5th. metatarsal shaft.

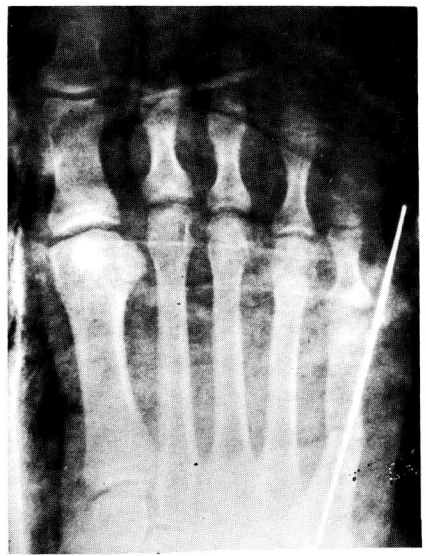

Fig. 6-21H. Post-operative x-ray shows fixation of osteotomy with Kirschner wire.

Metatarsus Varus (Pes Adductus)

Metatarsus Varus is essentially a positional (fetal) deformity. Although present at birth, the deformity sometimes goes unnoticed for months.

Clinically the patient will exhibit:

1. Adduction of the forefoot.
2. The lateral border of the foot will have a convexity resembling the letter "C".
3. The apex of this convexity will be the base of the fifth metatarsal.
4. On x-rays all metatarsal shafts will be in a varus position with a crowding of all of the bases.
5. The heel will be in valgus.
6. There is usually a bowing of the leg.
7. There is often a laterally displaced patella.

Before the child begins ambulating, the problem can be readily corrected with plaster of paris **serial casts.** It usually will take 3 to 6 casts to correct most cases. It is important that the child be followed up with **Brachman** bars, and orthosis if necessary.

The length of time that the cast is left on will depend on the age of the child:

One month or less . . . Change cast every week
One to three months . . . Change every ten days
Over three months . . . Change every two weeks

Casting Technique

Casting should begin as soon as the deformity is diagnosed. Time should not be wasted, as the child **will not outgrow the deformity.**

Casting of a small child is accomplished quite easily. In over a decade of casting children, I have **never** sedated a child to accomplish my work. Children will vary in personality as much as adults. Some are easy to work with and will respond to any attention you or your nurse can give them. Others will be difficult to work with and it is better to get the job over with rather than trying to play games with them.

I use **extra fast** setting 2" plaster of paris. First the foot and leg are covered with a small stockinette. Webril is then applied snuggly over the stockinette. A roll of plaster of paris is then rolled over back and forth into a 9 to 10 inch long strip, which will be used to form a platform.

Two rolls of plaster of paris are then quickly rolled over the foot distally, to below the knee. The heel is cupped in one hand and held in a neutral position to prevent movement when the forefoot is corrected.

The forefoot is then **forced** lateralwards at the same time a very small amount of eversion should be obtained to unlock the metatarsal bases. It is important to remember that:

1. The rear foot is held at a **neutral** position.
2. **Only** the forefoot is corrected.
3. During the first cast very little correction is obtained, but this will improve with the serial casting.

Incidentally, while you are holding the foot in its corrected position, your nurse should be cutting away the excessive cast and webril from the dorsum of the cast before the plaster sets.

After the correction is obtained, the plantar aspect of the cast is reinforced with the 9 to 10 inch long plaster strip that was prepared before. The cast is then finished in the usual manner.

The foot and leg are casted 2 to 3 times below the knee. After the lower deformity (foot and leg) begins to respond, then an **above the knee** cast is applied as follows:

1. Stockinette and webril are applied to above the knee.
2. The foot and leg cast (below the knee) is applied.
3. A roll of plaster is applied above the knee covering the patella.
4. After the cast dries, force is applied to **derotate** the upper (above the knee) cast from lateral to medial. This will bring the laterally displaced patella into its proper perspective (Figure 6-22).
5. At the same time the foot and leg cast is rotated from medial to lateral, and line-up with the patella.
6. The knee is **flexed slightly** (this position is more comfortable to the child).
7. The two casts are then held together in their corrected position, with another roll of plaster of paris.

Conclusion

The treatment of metatarsus adductus by plaster of paris castings, is simple and yields consistently good results. However, the following precautions should be observed:

1. Casting works best for **non-ambulating** children.
2. Children have a great amount of adipose tissues which must be compressed so that the cast must be applied snuggly if it is to work.
3. Have the mother take the cast off at home. She can do this by soaking it in water and peeling it layer by layer. This will require some time to do, but it is better than using an electric cast cutter to remove the cast.
4. Sedating a child for castings **is not** necessary.
5. It is important to follow up these patients with bars and orthosis for an adequate length of time to insure complete correction of the deformity.
6. **After** the child has begun ambulating, casting can be utilized, particularly if the condition is unilateral. However, the treatment will require a greater number of casts to obtain results.
7. Metatarsus varus in the older ambulating child can still be treated successfully with the use of the **Brachman** bar. When the patient is followed up with orthosis, torque-heels and proper shoes, it will be **seldom** if ever, that surgery will be required for these children.

Metatarsus Varus (Pes Adductus)

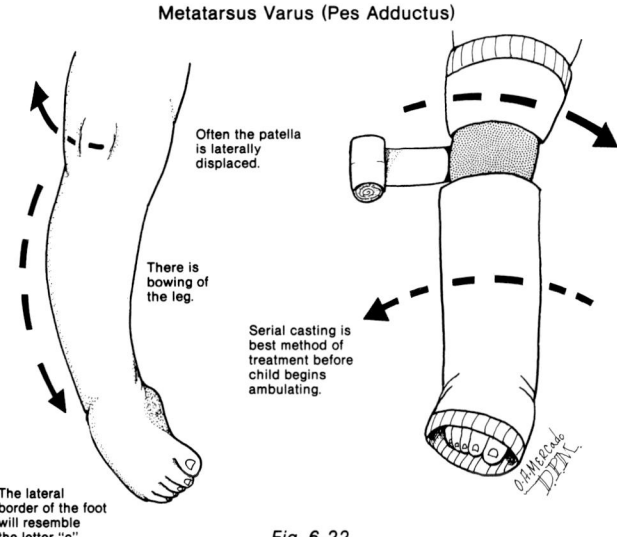

Fig. 6-22

Heyman, Herdon, and Strong (H. H. and S.) Technique

The **Heyman, Herdon,** and **Strong** technique is an operation used for the correction of metatarsus varus when the patient is too old for serial plaster of paris cast treatment and does not respond to Brachman bars, and other orthosis therapy.

The technique is used in children between the ages of 3 and 7 years. It calls for the soft tissue release of the intermetatarsal-base capsules and ligaments.

Technique

A transversed semi-elliptical incision is made on the dorsum of the foot extending from the dorsal-medial aspect of the first metatarsal-cuneiform-joint to the dorsal-lateral aspect of the fifth metatarsal-cuboidal-joint (Figure 6-23 A). The incision is carefully deepened to just past the superficial fascia. All vital nerves and tendons are preserved.

The first metatarsal-cuneiform-joint is first exposed. The large superficial vein (a branch of the dorsal cutaneous venous network) which is found in this area is carefully underscored and retracted with a Penrose drain. The extensor hallucis longus and tibialis anterior are carefully retracted so as to expose the joint capsule (Figure 6-23 B).

The first metatarsal is pulled distally and lateralwards and a number 15 blade is used to cut the joint capsule and ligaments from the dorsal-medial and lateral aspect. Care is taken when cutting the medial joint capsule and ligaments not to injure the tibialis anterior tendon.

The **neurovascular bundle** (containing the dorsalis pedis) is identified and retracted and the dorsal-medial and lateral joint capsule and ligaments of the second metatarsal-cuneiform-joint are cut. The ligaments on the joint capsule on the dorsal-medial and lateral aspects are also cut on the remaining metatarsal bases (Figure 6-23 C).

The forefoot is then pulled and planti-flexed and the plantar joint capsule and ligaments of all the metatarsals are cut on the medial aspect **only.** The lateral aspect is left intact to prevent displacement during manipulation. The foot is then **forced** lateralwards with some eversion (Figure 6-23 D).

The wound is closed in layers with the choice of suture material. An above the knee cast is applied with the foot in the corrected position.

The patient is discharged with a below the knee cast which is left on for 3 weeks. Physical therapy, orthosis, and adequate shoes are essential postoperatively to insure an excellent result.

Conclusion

1. The Heyman, Herdon, and Strong (H. H. and S.) technique is indicated in children between the ages of 3 to 7 who are too old for serial casting and **have not** responded to Brachman bars and orthosis.
2. I must **emphasize** that most metatarsus varus patients **will** respond to conservative therapy and that surgery is **seldom** necessary.
3. In the cases where surgery is indicated, the H. H. and S. technique as described here will give excellent results.

Heyman, Herdon and Strong (H.H. and S.) Technique

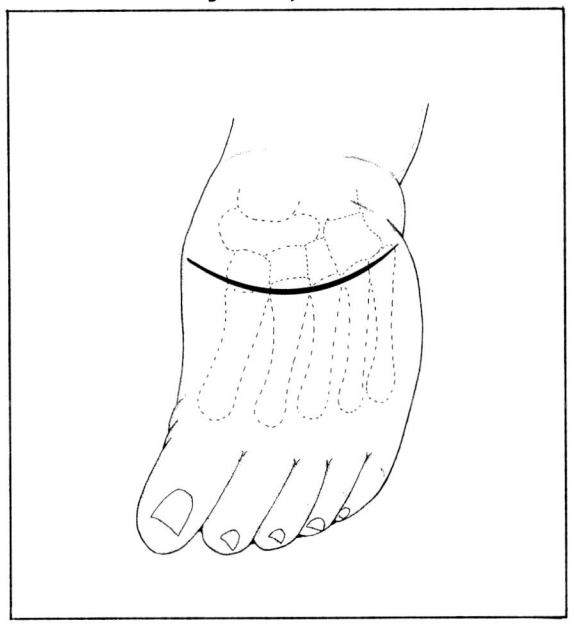

Fig. 6-23A

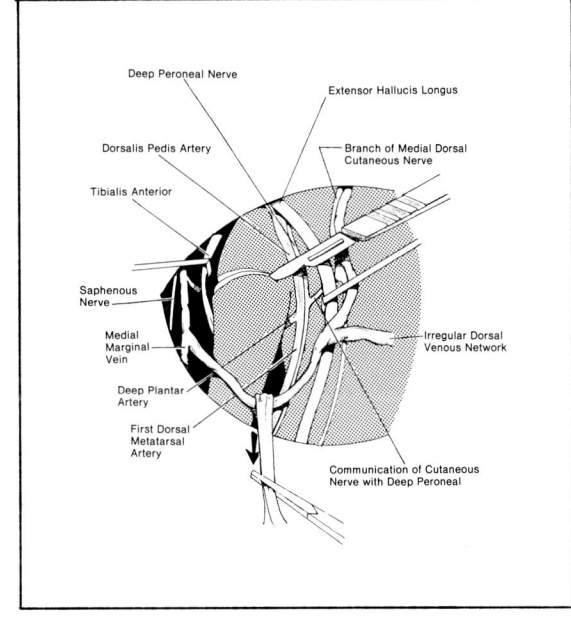

Fig. 6-23B

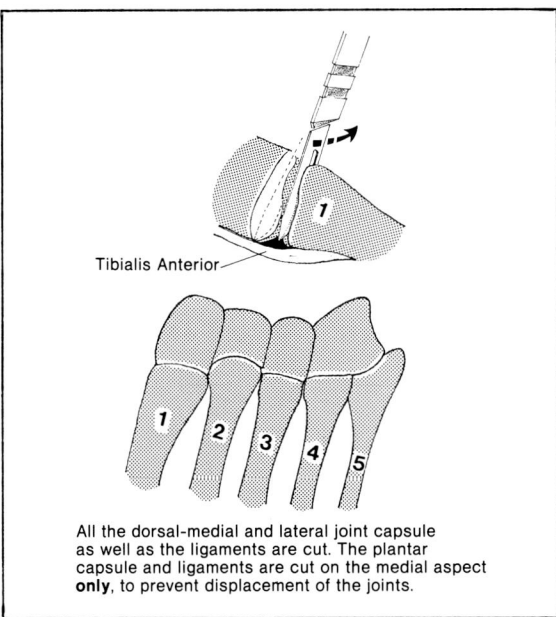

All the dorsal-medial and lateral joint capsule as well as the ligaments are cut. The plantar capsule and ligaments are cut on the medial aspect **only**, to prevent displacement of the joints.

Fig. 6-23C

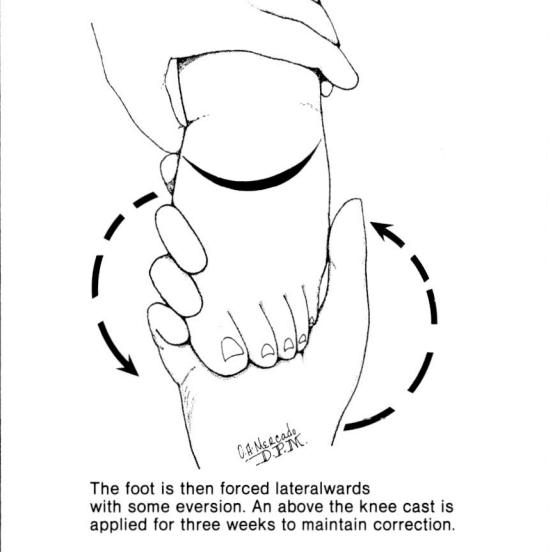

The foot is then forced lateralwards with some eversion. An above the knee cast is applied for three weeks to maintain correction.

Fig. 6-23D

Base Crescentic-Osteotomy for Metatarsus Varus

The Base Crescentic-Osteotomy for Metatarsus Varus is indicated when the child is over 8 years of age and has not responded to conservative therapy. The technique is also useful in the correction of **splay foot;** the only modifications in these cases is that a closing wedge is performed on the fifth ray since this ray is usually laterally deviated.

Technique

The metatarsal bases are approached by way of three longitudinal incisions. The first incision will lie immediately over the first metatarsal-cuneiform-joint, the second incision lies in between the second and third metatarsal bases; and the third incision is placed in between the fourth and fifth metatarsal bases (Figure 6-24 A).

The first incision is deepened and the tendon of extensor hallucis longus is retracted laterally. The capsule and periosteum are carefully peeled from the base of the metatarsal so as not to injure the deep plantar artery found lying in between the bases of the first and second metatarsal (Figure 6-8 C-D dorsi-flectory wedge in this chapter).

The **epiphyseal plate** is found near the joint line of the first metatarsal-cuneiform-joint (this can readily be seen in the x-ray) and it must be avoided. The osteotomy site is then marked with an osteotome.

The bases of all the other metatarsals are then exposed and underscored in a similar manner. The osteotomy sites are marked (approximately one cm. from the joint line). There are no epiphyseal plates in the lesser metatarsal bases, so we do not have to be concerned with them.

A crescentic blade is then chosen which will give the proper size cut. Crescentic blades are notoriously **fragile** and as we have pointed out elsewhere in this book, they must be used properly. Once the osteotomy site is located, the electric saw is started before the blade meets the bone.

The blade must be held at **90°** to the bone. The wrist is moved slightly from side to side to help the blade start the cut. Once the cut (actually the groove) is started, the blade will cut the bone without difficulties (Figure 6-24 B). It is important to continue cutting until the bone is cut all the way thru the plantar aspect as this will insure a smooth even cut which will allow the desired movement of the metatarsals. After all the metatarsal bases are cut, the foot is carefully placed in a corrected position. Care is taken so as not to cause dorsal (or plantar) displacement of the metatarsals.

A large Kirschner wire is then driven across, just proximal to all metatarsal heads. The wounds are closed in the usual manner. An above the knee cast is applied. A below the knee cast is applied before the patient is discharged.

The cast is removed in 4 to 5 weeks. Physical therapy, orthosis and proper shoes are essential to insure excellent results.

Conclusion

1. The base crescentic-osteotomy should only be used in the most recalcitrant cases of metatarsus adductus, and then only when all conservative therapy has failed.
2. The crescentic-osteotomy is as a rule very unstable. The osteotomy sites **should** be individually fixated (as in metatarsus varus correction for hallux valgus). When the osteotomy is fixated distally with a Kirschner wire, (as shown in our illustration) it can displace dorsally, plantarly, or even separate. For this reason, it is important to check and double check **all osteotomy sites** before closing the wound.
3. When all indications and precautions are followed, the crescentic-osteotomy technique will yield excellent results.

Base Crescentic-Osteotomy for Metatarsus Varus

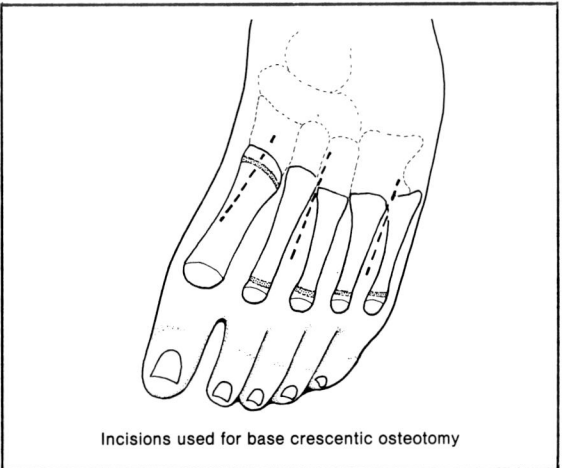

Incisions used for base crescentic osteotomy

Fig. 6-24A

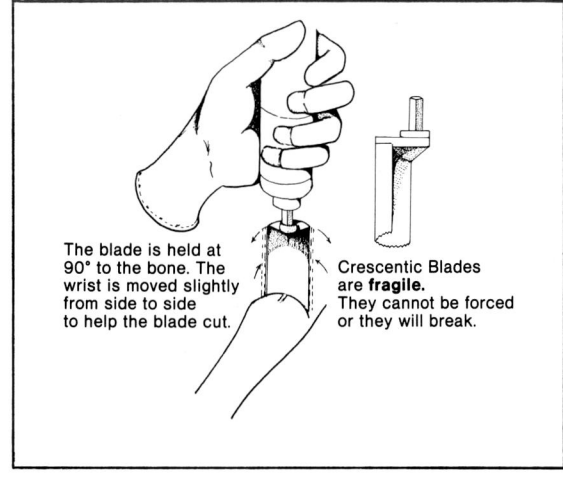

The blade is held at 90° to the bone. The wrist is moved slightly from side to side to help the blade cut.

Crescentic Blades are **fragile.** They cannot be forced or they will break.

Fig. 6-24B

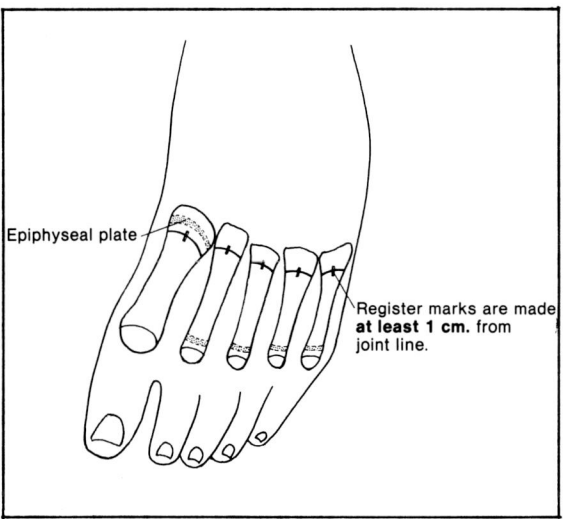

Epiphyseal plate

Register marks are made **at least 1 cm.** from joint line.

Fig. 6-24C

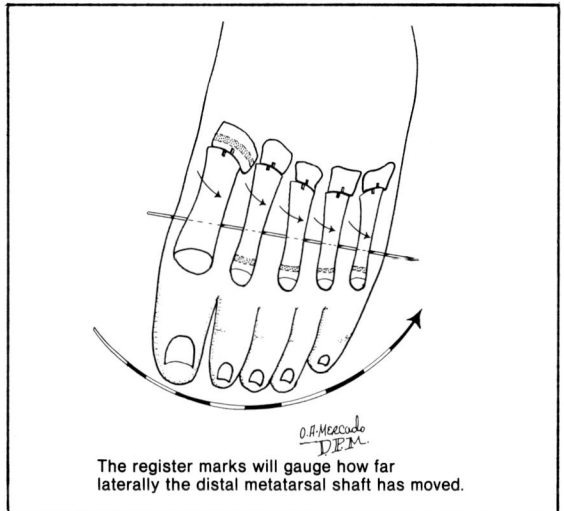

The register marks will gauge how far laterally the distal metatarsal shaft has moved.

Fig. 6-24D

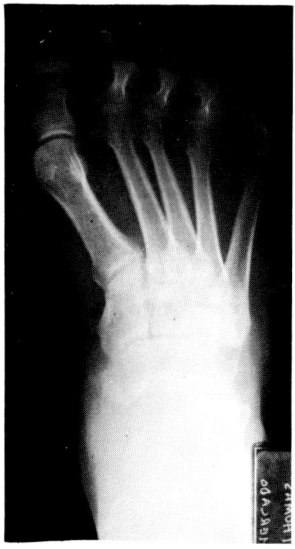 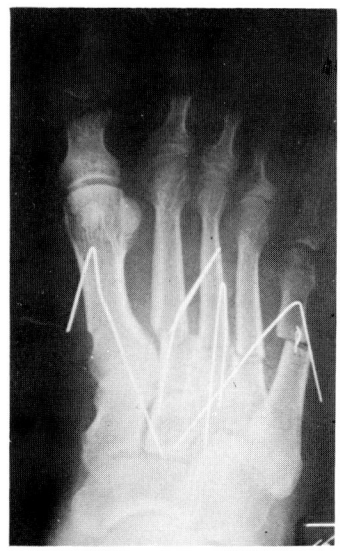

Fig. 6-24E. The Base Crescentic-Osteotomy can also be used for the correction of **splay-foot**.

Fig. 6-24F. Post-operative x-ray. Base crescentic-osteotomy was performed on the 1st., 2nd., 3rd. and 4th. metatarsals. A Closing Wedge Osteotomy was performed on the 5th.

Rheumatoid Arthritis

"Rheumatoid arthritis! What a terrible disease to have to live with. It immediately brings to mind a severely crippled patient, burdened with despair."

Leonard Marmor

Rheumatoid arthritis (R.A.) has been tormenting mankind since the early beginnings. Today, the disease is second only to heart disease as a major cause of chronic limitation to normal living. **No other** disease affects the feet so devastatively as does R.A. The rheumatoid foot is rigid and always **painful.** The resilience and elasticity necessary for normal walking is absent. The patients often walk with an unstable shuffling gait, shifting from one foot to another as though they had artificial feet.

Rheumatoid arthritis is essentially a disease causing non-specific **periarticular** changes (synovitis) with secondary changes to the joint structures. The synovium becomes thickened and progresses to invade into the sub-chondral bone and articular cartilage, forming a **pannus.** The invasion of the thickened synovium into the joint prevents normal extension and flexion of the joint, eventually leading to a flexion contraction deformity. As the disease progresses the sub-chondral bone is invaded and the joint is eroded (Figure 6-25 A-B-C-D).

Surgery in the rheumatoid should be performed as soon as possible. The surgery simply aims at removing the disease tissues (synovectomy) and disease bone (ostectomy). Almost every surgeon operating on the rheumatoid foot can tell of patients that have been an unqualified success, where the patients whole outlook on life was totally changed after the pain on the feet was gone (one of my patients went from barely being able to walk to where he is now in charge of the parole services for the state of Illinois); to the patient where the disease keeps progressing no matter what is done.

M.P.J. SURGERY

Sometimes the biggest stumbling block for the surgery is the patient that has become so totally defeated by the disease that they lack the motivation necessary for surgery. The surgeon should work with the patients family to motivate the patient, any relief that can be given will make the patients' existence more tolerable.

Joint Erosion Caused by Rheumatoid Arthritis

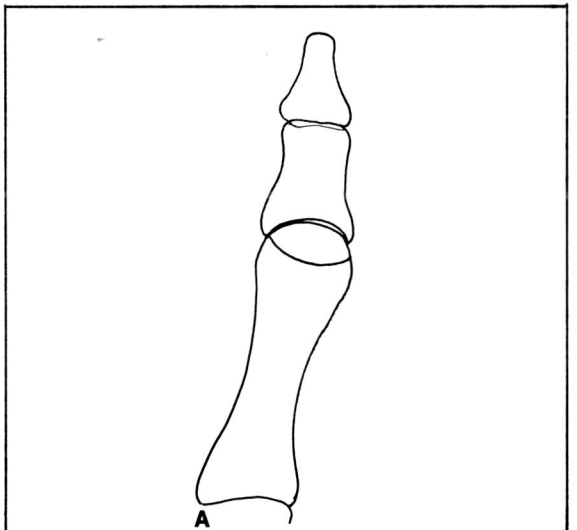

Fig. 6-25A. Normal 1st. metatarsal phalangeal joint.

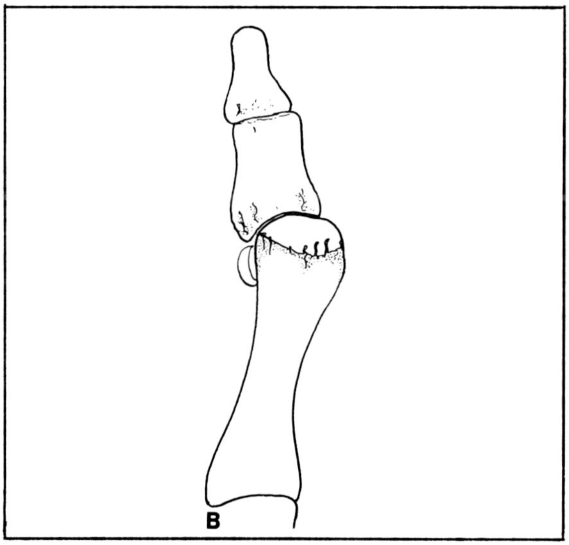

Fig. 6-25B. Mild erosion progresses to . . .

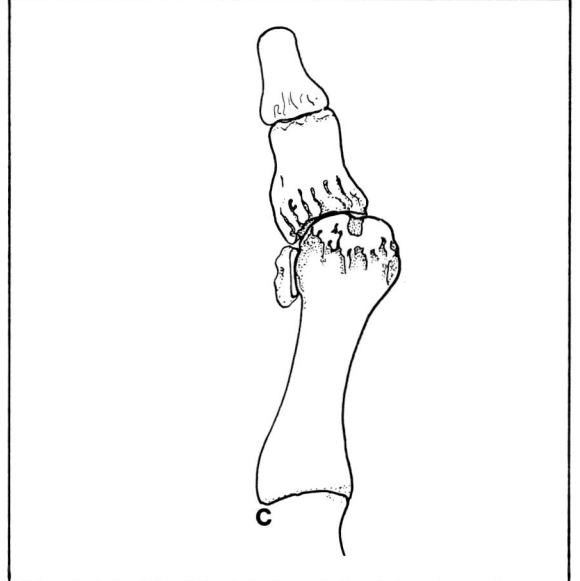
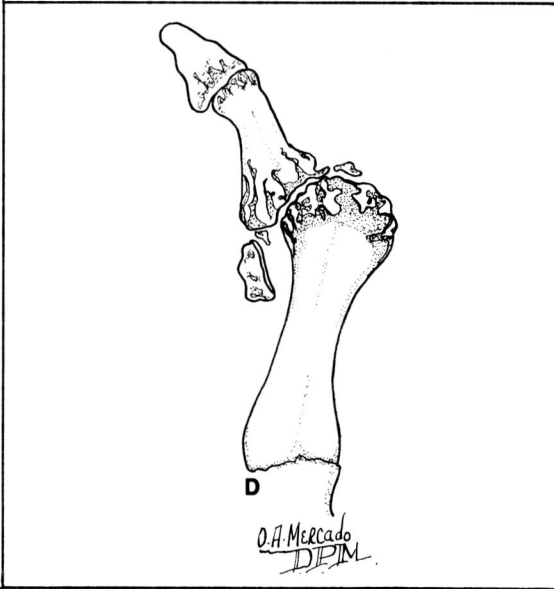

Fig. 6-25C. Moderate erosion and sub-chondral bone invasion leading to . . .

Fig. 6-25D. Complete erosion (destruction) of the joint.

Modified Clayton Pan-Metatarsectomy

Pan-Metatarsectomy for the severely crippled rheumatoid forefoot was described by **M. L. Clayton** in 1960. His technique calls for the resection of all of the metatarsal heads as well as the bases of the proximal phalanges.

Our technique of choice is essentially the same as Clayton's, however, the bases of the proximal phalanges **are not** removed. This results in a more stable and functional foot.

Technique

The metatarsal-phalangeal-joints can be approached by either a lineal incision over the first, metatarsal-phalangeal-joint and a transversed incision over the lesser metatarsal (Figure 6-26 A) or three lineal incisions over the first metatarsal-phalangeal-joint and in between the second and fourth intermetatarsal spaces (Figure 6-26 B).

The first metatarsal head is resected as shown in Figure 6-26 F. A transversed incision is then made and the superficial structures are carefully underscored and retracted. The tendon is underscored and the capsule is exposed.

The base of the proximal phalanx is usually laying over the dorsal aspect of the metatarsal head (Figure 6-26 C). Sometimes the joint is totally **sub-luxated.** The capsule is opened and preserved as much as possible. Usually the capsular tissues have penetrated so deeply into the sub-chondral bone that the capsule must be removed (Synovectomy). It is almost impossible to deliver the metatarsal head as is usually done during some metatarsal head surgery (Figure 6-10 E). Usually, the anatomical head is identified and the bone is resected and rasped smooth. This is about the **only time** that a complete resection of the metatarsal head is indicated.

The same procedure is then performed on the third, fourth, and fifth metatarsal heads. The **diseased** capsular tissue is removed as much as possible. The wound is then closed in layers using the suture material of choice.

Sometimes partial phalangectomies are performed with this technique to correct hammer toe deformities, if present.

Conclusion

1. Surgery on the rheumatoid foot should be done **as soon** as possible.
2. The results of this procedure vary from usually excellent to sometimes fair, depending on the status of the patients disease (how fast it is progressing).
3. The patient should have a **positive** motivation for the surgery.
4. The rheumatoid foot presents to the surgeons an interesting surgical challenge, sometimes frustrating, other times rewarding. Frustrating, because sometimes all that is accomplished is temporary relief of a progressive disease of unknown etiology; rewarding, because sometimes a patient's outlook on life will be totally changed once they can walk without pain.

M.P.J. Surgery

Modified Clayton Pan-Metatarsectomy

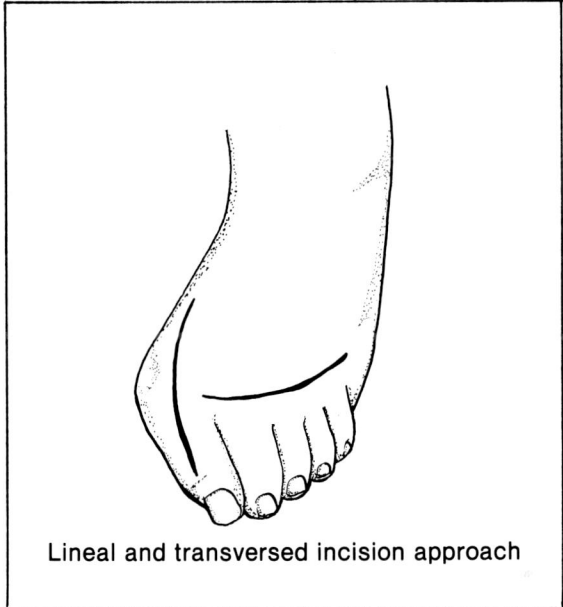

Lineal and transversed incision approach

Fig. 6-26A

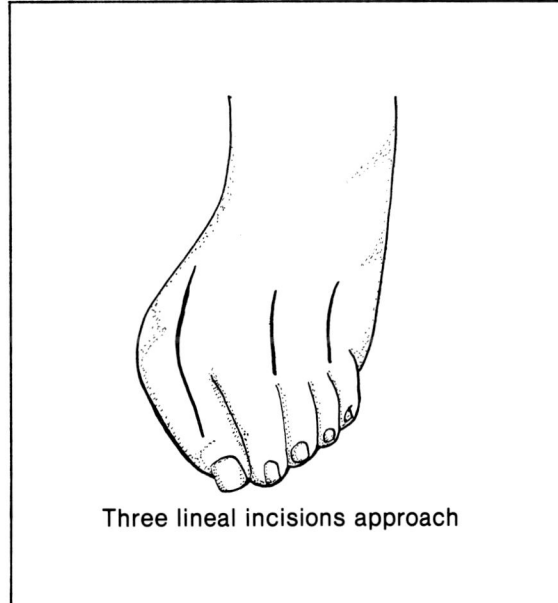

Three lineal incisions approach

Fig. 6-26B

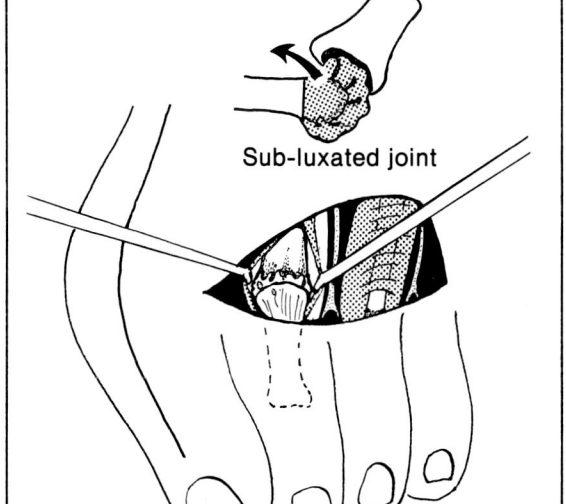

Sub-luxated joint

Fig. 6-26C

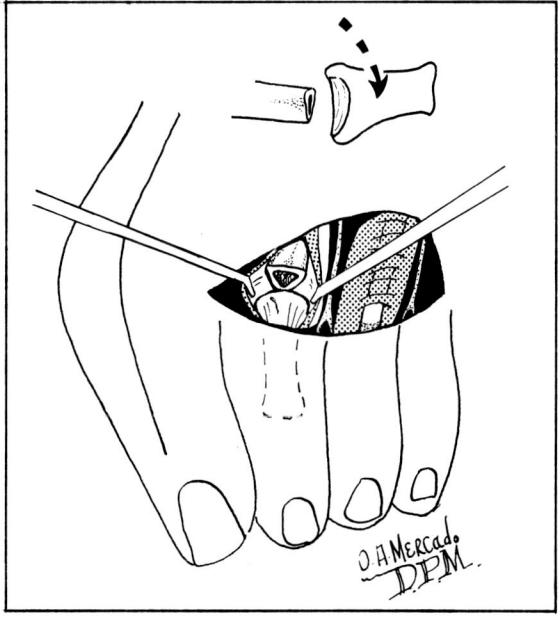

Fig. 6-26D

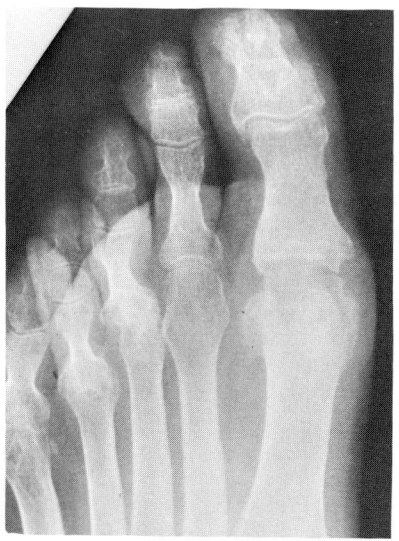 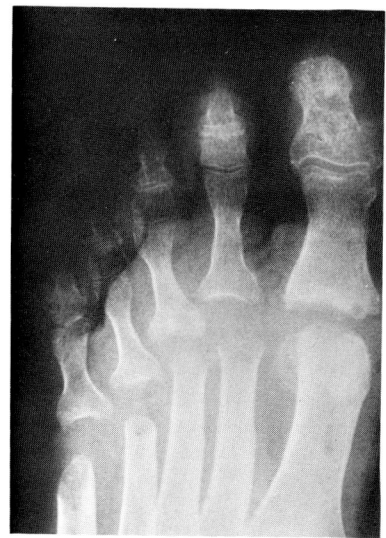

Fig. 6-26E. Pre-operative x-ray. Note R.A. destruction of metatarsal phalangeal joints.

Fig. 6-26F. Post-operative x-ray of pan-metatarsectomy.

Freiberg's Infraction

The **avascular necrosis** that is sometimes found on one of the inner (two, three, four) metatarsal heads was first described as an infraction by **A. H. Freiberg** in 1914. The etiology of this condition is linked to a vascular deficiency or perhaps an "... embolic obstruction of the epiphyseal end arteries by mildly virulent bacteria ..." (G. Auxen as quoted by Kelikian).

The condition is found in both females and males and can occur prior to or after epiphyseal closure. The involved head presents a flattened appearance and look quite **"abnormal"** in relationship to the other metatarsal heads (Figure 6-27 A). Clinically, the area over the affected metatarsal head appears swollen and painful (Figure 6-27 B).

Some authorities advocate the use of a surgical wooden shoe for the management of the younger (pre-epiphyseal closure) patients, surgery is the treatment of choice once the epiphysis has closed.

Technique

A lineal incision approximately 4.5 cm. long is made over the involved metatarsal head. The incision is deepened and the dorsal tendon are retracted to expose the metatarsal-phalangeal-joint capsule.

An incision is made over the joint and the capsule is carefully retracted. Sometimes an **osteophyte** is found lying over the metatarsal head (Figure 6-27 C and E). If one is found it is resected in-toto. The collateral ligaments are then cut and the deformed metatarsal head is exposed. A partial or complete metatarsal head resection is performed (Figure 6-27D).

The bone is rasped smooth, the capsule, deep and superficial tissues as well as the wound are closed with the suture material of choice. Healing is usually uneventful.

Conclusion

1. Pre-epiphyseal closure patients can be treated conservatively.
2. Surgery is indicated once the epyphysis has closed.
3. Surgery should consist of the partial or complete removal of the metatarsal head. If the base of the proximal phalanx is enlarged, the hypertrophic bone around the articular facet should be trimmed. If the base is so enlarged that it required resection, then Silastic® implant should be inserted to prevent undue shortening and deformity (accordion toe) (Figure 6-28 A-B-C-D).

Freiberg's Infraction

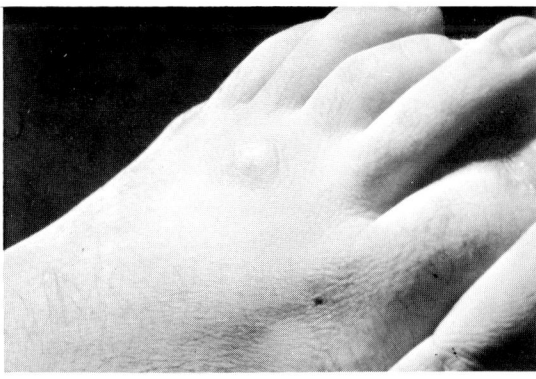

Fig. 6-27A. Freiberg's Infraction is seen on a 3rd. metatarsal head.

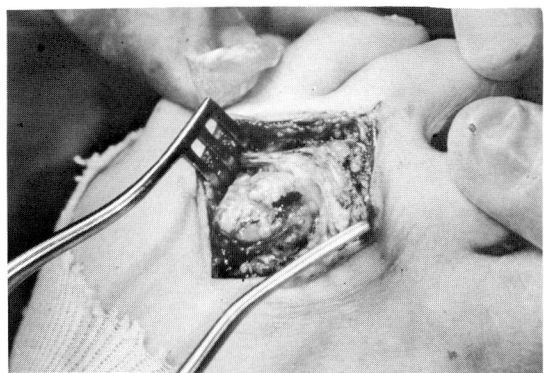

Fig. 6-27B. Large osteophyte is seen laying over the metatarsal head.

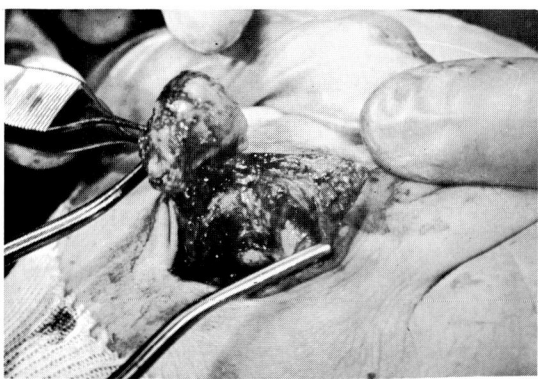

Fig. 6-27C. The metatarsal head is resected.

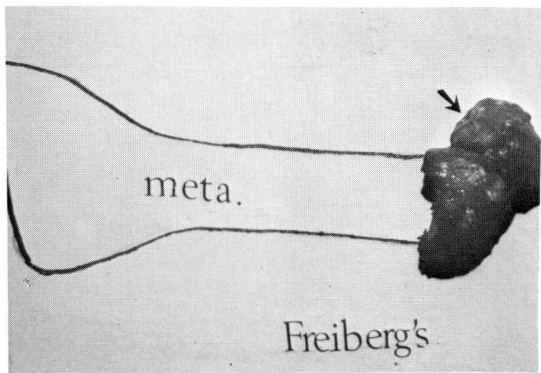

Fig. 6-27D. Drawing done at time of surgery shows actual bone removed. Arrow points to osteophyte overlaying metatarsal head.

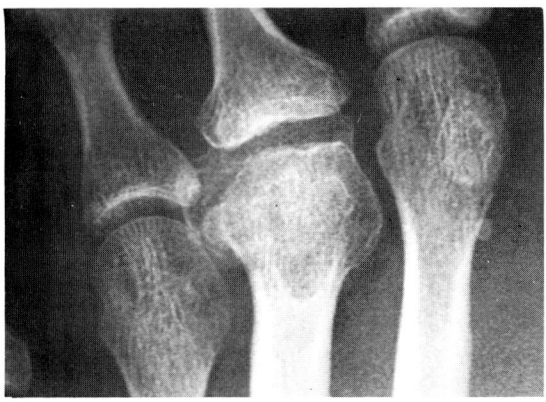 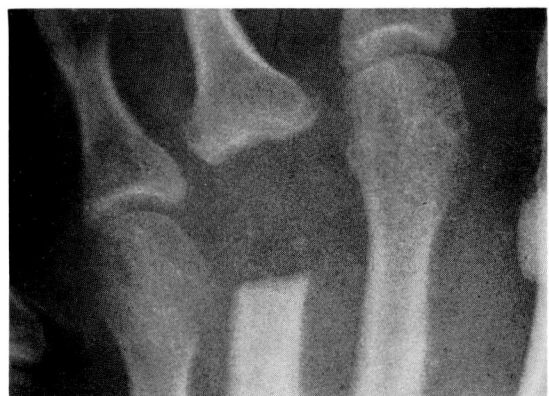

Fig. 6-27E. Pre-operative x-ray shows Freiberg's Infraction of the 3rd. metatarsal head.

Fig. 6-27F. Post-operative x-ray reveals resection of **diseased** bone.

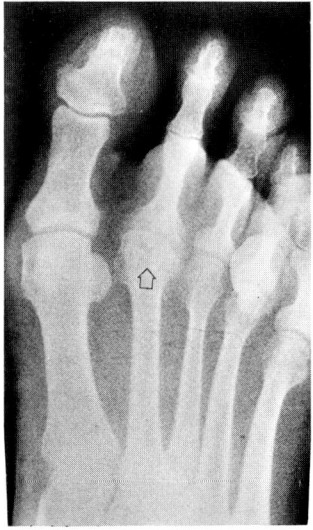 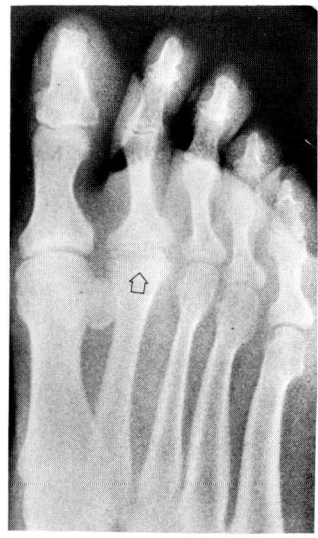

Fig. 6-28A. Pre-operative dorsal-plantar view. Freiberg's infraction of 2nd. metatarsal and base of proximal phalanx.

Fig. 6-28B. Pre-operative x-ray — oblique view.

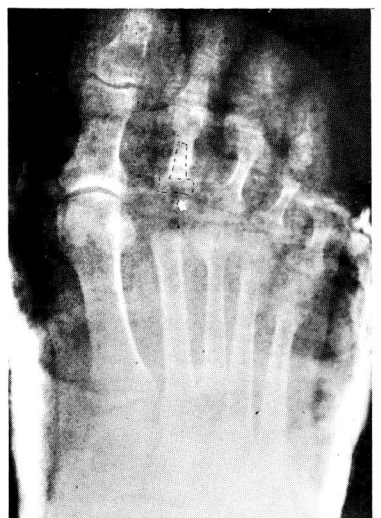 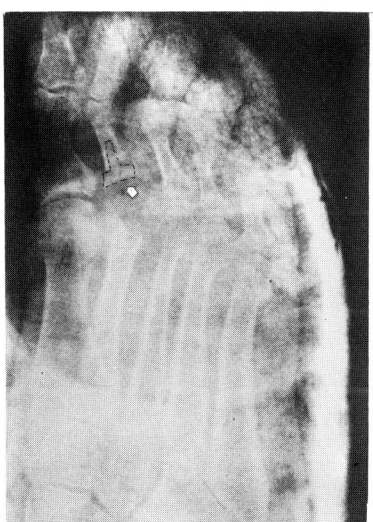

Fig. 6-28C. Post-operative dorsal-plantar view. Arrow points to Silastic® Implant used to replace the hyperthrophic phalangeal base.

Fig. 6-28D. Post-operative x-ray — oblique view. Arrow points to Silastic® Implant (dotted line).

Bone Tumor (Osteoma)

The incidence of bone tumors in the foot is rare. The occurrence of a **malignant bone tumor** is rarer still. In fact, in all of my years in practice I have only seen three patients with a malignant tumor in the foot. Incidentally, some researchers have become interested as to why there is such a **low** incidence of malignant tumors in the foot. Their findings and conclusion should prove interesting reading.

Technique

Obviously, bone tumors should be **excised** and studied by the pathologist. The surgeon's main role is to remove the tumor as carefully as possible while paying attention to the post-surgical function of the foot.

The osteoma seen in Fig. 6-29A, caused a great deal of pain to the patient and created a problem in shoe fitting — since any compression of the metatarsal heads caused extreme pain.

In our surgery (Fig. 6-29B), we were careful to preserve as much of the metatarsal shafts as possible, while removing the tumor.

The surgeon called to operate on a bone tumor should take the following precautions:

1. Be honest with the patient. Explain to them that while there is a **low** incidence of malignancies in the foot, it is important that the tumor be removed and studied microscopically.

2. Try to preserve as much as the anatomical structures as possible.

3. **When removing the tumor, take care to remodel the bone so that the least amount of function is impaired.**

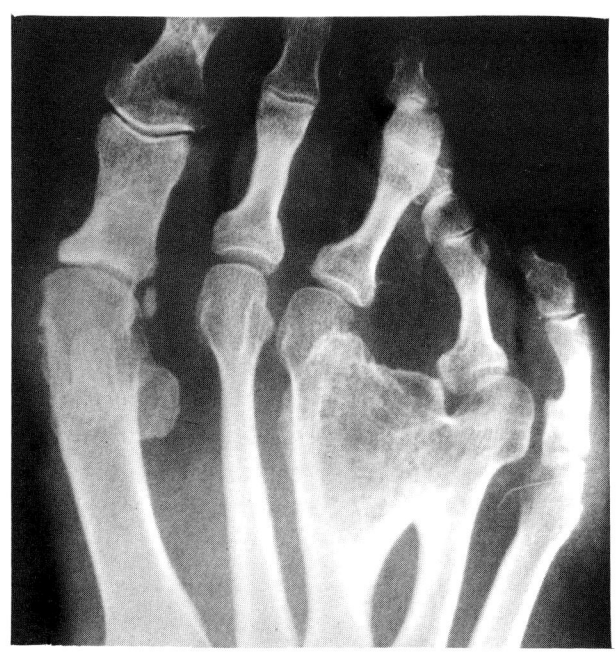

Fig. 6-29A. Pre-operative x-ray of metatarsal **osteoma.**

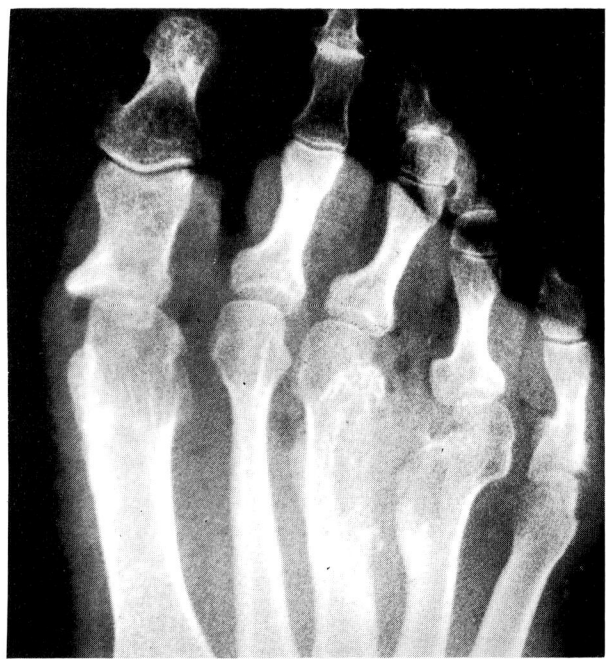

Fig. 6-29B. Post-operative x-ray. Note that metatarsal shafts were preserved. Also note decrease width of foot and improved articulation of the 4th. metatarsal phalangeal joint.

CHAPTER 7
HALLUX VALGUS SURGERY

I. **History of Hallux Valgus Surgery**

II. **Criteria for Hallux Valgus Surgery**

III. **Techniques for the Correction of Simple Hallux Valgus**
    A. Mini-Bunion Operation
    B. Basic (simple) bunionectomy

IB **Interphalangeal Hallux Valgus** — The Akin Operation

V. **Techniques for the Correction of Moderate Hallux Valgus**
    A. Basic Bunionectomy with Lateral Sesamoidectomy (McBride Type Bunionectomy)
    B. The Reverdin Operation
    C. Distal Crescentic Osteotomy

VI. **Techniques for the Correction of Severe Hallux Valgus (Metatarsus Primus Varus Techniques)**
    A. Closing Wedge Osteotomy
    B. Proximal Crescentic Osteotomy
    C. The Lapidus Operation

VII. **Techniques for Implant Surgery**
    A. Hemi-Implant
    B. Total Joint Implant

CHAPTER 7

HALLUX VALGUS SURGERY

History

Perhaps the first surgeon to report an operation for the correction of hallux valgus was **Hueter** in 1877, his technique consisted of the resection of the head of the first metatarsal. Since that time, the first metatarsal-phalangeal-joint has been surgically osteotomized, resected, wedged, rasped, pinned, and wired more often than any other joint in the human body (see Figure 7-1).

Some surgeons advocated the removal of the base of the proximal phalanx **(Olivecrona, Keller)**; some wanted to remove at least half of the phalanx **(Brauneck)**; others wanted to leave the base but remove the rest of the phalanx **(Girdlestone and Spooner)**; while still others were satisfied with nothing less than the removal of the entire phalanx **(Alsberg)**.

Medial ostectomy of the first metatarsal head **(M. Schede, Barker, Hohmann)** had its vogue, as well as the complete resection of the metatarsal head **(Mayo, R. Jones, Muhsam)**. Intricate wedge osteotomies for the metatarsal head **(Reverdin, Hawkins, Mitchell, Hedrick)**; and base of the metatarsal **(Loison-Balacescu, Juavara)**; and the first cuneiform **(Albrecht, Breuner, Lapidus)** were also in style.

Today, surprisingly as it may seem, the techniques most commonly used for the correction of hallux valgus are updated versions of those described forty, fifty, and even ninety years ago! Indeed, some of the thinking of the early surgeons was remarkable.

In the 1930's, the classical works of **Dudley Joy Morton** and **Frederick Wood-Jones,** gave the world the first truly scientific understanding of the evolution, anatomy and physiology of the human foot. Their writings along with those of men like **Silver, McBride, Lapidus,** and later on, **DuVries,** did much to illuminate the way towards the comprehension of the patho-mechanics and causation of bunions.

HALLUX VALGUS SURGERY—Historical Review

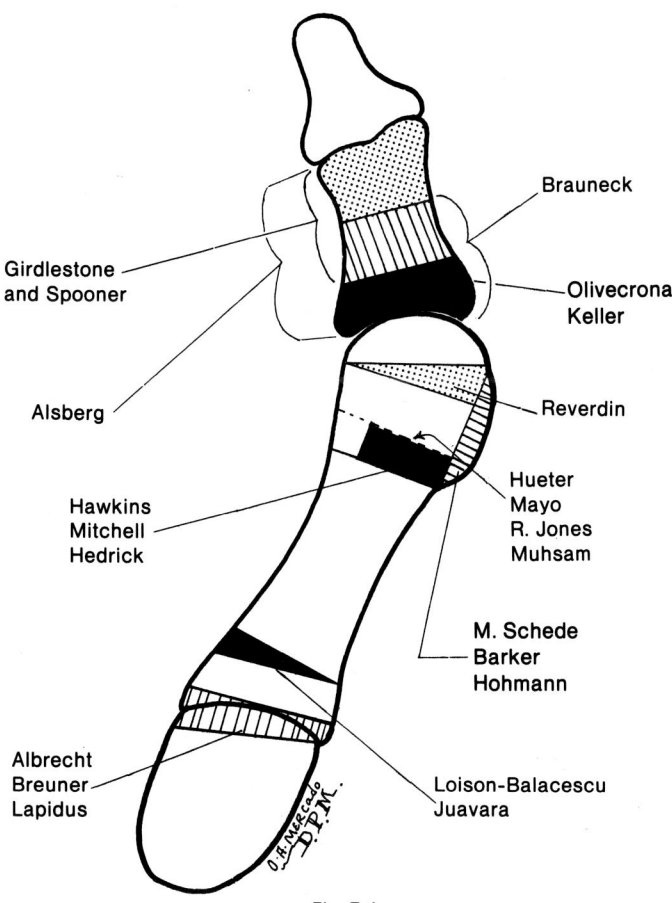

Fig. 7-1

Etiology of Hallux Valgus

Today the general consensus as to the etiology of hallux valgus is that it does have strong familial tendencies, perhaps, even a philogenetical predisposition. Lapidus explained that this philogenetical influence is observed in the human embryo where the varus of the first metatarsal is usually 32° in an eight-week human fetus and diminishes to 6°-8° in an adult. In other words, the hallux of the human embryo has **simian** features that are gradually lost with growth.

The simian features that Lapidus refers to are the shape of the first cuneiform-metatarsal-joint, which is more ball and socket like in the movable hallux of the lower primates and becomes flattened in higher primates — specially in man with the loss of mobility of the first metatarsal-ray. This philogenetical predisposing factor is then aggravated by modern foot gear, particularly in women, and leads to the formation of the hallux valgus.

Criteria for Hallux Valgus Surgery

Before we setup a criteria for hallux valgus surgery, it is essential that we review; (1) First metatarsal-phalangeal-joint shapes (2) First metatarsal-cuneiform-joint shapes, and (3) Some basic measurements.

First Metatarsal-Phalangeal-Joint Shapes

The variety of **shapes** found in the first metatarsal-phalangeal-joint can be readily appreciated just by looking at the x-rays of various patients. After looking at the x-rays for some time, it will become apparent that there is a certain pattern to the joint shapes. Basically, these joint shapes can be divided into three categories: **round, square,** and **deviated** (Figure 7-2).

The **round shaped** joint is the most common. In patients with hallux valgus occuring on a round shaped joint with little or no metatarsus primus varus, the surgical technique used will usually aim at the remodeling of the hypertrophic bone formed on the metatarsal head. If metatarsus varus is present, the intermetatarsal angle can be decreased with the appropriate technique (closing wedge, proximal crescentic, or Lapidus) so as to properly realign the metatarsal-phalangeal-joint.

The **square shaped** joint is the most stable type of joint, Hallux Valgus does not usually develop in these joints. What can develop is traumatic arthritis in the form of hallux rigidus.

The **deviated shaped** joint occurs more frequently than most surgeons realize. It can occur as a true anatomical variation of the metatarsal head or as a functional adaptation of the cartilage. I tend to believe that **cartilage adaptation** is the most common reason for a deviated shaped joint.

Deviated shaped joints presents one of the biggest pitfalls in hallux valgus surgery. Too often, the unwary surgeon attempts correction of hallux valgus on a deviated joint by mere remodeling of the hypertrophic bone. If the cartilage is not realigned by sub-capital (Reverdin) osteotomy, the end result will be a recurrent hallux valgus, or worse, a hallux varus.

When metatarsus primus varus is present in a deviated joint, then a double osteotomy (closing wedge at the metatarsal base and a Reverdin) will usually be required to correct the problem.

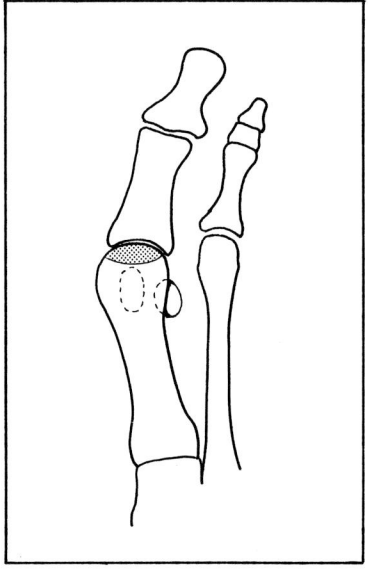
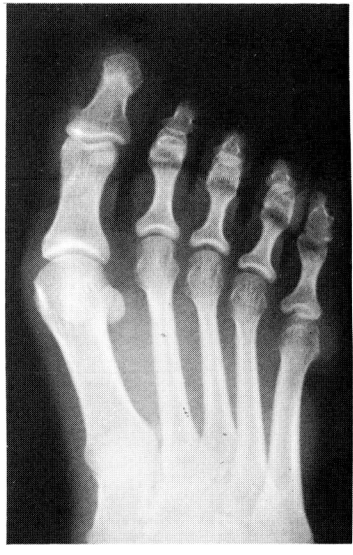

Fig. 7-2A. Round shaped joint.   *Fig. 7-2B.* X-ray of round shaped joint.

HALLUX VALGUS SURGERY

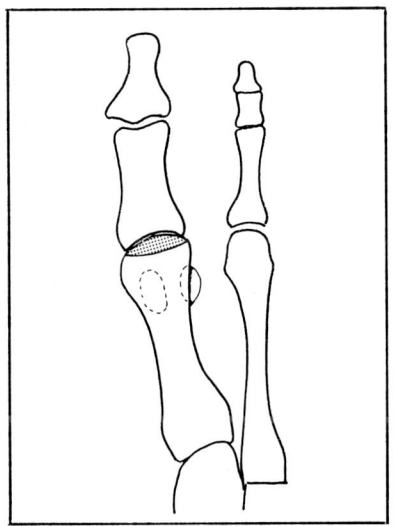

Fig. 7-2C. Square shaped joint.

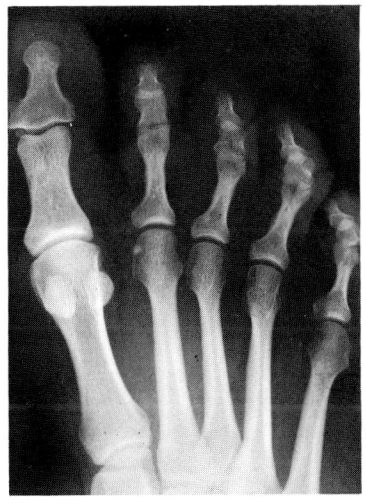

Fig. 7-2D. X-ray of squared shaped joint.

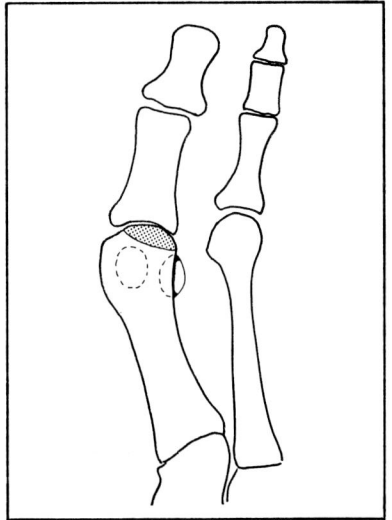

Fig. 7-2E. Deviated shaped joint.

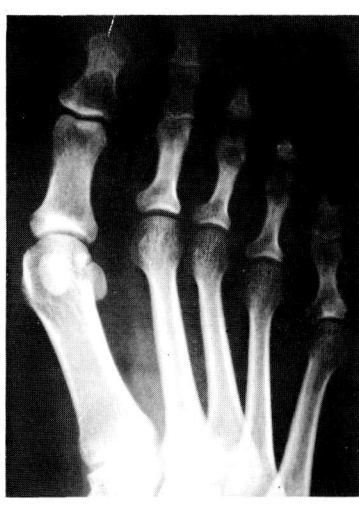

Fig. 7-2F. X-ray of deviated shaped joint.

First Metatarsal-Cuneiform-Joint Shapes

The first metatarsal-cuneiform-joint is **concavo-convex** in shape and it is one of the most important and interesting joints in the foot. The only other concavo-convex joint in the foot is the calcaneo-cuboidal joint. This concavo-convex shape allows adequate movement on a dorsal-plantar plane and some movement on a medial-lateral plane. The joint is larger than any of the other metatarsal base joints, usually achieving an average length of 3.5cm in the adult.

The shape of the first metatarsal-cuneiform-joint will determine the amount of **metatarsus primus varus** that can occur. A **stable joint,** such as the one shown in fig. 7-3A, will not allow the first metatarsal to migrate to a varus position. On the other hand, a **medially deviated joint,** as shown in fig. 7-3B, is predestined towards metatarsus primus varus.

Sometimes, the metatarsal-cuneiform-joint is stable but a metatarsus primus varus is present due to a **deviated shaft** (fig. 7-3C). The surgeon correcting a metatarsus primus varus must take into account the shape of the joint as well as the relative configuration of the shaft itself, in order to choose a satisfactory technique.

FIRST METATARSAL-CUNEIFORM-JOINT SHAPES

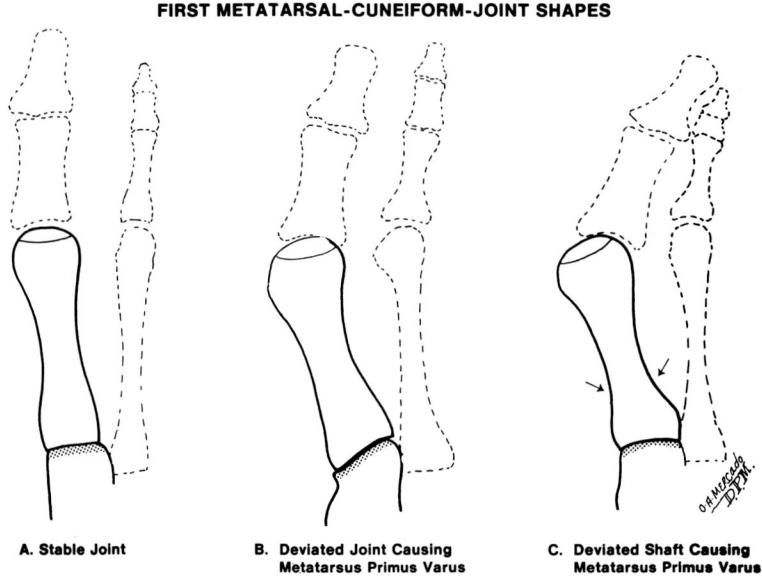

A. Stable Joint   B. Deviated Joint Causing Metatarsus Primus Varus   C. Deviated Shaft Causing Metatarsus Primus Varus

Fig. 7-3A, B and C

Basic Measurements

There are a number of measurements that have been advocated by various writers, including **Hardy, Clapman, Piggott, Sgarlato, Weil** and **Smith.** Of all the measurements advanced, the two most important are the intermetatarsal angle and the hallux abducto angle.

The **intermetatarsal angle** measures the amount of varus in the first metatarsal in relationship to the second metatarsal. Normally, this angle should be 6-8°. Anything **over 15°** is considered **metatarsus primus varus** (see Figure 7-3D).

HALLUX VALGUS SURGERY

This is not to say that when a patient exhibits an intermetatarsal angle of 15° or more, a closing wedge osteotomy is automatically performed. On the contrary, the I.M. angle is just a useful piece of information that, when placed in its proper perspective (I.E. its relationship to the metatarsal-cuneiform and metatarsal-phalangeal-joints; the severity of the deformity, the age and occupation of the patient, the length of the metatarsals, etc.) will guide the surgeon in selecting the proper technique.

The **hallux valgus angle** measures the amount of lateral deviation of the hallux as related to the metarsal head (see Figure 7-3E). There is normally an angle of 5°-20° present. When the angle is more than **30°**, it is not unusual to have some inward rotation (hallux abducto valgus) of the great toe.

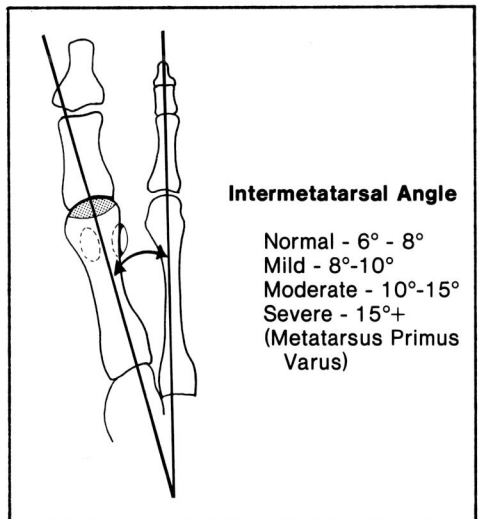

Intermetatarsal Angle

Normal - 6° - 8°
Mild - 8°-10°
Moderate - 10°-15°
Severe - 15°+
(Metatarsus Primus Varus)

Fig. 7-3D

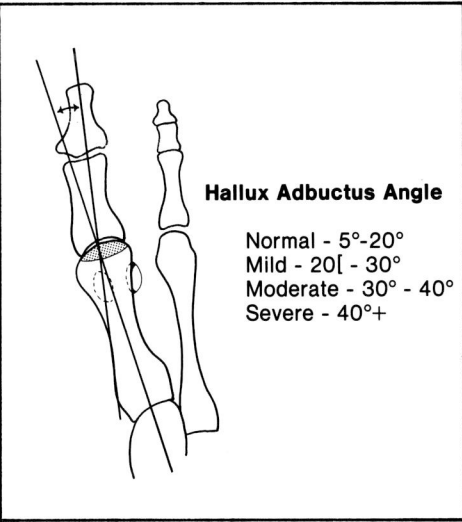

Hallux Adbuctus Angle

Normal - 5°-20°
Mild - 20[- 30°
Moderate - 30° - 40°
Severe - 40°+

Fig. 7-3E

Selecting the Proper Technique

Perhaps the most dangerous pitfall in hallux valgus surgery is the deplorable habit of performing the same procedure for every case. The surgeon who clings to this practice is courting failure in his work. **Henri DuVries** wrote, "The surgeon must study each individual case of hallux valgus, and apply a procedure or combination of procedures to that particular case." Kelikian put it another way, "The imaginative surgeon does not cling to any stereotyped procedure."

At Franklin Boulevard Community Hospital, we have developed a simple criteria to help the surgeon in choosing a technique, and at the same time avoid overutilization of any one procedure. This criteria has been in use for a good number of years and has worked consistently well.

We classify all hallux valgus into three categories;

1. Simple hallux valgus
2. Moderate hallux valgus
3. Acute hallux valgus (hallux abducto valgus)

CLASSIFICATION OF HALLUX VALGUS

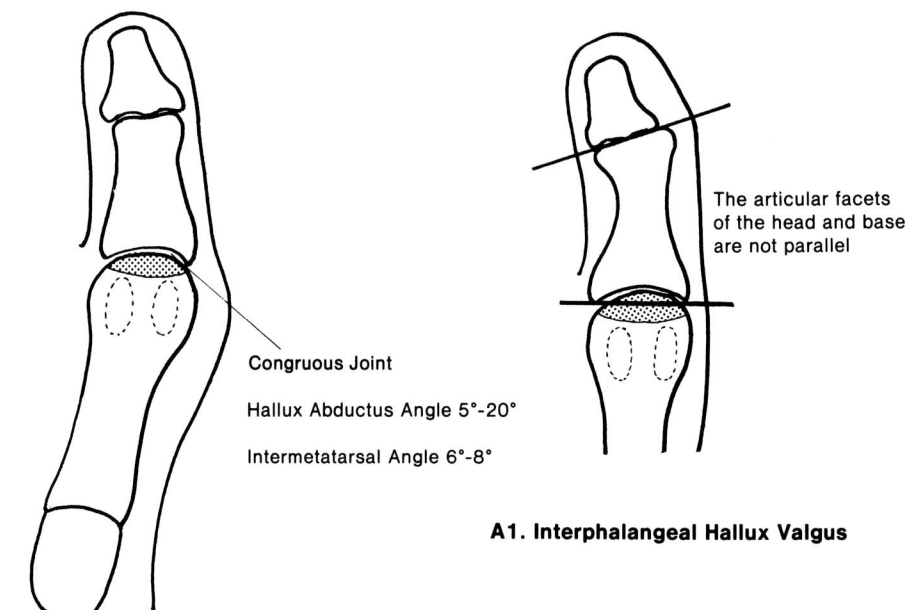

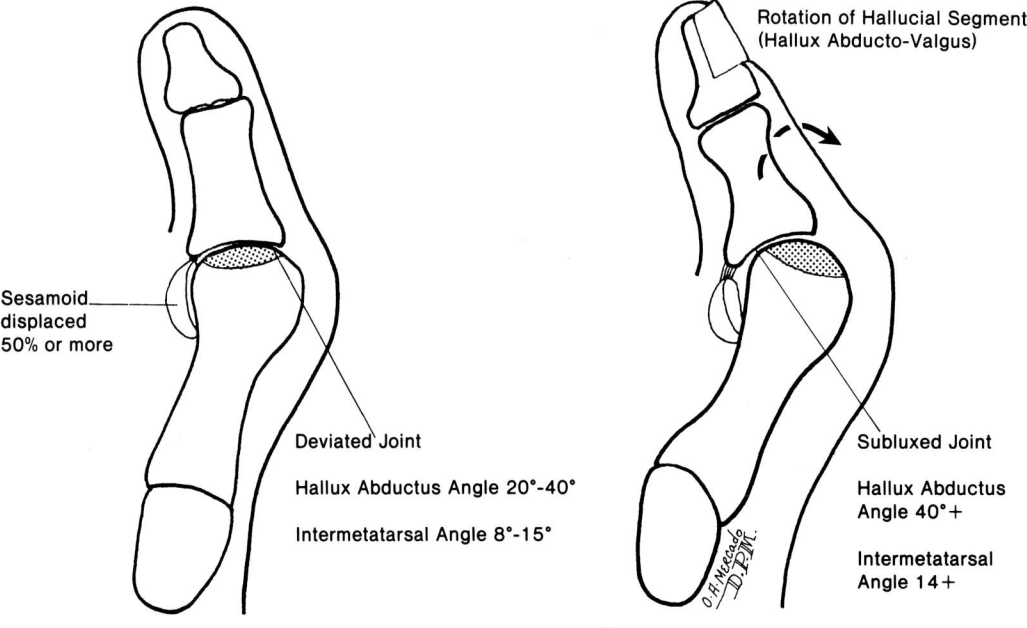

Fig. 7-4A, B and C

Simple Hallux Valgus

In category one, simple hallux valgus (fig. 7-4A), we find the following;
—A **hyperostosis** on the medial aspect of the metatarsal head.
The joint is **congrous.**
—The hallux abductus angle is usually normal (5°-20°).
—The intermetatarsal angle is **normal** (6°-8°).
—The lateral sesamoid **is not** deviated.

Under the classification of simple hallux valgus, we should include as a **subcategory,** interphalangeal hallux valgus

An **interphalangeal hallux valgus** (Fig. 7-4A1), is usually the result of an extremely long proximal phalanx. Upon close examination, it will be noted that the articular facets of the proximal phalangeal base and head are **not** parallel.

An interphalangeal hallux valgus can also occur in conjunction with moderate and acute hallux valgus. When it does, the hallucial deviation can be misleading during surgery. Often, the valgus of the hallux is corrected only to have the patient unhappy because her toe is "still crooked."

The surgeon should always keep in mind that interphalangeal hallux valgus occurs, as its name implies, at the interphalangeal joint, so that no amount of correction at the M.P.J. level is going to repair the deviation of the interphalangeal joint. The correction of interphalangeal hallux valgus requires specific osteotomy (**Akin** procedure).

Moderate Hallux Valgus

Category two, moderate hallux valgus (Figure 7-4B), consists of:
—A **hyperostosis** on the medial aspect of the metatarsal head.
—The joint is **deviated.**
—The hallux abductus angle is **mild** (20°-30°), to **moderate** (10°-15°).
—The lateral sesamoid is **usually** deviated 50% into the intermetatarsal space.

Acute Hallux Valgus (Hallux Abducto-Valgus)

Category three, acute hallux valgus (Fig. 7-4C) consists of:
—Marked hyperostosis and **osteophytic** changes around the medial, dorsal and sometimes lateral aspect of the metatarsal head.
—The joint is **subluxed.**
—The hallux abductus angle is **moderate** (30°-40°), to **severe** (40°+).
—The intermetatarsal angle is **14+.**
—Usually there is marked **rotation** of the hallucial segment (hallux abducto valgus).
—The lateral sesamoid is **totally** in the intermetatarsal space.

TECHNIQUES OF CHOICE

Simple Hallux Valgus

The underlying problem in simple hallux valgus is the hypertrophic bone on the medial aspect of the metatarsal head. Surgery aims at the reduction of the excessive bone.

The techniques of choice are:

(1) The Mini-Bunion operation
(2) Basic (simple) bunionectomy

Interphalangeal Hallux Valgus

The technique of choice for interphalangeal hallux valgus is the Akin operation.

Moderate Hallux Valgus

The techniques of choice for moderate hallux valgus are:

(1) Basic bunionectomy with lateral sesamoidectomy (McBride type bunionectomy)
(2) The Reverdin operation (if the articulate facet is laterally deviated)
(3) Distal crescentic osteotomy (used for a short ray with a laterally deviated articular facet)

Acute Hallux Valgus

There are a number of techniques that are used to correct acute hallux valgus. As a rule a combination of two or more techniques are used.

The **positional** (M.P.J.) deformity is corrected with either a simple bunionectomy, McBride type bunionectomy or Reverdin operation; the **metatarsus primus varus** is reduced by means of:

(1) Closing wedge osteotomy — used on average to long metatarsal rays, or deviated shafts (Fig. 7-3C).
(2) Crescentic osteotomy — used on short metatarsal rays.
(3) Lapidus Operation — used on deviated shaped first metatarsal-cuneiform joint (Fig. 7-3B).

The Mini-Bunion Operation

The Mini-Bunion operation is one of the techniques used for a simple hallux valgus. When used properly it will remove the hyperostosis (or bump) on the medial aspect of the metatarsal head and correct a mild amount of lateral hallucial deviation. The operation aims at:

1. Intracapsular reduction of the hyperostosis by **osteotripsy** (rasping).
2. Intracapsular release of the lateral contracted capsular ligament, adductor hallucis, and lateral head of flexor hallucis longus.

HALLUX VALGUS SURGERY

Technique

A transversed incision 1.5cm. in length is made immediately over the medial aspect of the first metatarsal-phalangeal-joint line. The incision is then deepened to the joint space **without** underscoring (fig. 7-5A).

A thumb and finger forceps is used to pick up the anterior margin of the incision where the skin, fatty layer, and capsular ligament are easily identifiable. A periosteal elevator is inserted in-between the joint capsule and bone. With great care, the capsule is freed (separated) from the hyperostosis (see Fig. 7-5B).

Once the capsule is freed, a rasp is introduced under the capsule and the exostosis is rasped smooth. The rasping is done **vigorously** and is easily guided by first feeling the exostosis through the skin and then rasping until the area feels smooth. The bone dust (or toothpaste like material) is removed with the outstrokes of the rasp (fig. 7-5C). After the exostosis is rasped smooth, the wound is thoroughly flushed with saline solution to insure complete removal of the bone dust.

The great toe is then pulled distally (fig. 7-5D) so as to increase the joint space. A number 15 blade is inserted into the joint space and the lateral capsule, the lateral half of the plantar capsule, the lateral head of flexor hallucis brevis and the adductor hallucis tendon are cut (fig. 7-5E). When cutting the plantar capsule and lateral head of flexor hallucis brevis, care is taken so as not to go **too far** medially as the flexor hallucis longus tendon lies in between and below the sesamoids. The cutting of the lateral head of flexor hallucis brevis will allow the lateral sesamoid to return (since the muscle will retract) to its normal position (fig. 7-5F).

The hallux is then held in the desired corrected position and the wound is closed with the suture material of choice. The wound is dressed with vaseline gauze and kling bandages reinforced with ½" strips of adhesive tape to maintain the correction.

The Mini-Bunion Operation

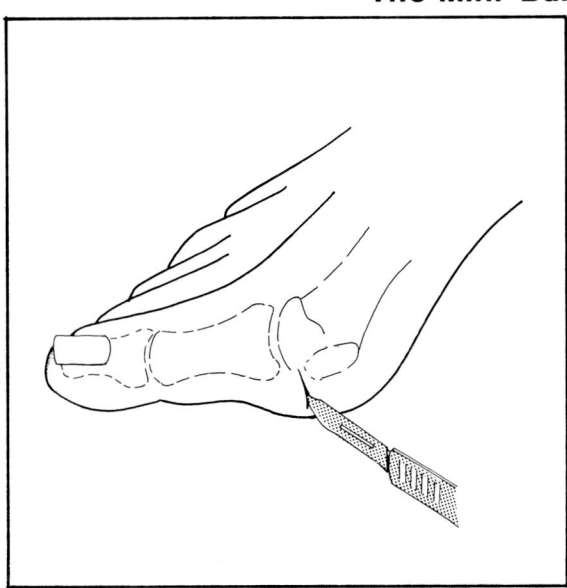

Fig. 7-5A. A small incision is made over the joint.

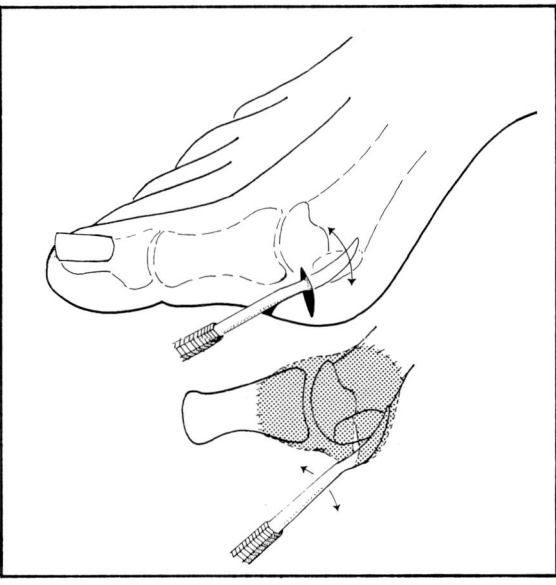

Fig. 7-5B. The capsule is carefully freed (separated) from the hyperostosis with a periosteal elevator.

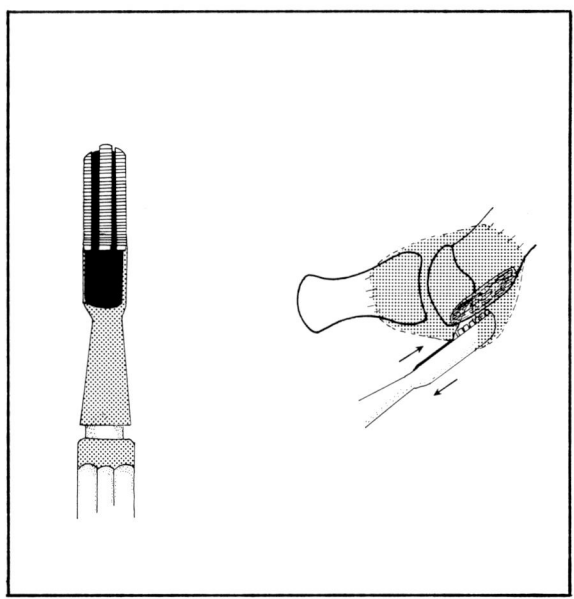

Fig. 7-5C. A rasp is introduced under the capsule. The exostosis is rasped smooth.

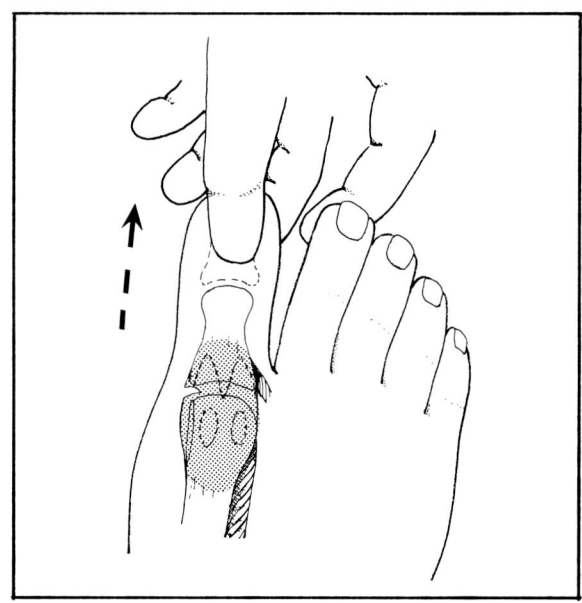

Fig. 7-5D. The hallux is then pulled distally so as to increased the joint space.

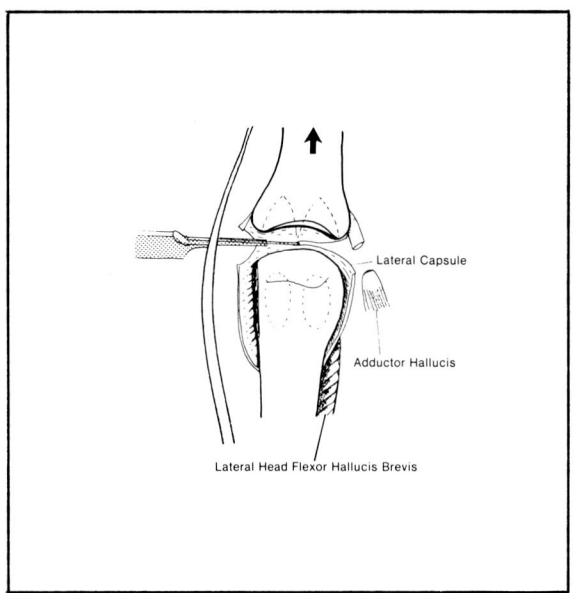

Fig. 7-5E. A No. 15 blade is inserted into the joint space and the lateral capsule, the lateral head of flexor Hallucis Brevis and adductor Hallucis tendon are cut.

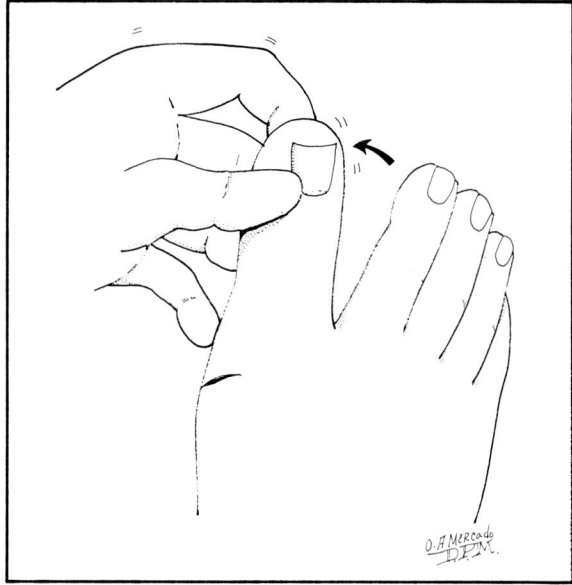

Fig. 7-5F. The hallux is held in the corrected position and the wound is closed with 5-0 nylon.

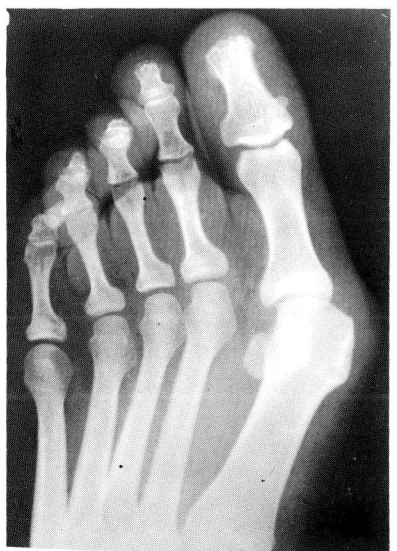 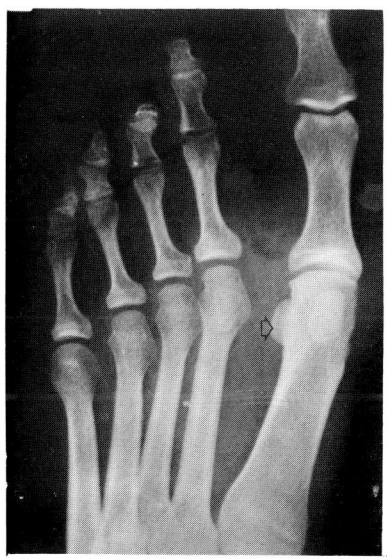

Fig. 7-5G. Pre-operative x-ray.

Fig. 7-5H. Post-operative x-ray. Note resection of medial exostosis — also note how lateral sesamoid has returned to a more normal position.

Conclusion

1. The Mini-Bunion operation will work consistently well when the underlying problem is a hyperostosis on the medial aspect of the metatarsal head with little or no lateral deviation of the hallux.
2. The incision must be placed immediately over the joint space (on the medial aspect) to allow access to the lateral joint capsule.
3. Power equipment can be used instead of a hand rasp.

THE BASIC (SIMPLE) BUNIONECTOMY

Our standard approach for the correction of a hallux valgus is as follows. First, we straighten the toe out as much as possible to ascertain a long straight incision. Our incision as you can see in figure 7-6A is medial to the tendon of extensor hallucis longus.

There is always a tendency to make incisions **too short.** When an incision is underscored and retracted, it loses almost 30% of its visualization capabilities. Also, and this may sound ridiculously fundamental, keep the blade at 90° to the skin, don't bevel the skin as this will lead to poor healing. **Remember** wound healing begins with the first incision.

The dotted line that we show in our drawing in figure 7-6A is used to extend our basic incision to expose the first metatarsal-cuneiform-joint. Note that the dotted line curves dorsally and lateralwards. We experimented with a number of approaches for exposing the first metatarsal-cuneiform-joint area and found that this incision gives us the **best exposure** when we perform a closing wedge, a crescentic osteotomy or a Lapidus technique.

Once we have made our incision, we then carefully deepen it and underscore around the medial aspect of the first metatarsal-phalangeal-joint taking care to preserve the **neurovascular bundle** that lies immediately underneath the skin. This bundle, which we can see in our telescopic view (figure 7-6B), contains a **nerve** (the medial dorsal cutaneous and end of the saphenous nerve); an **artery** (the medial digital branch of the first dorsal metatarsal artery) and a **vein,** which becomes continuous, proximally with the medial marginal vein.

Years ago when I was a resident in training, we never used to worry about the neurovascular bundle. This resulted in a great deal of numbness (parasthesia) post-operatively. Today, we are careful with our dissection and the patient who complains of post-operative parasthesia is rare indeed.

Lying proximal and lateral to the neurovascular bundle is the muscle belly of **abductor hallucis.** This muscle is the most medial of the first layer of the plantar muscles and it is a strong muscle. Actually, it is **90%** muscle belly and **10%** tendon. Some drawings show the abductor hallucis inserting into the medial aspect of the proximal phalanx as a long slender tendon. In reality, its insertion is by way of an **aponeurosis** which blends in with the medial capsule of the first metatarsal-phalangeal-joint.

In our drawings we can also see the very important **hood ligament.** The purpose of the hood ligament is to tack down the tendon of **extensor hallucis longus** and prevent bow-stringing. When we make our capsular incision, as we will see later, we try to preserve the hood ligament as much as possible.

Running parallel and medial to extensor hallucis longus is the so-called accessory slip of extensor hallucis longus which is often confused with a cutaneous nerve. In reality, this accessory slip is not only present almost **100%** of the time, but has a very definite capsular function and a most interesting name — it is called **extensor hallucis capsularis.**

A couple of years ago at the Illinois College of Podiatric Medicine, **Drs. Russel Tate** and **Randy Pachnik** dissected 100 cadavers and found the accessory slip of Extensor Hallucis Longus present 95 times.!

Their study showed that the tendon inserts into the joint capsule and functions by pulling the capusle away from the articulation during dorsi-flexion, thus preventing **impingement** of the capsule. If this sounds far-fetched, one only has to go to the knee to find the tendon of **articularis genu** performing the same function during extension of the knee. In our illustration (figure 7-6C), we can see a line drawing of our photograph. The tendon of extensor hallucis longus, the top tendon, is tacked down by the hood ligament and inserts into the distal phalanx. The tendon of extensor hallucis capsularis inserts into the joint capsule.

Function of Extensor Hallucis Capsularis

When extensor hallucis longus contracts, a couple of things happen. First, the hood ligament holds the tendon down so that it will not **bow-string.** Secondly, the extensor hallucis capsularis contracts, synergistically, pulling the capsule away from the joint line.

Because of its **important function,** we try to preserve extensor hallucis capsularis when we make our capsular incision during hallux valgus surgery. There are a number of capsular incisions which may be used, such as the Silver "V" Capsule and the Washington Monument Capsule — a long, slender V-shaped capsule with its apex directed distally. The one that is used the most frequently is the "L" shaped capsular incision (figure 7-6D).

Capsular Incision

The capsular incision is made in between the tendon of extensor hallucis longus and extensor hallucis capsularis and carried to the joint line. Incidentally, during actual surgery, what I tell the students to do in order to find the joint line is to pull the hallux back and forth a number of times. This causes **puckering** of the **joint capsule** making it easier to find the joint line. Once the incision is made to the joint line, the toe is pulled distally to increase the joint space and a second incision is made from plantar to dorsal.

In our illustration in figure 7-6E, we can see the plantar extension of the **L-shaped** capsular incision. We can also see the muscle of **Abductor Hallucis** and how it blends in, as we pointed out before, into the capsule, below this we can see the **medial head of Flexor Hallucis Brevis.**

Once we have our incision made, we carefully dissect the capsule from the metatarsal head without **tearing** or **injuring** it. **Capsular preservation** is a very important concern. In fact, there is an old adage in hallux valgus surgery that says; "the better the **capsular dissection** . . . the better **the correction."**

Getting a good capsule is no **accident.** In spite of the fact that some surgeons still insist that some capsules are **thin** while others are **thick.** If we are dealing with healthy individuals, all capsules are about the same thickness. Even if the capsule were **thin,** the method that we use for its dissection will guarantee a **viable capsule.**

Dissecting the Capsule

Here's how we do it . . . (figure 7-6F) once we have completed our L-shaped capsular incision, we begin our dissection on the dorsal aspect. The capsule and periosteum are dissected (actually peeled) from the dorsum of the metatarsal head. When we peel the capsule and periosteum, we find pin-points of bleeding on the bone. The periosteum sends tiny nutrient vessels into the **Volkman's canals** of the bone and when the capsule and periosteum are dissected away, it causes the pin-points of bleeding that we see.

Once we have dissected the **capsule** from the dorsal aspect of the metatarsal head, we pull the capsule **medialwards** and, with a number 15 blade turned so that the blade is facing up, we find the **Student Hole.**

Student Hole

The student hole is the space found in between the medial collateral ligament and the metatarsal head. By inserting the tip of the blade into the hole and cutting from plantar to dorsal we get a **consistently thick capsule.** It is important that we only use the tip of the blade and follow the contour of the metatarsal head.

In our illustration on figure 7-6G, we see an anterior view of the **student hole.** Notice that we are only using the tip of the blade to dissect the capsule away from the bone. If the blade is buried too deeply, there will be a great likelihood of tearing or, what we call "button-holing", the capsule. Incidentally, most of the **capsular button-holing** occurs at the level of the metatarsal anatomical neck where the shaft expands into the head. The surgeon buries his blade and forgets to follow the contour of the bone and before he knows it, he has a gaping **button-hole** in the capsule. Remember, to obtain a consistently **thick capsule,** first find the **student hole,** then use only the tip of the blade for dissection, and finally, follow the contour of the bone.

Now that we have our nice **thick capsule** dissected from the medial aspect of the metatarsal head, we start dissecting the dorsal lateral aspects (figure 7-6H). The toe is held slightly planti-flexed, as our illustration shows, we then **pull** the capsule dorsally, away from the bone. This will create a space in between the capsule and the articulate cartilage; the blade is inserted into this space and the capsule and periosteum are freed from distal to proximal.

Lateral Collateral Ligament

We are now ready to locate and cut the **lateral collateral ligament** (figure 7-6I). It is important to cut the lateral collateral ligament for two reasons. **First,** by cutting this ligament, we will be able to retract the metatarsal head outside the wound, thus allowing us **greater accessibility** when the ostectomy is performed.

Secondly, in hallux valgus, the lateral collateral ligament is contracted, thus helping to maintain the deformity.

We cut the lateral collateral ligament in the following manner. The **capsule is retracted** lateralwards and dorsally, as it is shown in our top illustration (figure 7-6I), using the sharp end of a **Senn retractor.** The **blunt end** of another Senn retractor is placed around the anatomical neck of the metatarsal and pulled medialwards. The surgeon will then pull the toe distally and the **lateral collateral ligament** will be readily seen. Remember, that in the metatarsal-phalangeal-joints, the collateral ligaments are inside the capsule.

A number 15 blade is then inserted in between the collateral ligament and the bone, and then the ligament is cut from **plantar to dorsal** as is shown in our lower illustration (figure 7-6I). The collateral ligament is extremely thick and wide, so that it is important to cut all of the ligament from its attachment to the metatarsal head. Once this is done, a Seeburger retractor is used to expose the metatarsal head.

Cartilage

With the metatarsal head exposed (figure 7-6J), the surgeon can **note** the **color** of the **cartilage** which is a good indication of its viability. **Cartilage** has **no circulation** of its own, it depends on the **subchondral bone** for its **nutrition.** Also, cartilage **needs** activity to survive. The surgeon's aim should be to preserve as much of the **cartilage** as possible and to realign the joint in such a fashion so that it will function as **normally** as **possible.**

Crista

The illustration on figure 7-6K, shows how the osteotomy is placed so as to preserve the articulate fascet, the **crista** for the **medial sesamoid.** Notice how we are taking very **little bone** from the plantar aspect.

If too much bone is removed and the **crista** is destroyed, the joint will be unstable and there will be a great likelihood that the medial sesamoid will become displaced. This in turn, leads to an excessive pull from the medial head of flexor hallucis brevis and the tendon of abductor hallucis resulting in a hallux varus.

HALLUX VALGUS SURGERY

Ostectomy

In figure 7-6L, we see a dorsal view of the **hyperostosis** being removed. Notice how the osteotome is aimed so that it removes the hyperostosis even with the metatarsal shaft.

An important point to remember here is that on an **anterior** plane, the osteotome is aimed so as to remove more bone from the dorsal-medial aspect and less from the plantar-medial aspect, thus preserving the crista, the articulating facet for the medial sesamoid. From a **dorsal plane,** the hyperostosis is removed even with the metatarsal shaft. The hyperostotic ridge which is left on the dorsal-medial aspect of the head after the removal of the medial hyperostosis, is resected with an osteotome (figure 7-6M).

The hyperostosis on the dorsal (and sometimes lateral) aspect of the head is resected in order to increase dorsiflexion (figure 7-6N). The surgeon aims to create a **normal looking** and **functioning** metatarsal head. The plantar medial ridge is resected with bone forceps (figure 7-6O).

The bone is then rasped smooth. Care is taken not to injure the articulate cartilage (figure 7-6P). Bone has different **consistency** depending on the age and health of the patient. As an example, Osteoporotic bone is very fragile and improper technique in rasping can cause grooving and excessive removal of bone. On the other hand, normal bone can stand rigorous rasping. Any cartilogenous ridging left can be easily removed (trimmed) with a number 15 blade without injuring the articulate fascet (figure 7-6Q).

The actual amount of **bone removed** is shown by the dotted line in figure 7-6R. Note that the hyperostosis was removed on the medial, dorsal and lateral aspect of the head. Note also, that the **crista** was left intact, thus preserving the articulate fascet for the medial sesamoid.

The metatarsal-phalangeal-joint is rearticulated and the joint capsule is closed with 2-0 Dexon. While the joint capsule is being sutured, the toe is held in the corrected position.

We start by closing the proximal end of the capsular incision first (figure 7-6S). The distal (plantar) end of the L shaped capsule is sutured as shown in our telescope view in figure 7-6S. Sometimes a small portion of the capsule has to be resected from the distal end to insure a tight capsular closure.

The important points to remember during any hallux valgus capsular closures are:

1. If the **proper** technique has **not** been performed, then no amount of over correction or splinting will correct the hallux valgus deformity.
2. **Overcorrection** of the capsule will result in an improperly functioning joint and can lead to a **hallux varus.** Once the capsule is sutured, the first metatarsal-phalangeal-joint will move through a good range of motion. Also, when the foot is loaded, the toe will remain in its corrected position. The deep and superficial fascias are then closed with 4-0 Dexon. The skin is then closed with the suture material of choice.

Precautions

The surgeon should always remember that the basic (simple) bunionectomy will **only** correct a simple hallux valgus. It **will not** correct a moderate or severe (acute) hallux valgus, no matter how much capsular overcorrection or hallucial splinting is done; in such cases the surgeon should use the appropriate technique indicated as outlined in this chapter.

The Basic (Simple) Bunionectomy

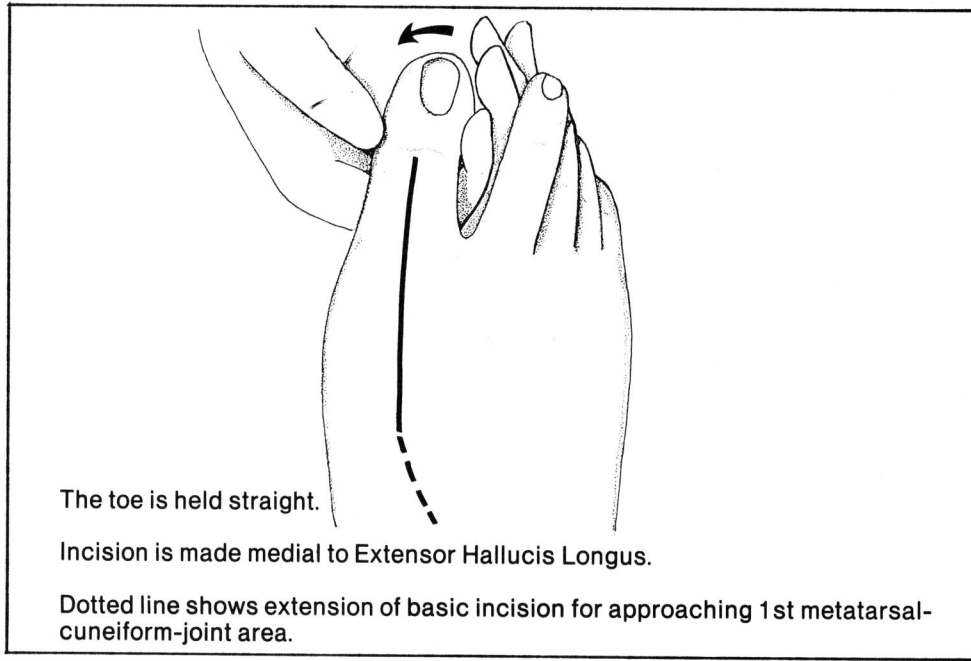

The toe is held straight.

Incision is made medial to Extensor Hallucis Longus.

Dotted line shows extension of basic incision for approaching 1st metatarsal-cuneiform-joint area.

Fig. 7-6A

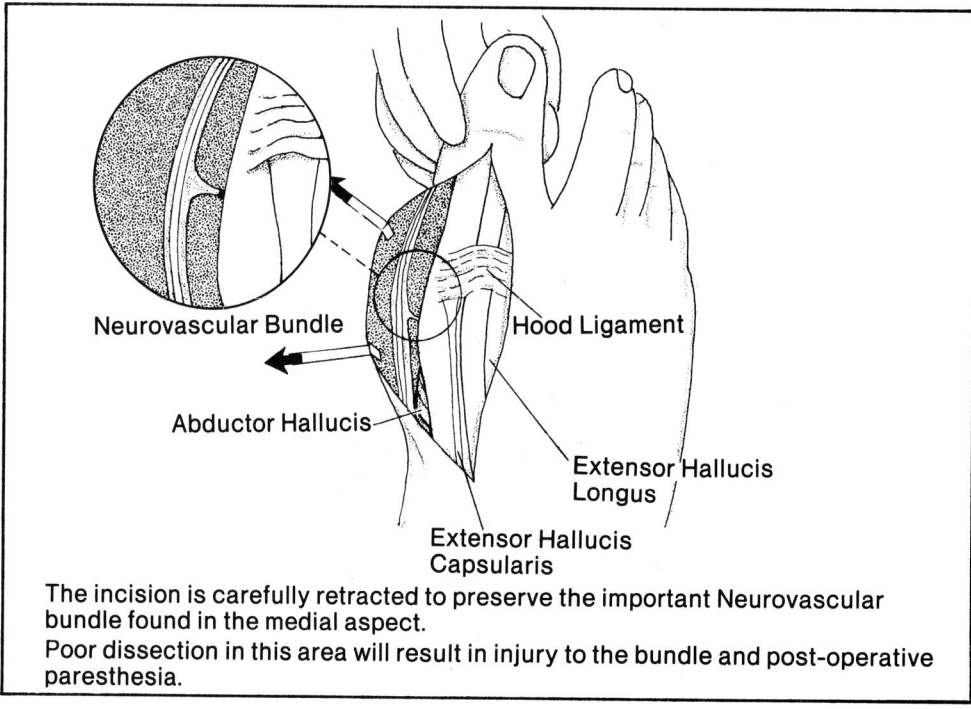

The incision is carefully retracted to preserve the important Neurovascular bundle found in the medial aspect.
Poor dissection in this area will result in injury to the bundle and post-operative paresthesia.

Fig. 7-6B

HALLUX VALGUS SURGERY

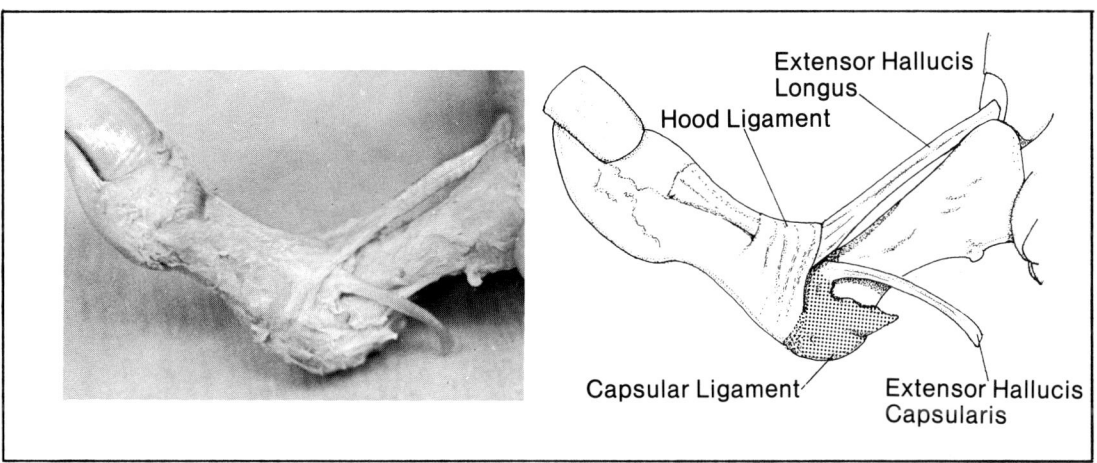

Fig. 7-6C

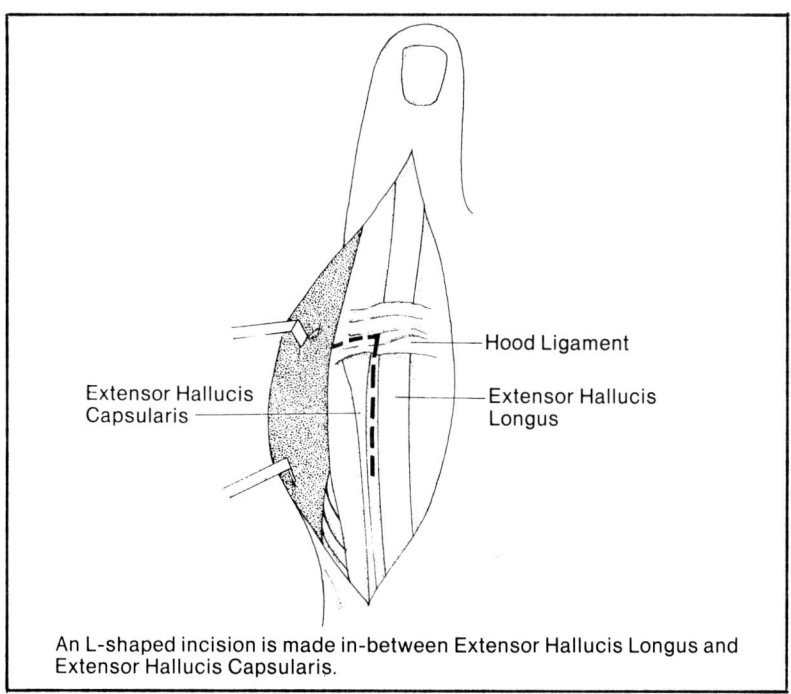

An L-shaped incision is made in-between Extensor Hallucis Longus and Extensor Hallucis Capsularis.

Fig. 7-6D

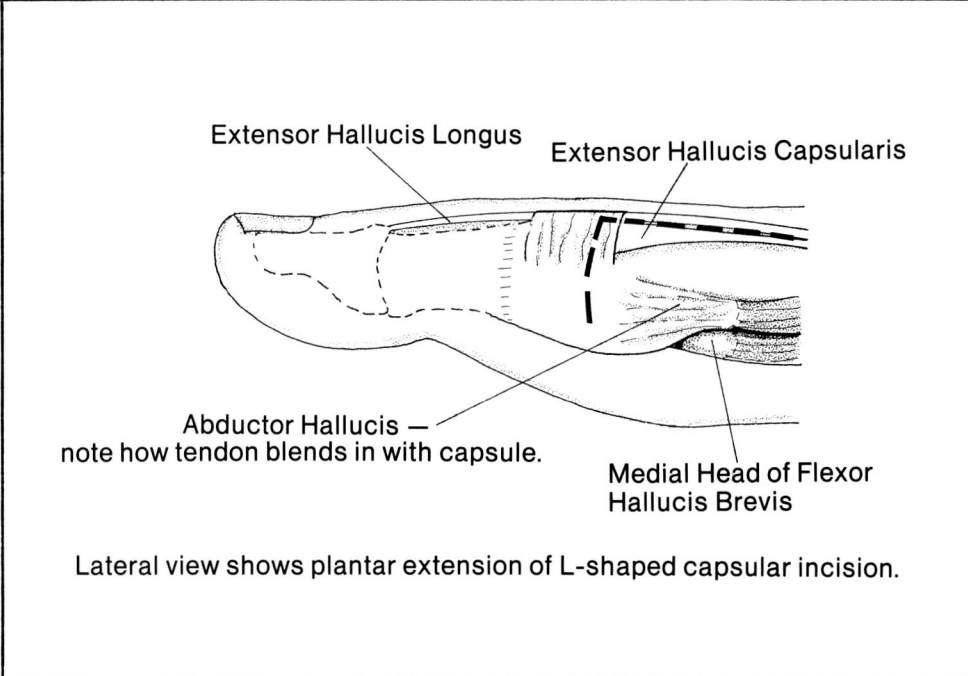

Fig. 7-6E

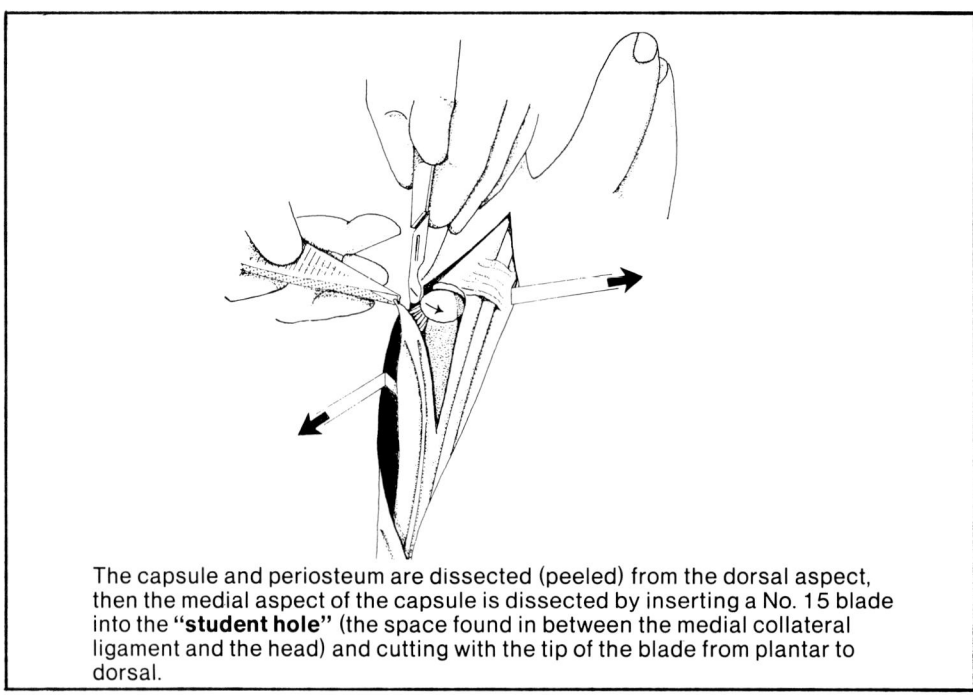

Fig. 7-6F

HALLUX VALGUS SURGERY

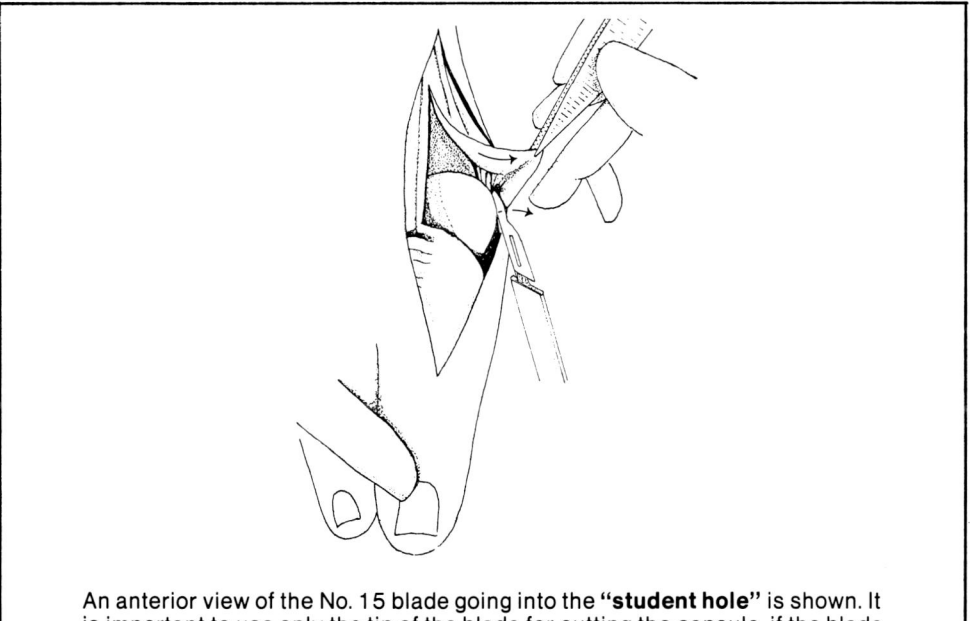

An anterior view of the No. 15 blade going into the **"student hole"** is shown. It is important to use only the tip of the blade for cutting the capsule, if the blade is buried there will be a great likelihood of **"button-holing"** the capsule.

Fig. 7-6G

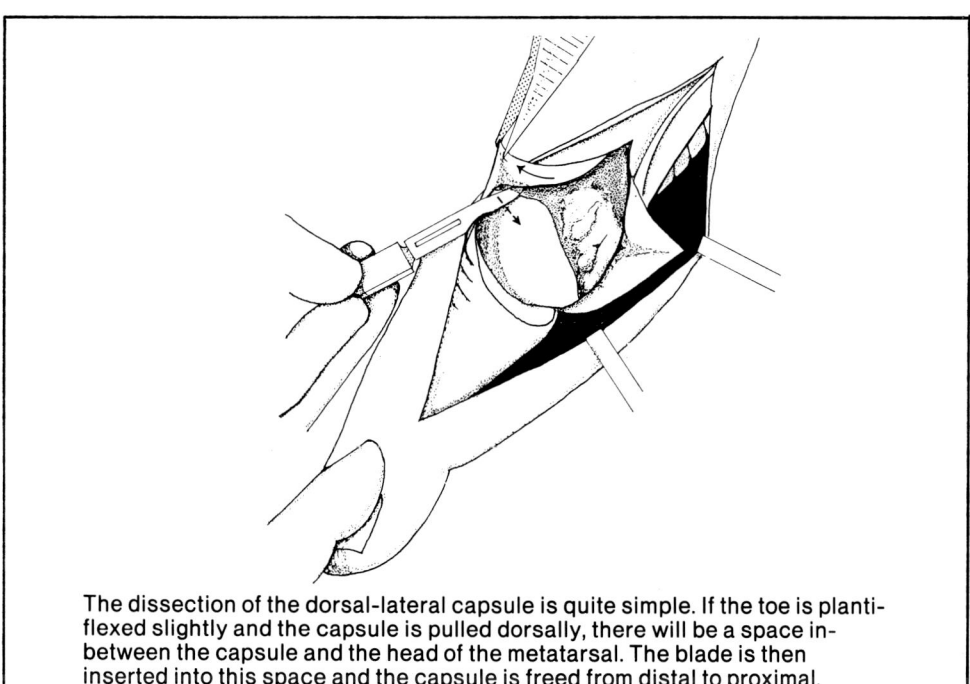

The dissection of the dorsal-lateral capsule is quite simple. If the toe is planti-flexed slightly and the capsule is pulled dorsally, there will be a space in-between the capsule and the head of the metatarsal. The blade is then inserted into this space and the capsule is freed from distal to proximal.

Fig. 7-6H

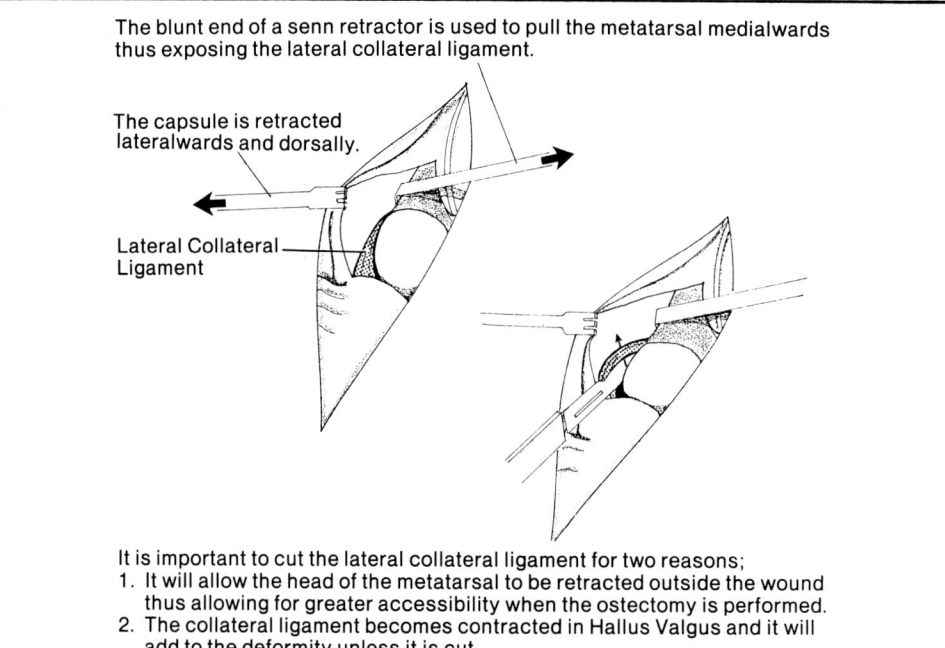

Fig. 7-6I

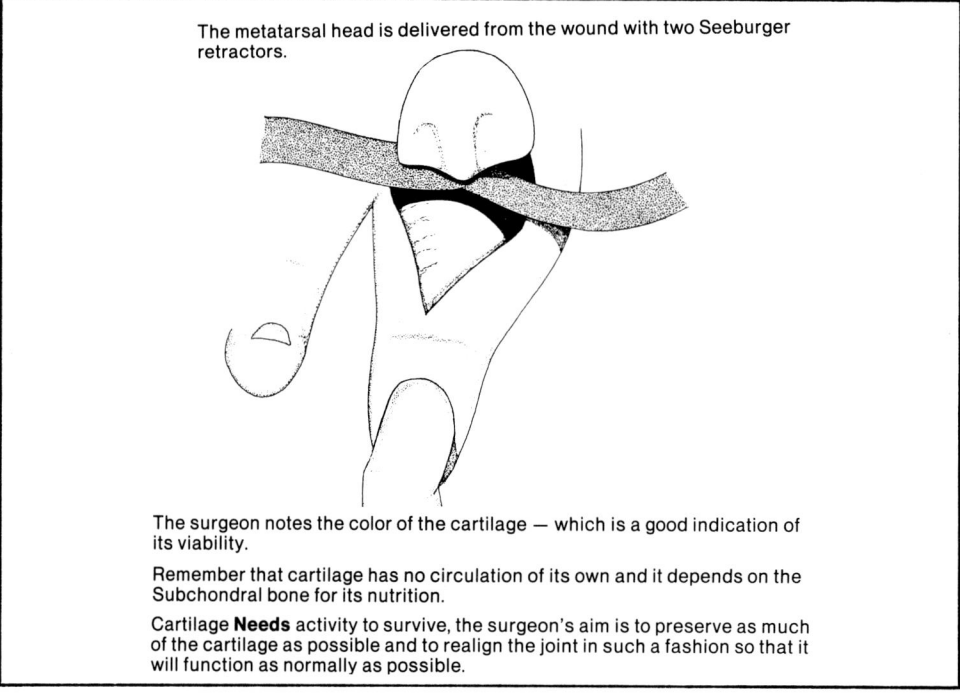

Fig. 7-6J

HALLUX VALGUS SURGERY

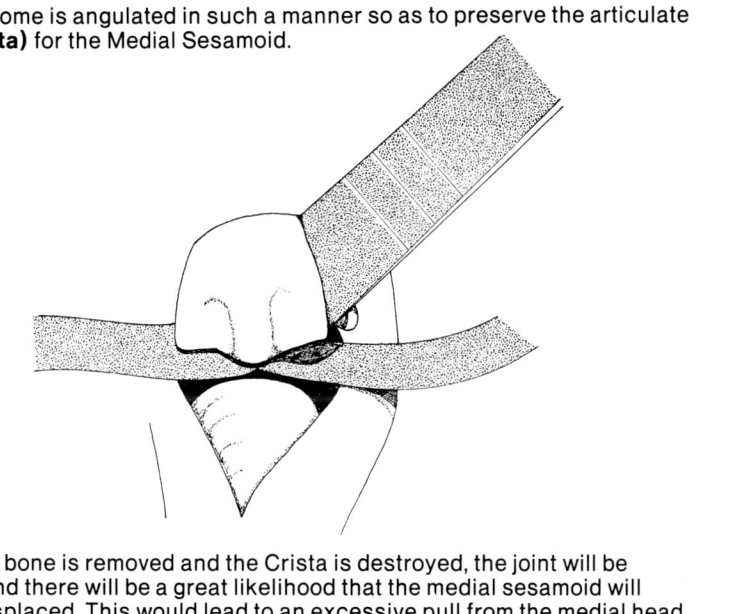

The Osteotome is angulated in such a manner so as to preserve the articulate facet **(Crista)** for the Medial Sesamoid.

If too much bone is removed and the Crista is destroyed, the joint will be unstable and there will be a great likelihood that the medial sesamoid will become displaced. This would lead to an excessive pull from the medial head of Flexor Hallucis Brevis and Abductor Hallucis resulting in a **Hallux Varus.**

Fig. 7-6K

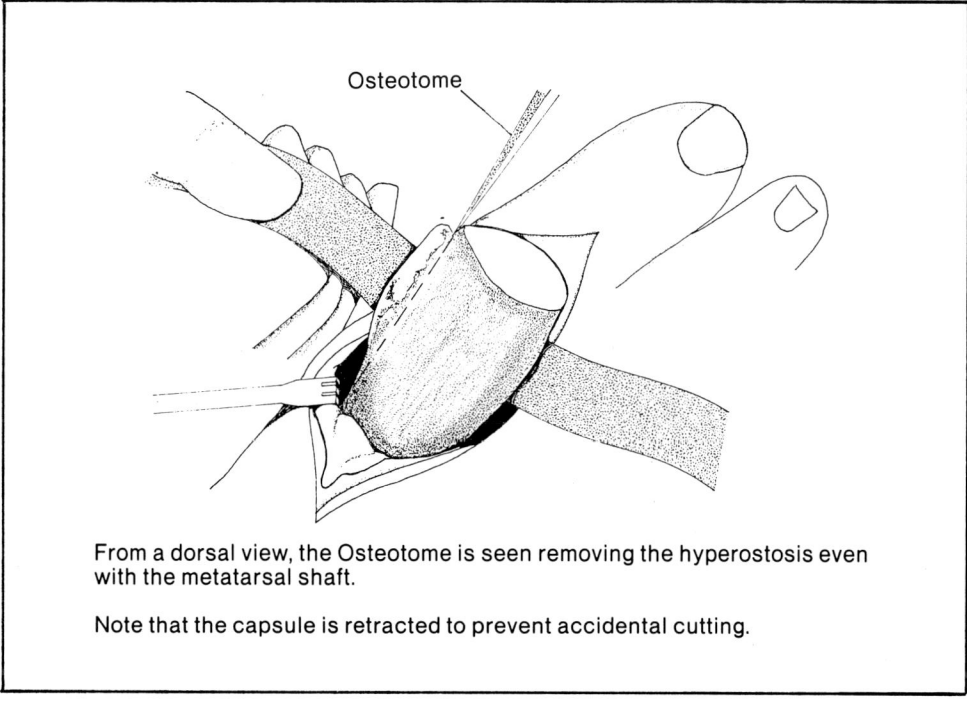

From a dorsal view, the Osteotome is seen removing the hyperostosis even with the metatarsal shaft.

Note that the capsule is retracted to prevent accidental cutting.

Fig. 7-6L

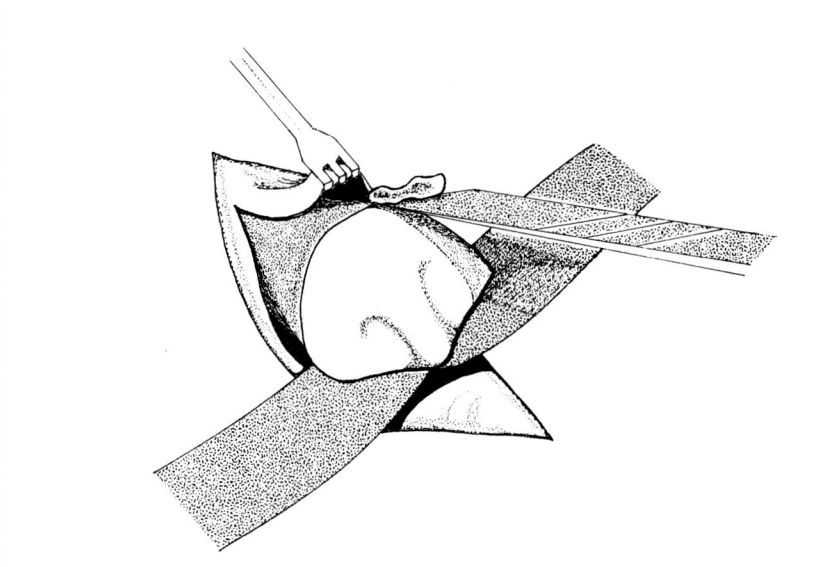

The hyperostotic ridge on the dorsal-medial aspect of the head is resected.

Fig. 7-6M

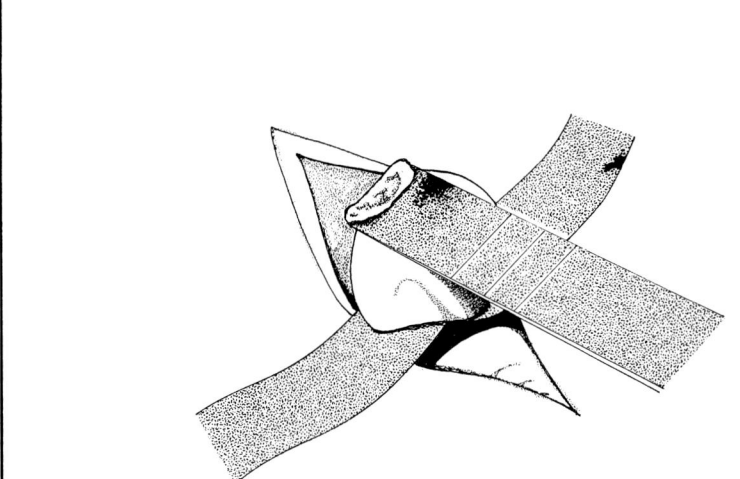

The hyperostosis on the dorsal (and sometimes the lateral) aspect of the head is also resected.

The surgeon aims to create a **normal** looking and functioning metatarsal head.

Fig. 7-6N

HALLUX VALGUS SURGERY

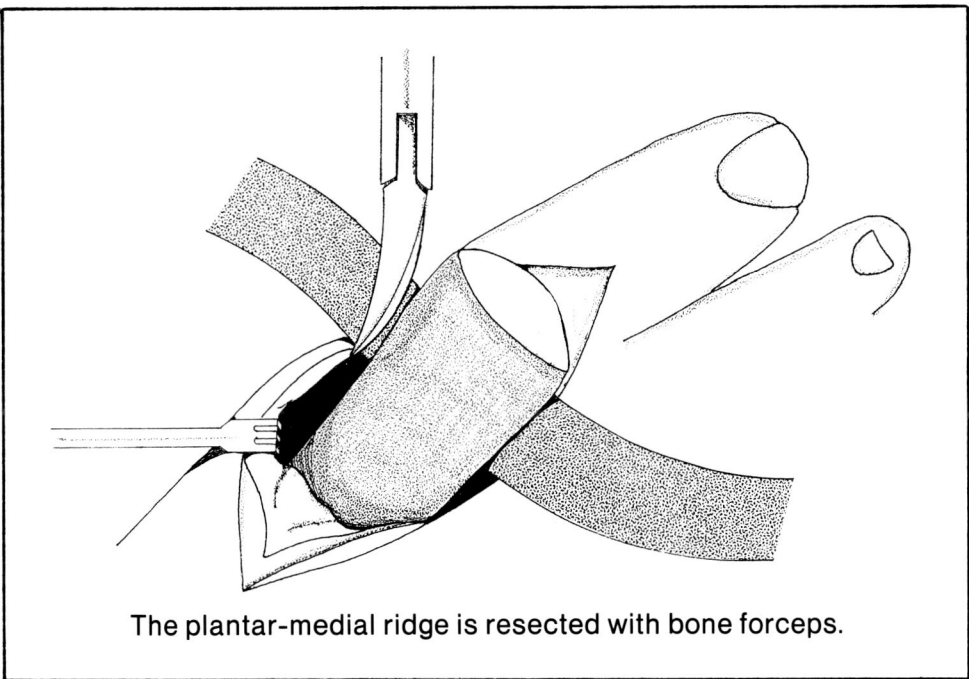

The plantar-medial ridge is resected with bone forceps.

Fig. 7-6O

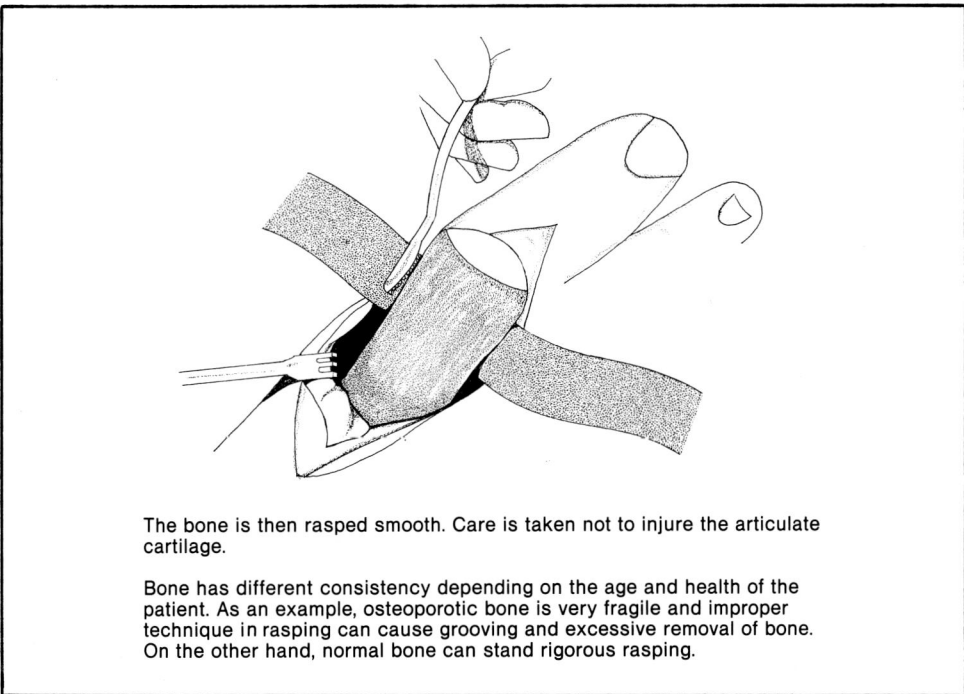

The bone is then rasped smooth. Care is taken not to injure the articulate cartilage.

Bone has different consistency depending on the age and health of the patient. As an example, osteoporotic bone is very fragile and improper technique in rasping can cause grooving and excessive removal of bone. On the other hand, normal bone can stand rigorous rasping.

Fig. 7-6P

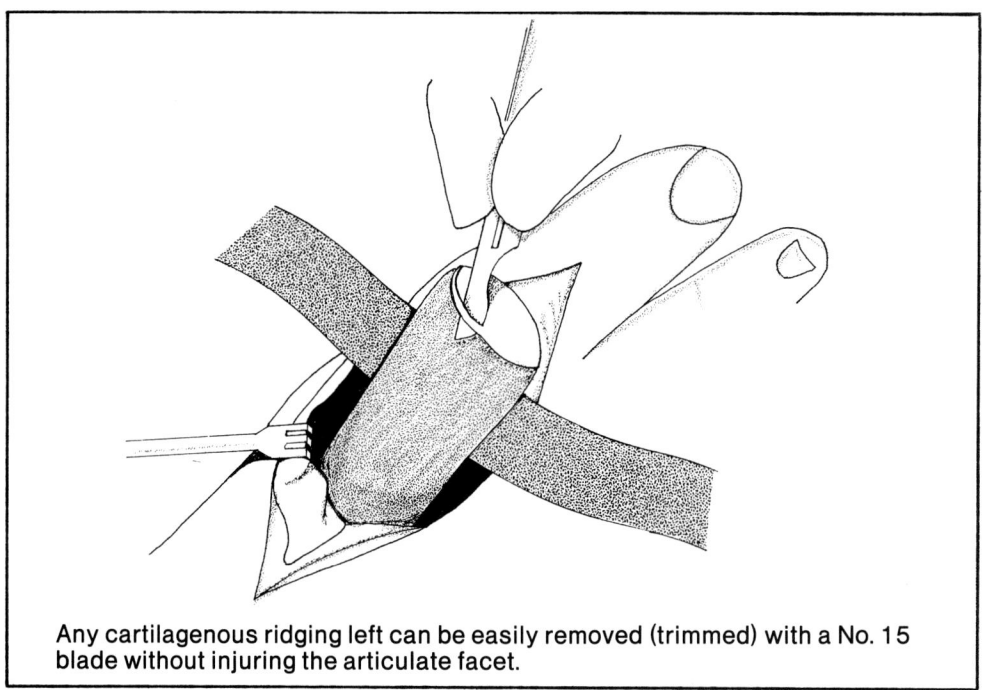

Any cartilagenous ridging left can be easily removed (trimmed) with a No. 15 blade without injuring the articulate facet.

Fig. 7-6Q

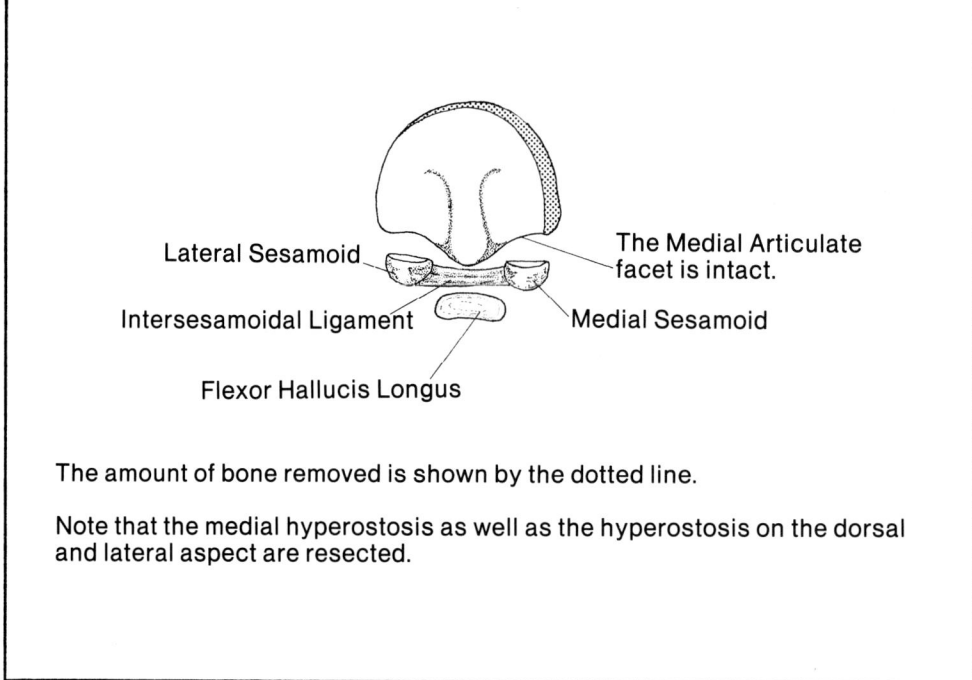

Fig. 7-6R

HALLUX VALGUS SURGERY

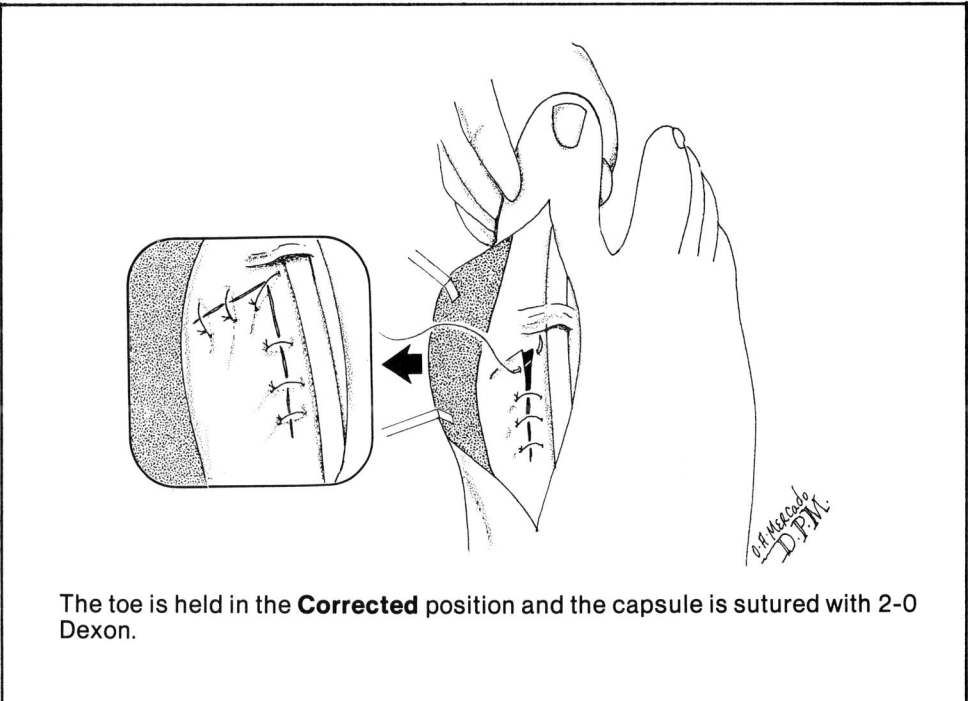

The toe is held in the **Corrected** position and the capsule is sutured with 2-0 Dexon.

Fig. 7-6S

The Akin Operation

The best technique for the correction of an interphalangeal hallux valgus is the operation described by **O.F. Akin** in 1925. Essentially, the Akin operation consists of a wedge ostectomy on the phalangeal shaft to realign the articulate facet of the head and base of the proximal phalanx.

The Akin operation can be performed as an independent procedure or in conjunction with hallux valgus surgery.

Technique

If the Akin operation is to be performed in conjunction with hallux valgus surgery, the bunionectomy is performed first.

When the Akin operation is performed as an independent procedure, it is done as follows:

A lineal incision is made immediately over the first metatarsal-phalangeal-joint extending distally to the head of the proximal phalanx. The incision is deepened and carefully retracted. The tendon of extensor hallucis longus is underscored and retracted laterally so as to expose the capsule.

A lineal incision is made and the capsule and periosteum over the shaft of the phalanx are carefully underscored and retracted. Two cuts forming a wedge are made on the shaft.

The **first** (proximal) cut is made parallel to the articulate fascet of the phalangeal base. It is important to have enough bone between the osteotomy line and the joint to insure the viability of the articulate cartilage. (fig. 7-7C).

The **second** (distal) cut is made somewhat parallel to the articulate facet of the phalangeal head, thus forming a wedge when it joins the first cut laterally. The two osteotomy lines **do not** go through the lateral cortex of the phalangeal shaft. When the wedge of bone is resected, a lateral hinge is left behind. The importance of this hinge is to allow lateral-to-medial movement, thus closing the wedge, but preventing dorsal or plantar displacement of the bone (fig. 7-7C).

The hinge is thinned out ever so carefully so as to allow the osteotomy site to close easily. The osteotomy line can be fixated by external (Kirschner wire) fixation; the wire is introduced somewhat obliquely from medial to lateral, taking care not to go through the articulate cartilage (see fig. 7-7D and x-rays 7-8A-B-C).

A short cast (above the ankle) is applied. The cast is removed in three weeks as are all sutures and Kirschner wire. Healing is usually uneventful.

Internal fixation can also be used. The method that we have devised is quite effective and is shown in figures 7-9A through L.

Essentially what is done is to drill a small hole on either side of the osteotomy line (fig. 7-9 G-H). A small half-circle needle with 3-0 mono-filament surgical steel suture material (available from Ethicon) is then passed through the holes from proximal to distal (fig. 7-9I). The needle is passed through two more times so that we have a total of three strands of the 3-0 wire (fig. 7-9J).

The three strands of 3-0 wire are gathered together with a **Kocher** forceps. The kocher forceps is then slowly turned, thus twisting the wires and closing (coaptating) the osteotomy site (fig. 7-9K). Care is taken not to tighten the wires **too** tight as they may break. The capsule and tissues are closed in the usual manner — a cast is **not** necessary.

Precautions

1. The Akin operation is indicated for the correction of interphalangeal hallux valgus.
2. It is important to leave a **hinge** on the lateral cortex of the shaft to avoid dorsal or plantar displacement.
3. If Kirschner wire fixation is used, the foot should be immoblized with a cast for three weeks.
4. If internal stainless steel wire fixation is used, a cast is not required.

HALLUX VALGUS SURGERY

AKIN OPERATION

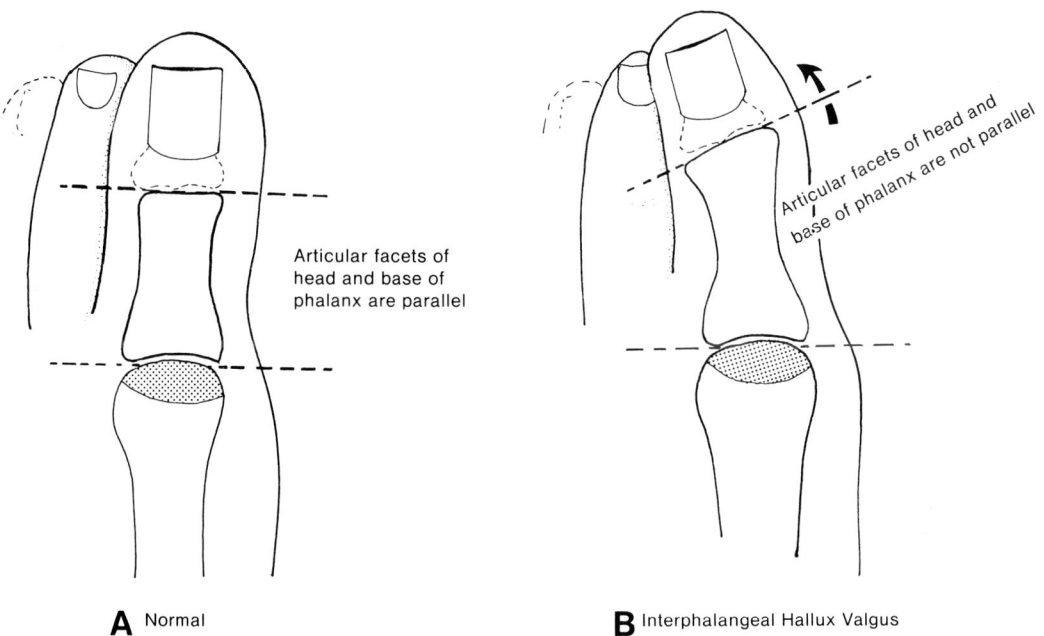
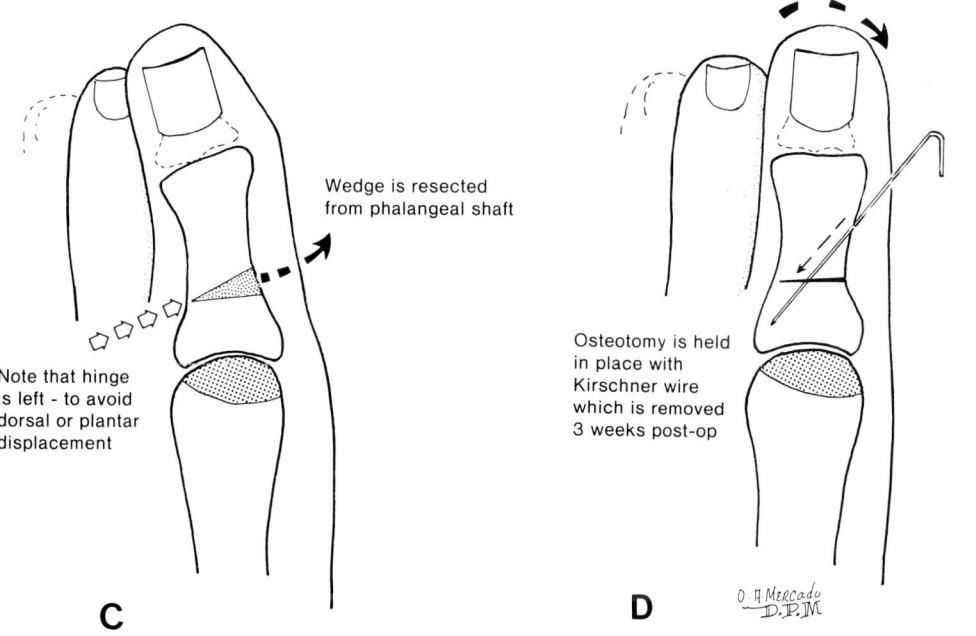

Fig. 7-7

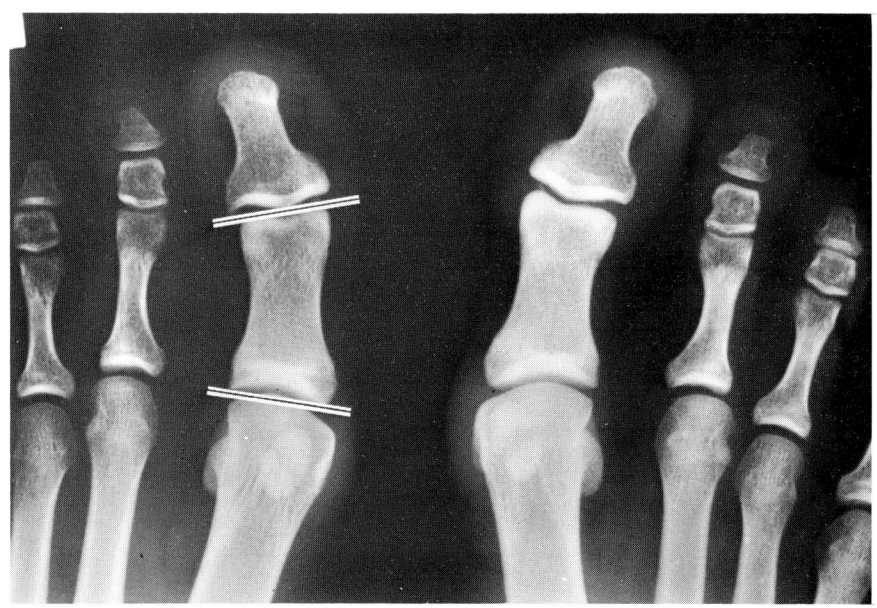

Fig. 7-8A. Pre-operative x-ray. Note that the articular facets of the proximal phalanges are not parallel.

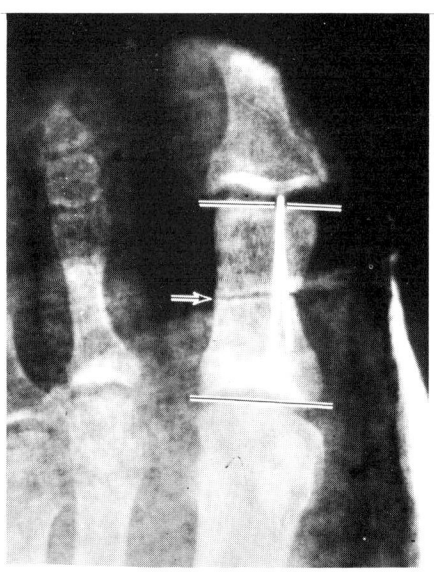

Fig. 7-8B. Post-operative x-ray. Akin procedure performed and externally fixated with Kirschner wire.

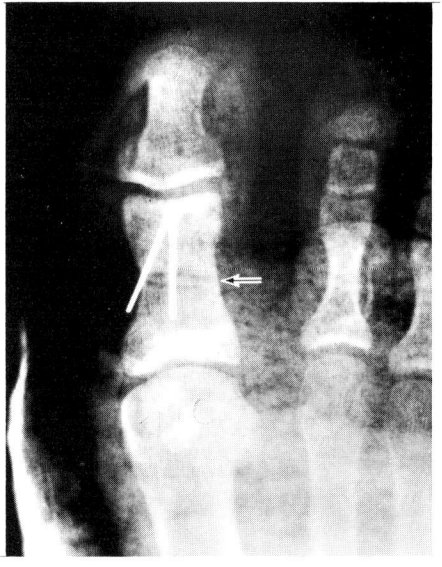

Fig. 7-8C. Arrow points to lateral hinge. The Kirschner wire and cast are removed in three weeks.

The Akin Operation

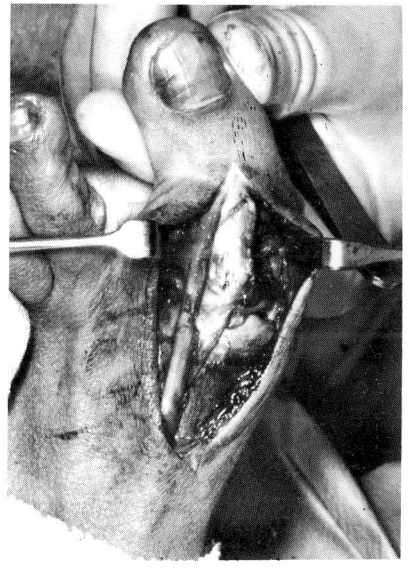

Fig. 7-9A. Note **lateral** deviation of interphalangeal joint.

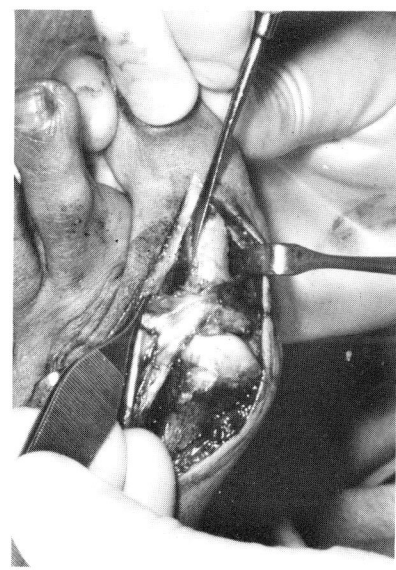

Fig. 7-9B. Periosteum is peeled from shaft of proximal phalanx.

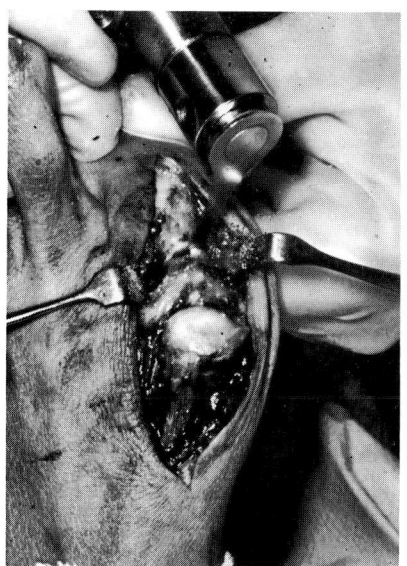

Fig. 7-9C. The **first** (proximal) cut is made parallel to the articulate fascet of the phalangeal base.

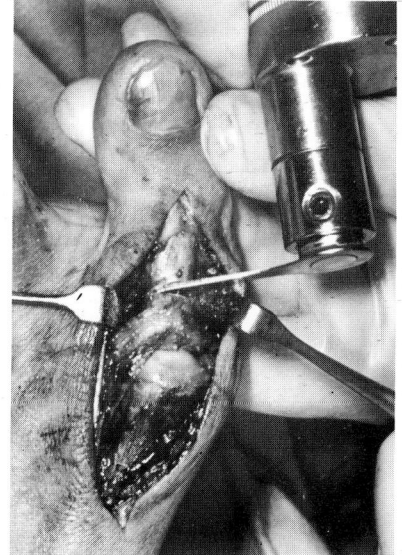

Fig. 7-9D. The **second** (distal) cut is made somewhat parallel to the articulate fascet of the phalangeal head — thus forming a wedge when it joins the first cut laterally.

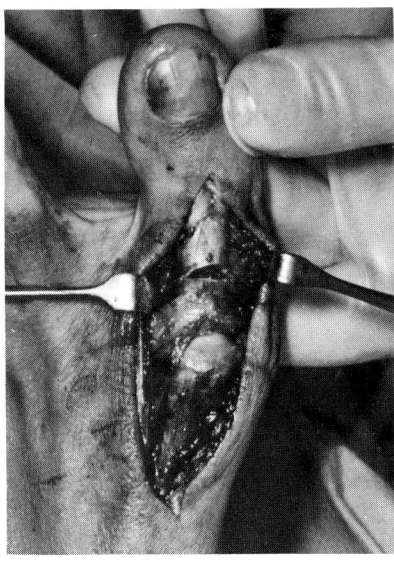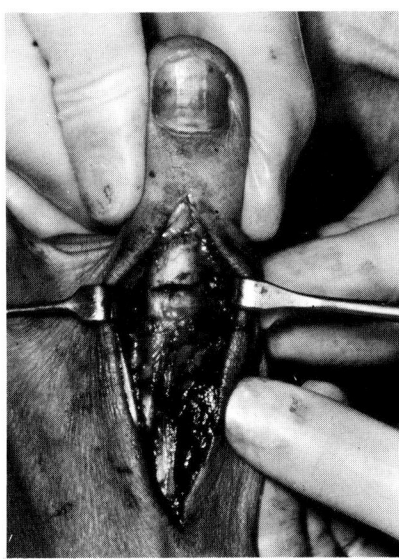

Fig. 7-9E. Note lateral hinge. This will allow lateral to medial movement — closing the wedge — but prevent dorsal or plantar displacement.

Fig. 7-9F. The osteotomy site is closed, thus correcting the deformity.

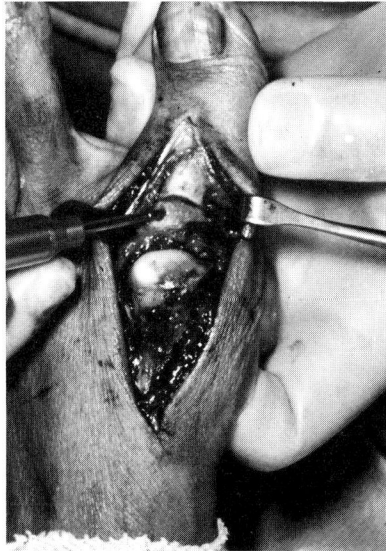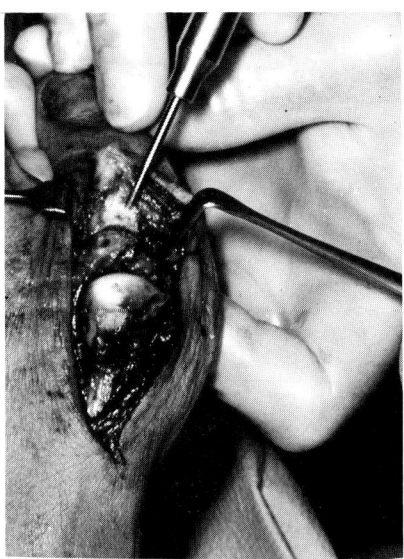

Fig. 7-9G. To internally fixate the osteotomy line a small hole is drilled proximal to the osteotomy line . . .

Fig. 7-9H. A second hole is then drilled distal to the osteotomy line.

HALLUX VALGUS SURGERY

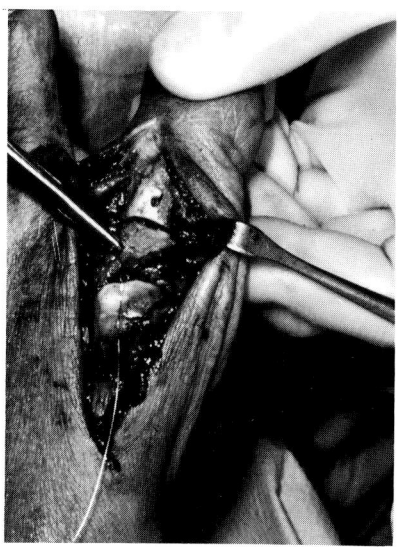

Fig. 7-9I. A small 3-0 mono-filament wire suture in a half-circle needle (available from **Ethicon**) is passed through the holes from proximal to distal.

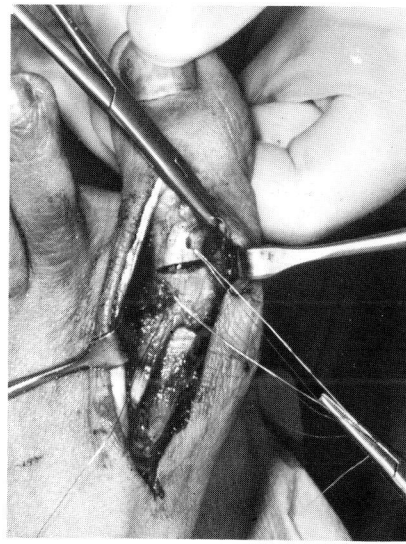

Fig. 7-9J. The needle is passed through two more times so that we have a total of three strands of 3-0 wire.

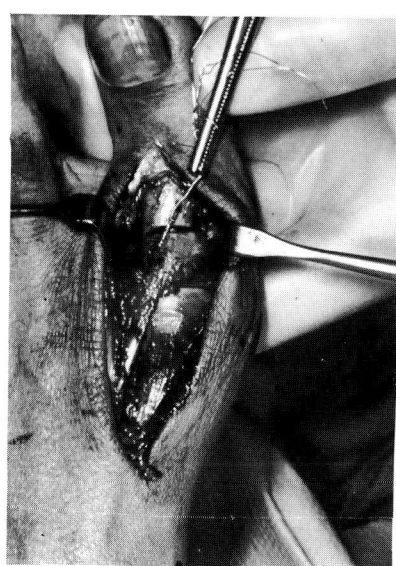

Fig. 7-9K. The three strands are gathered together — using a Kocher forceps — and slowly twisted until the osteotomy line is closed.

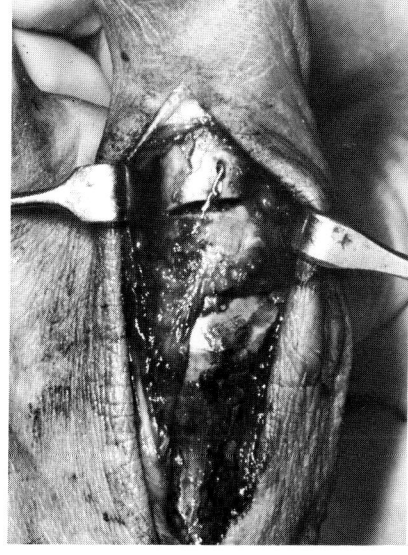

Fig. 7-9L. The twisted wires are cut and its end is carefully buried in one of the drilled holes.

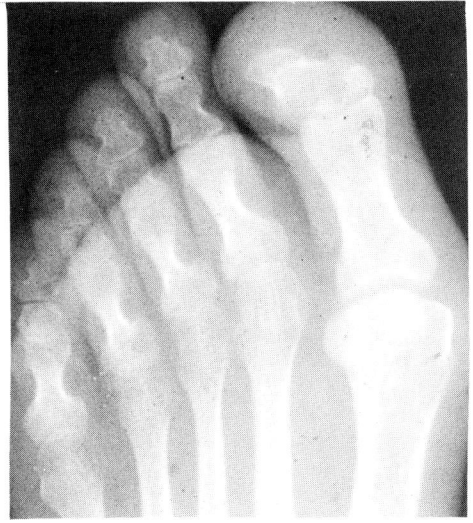 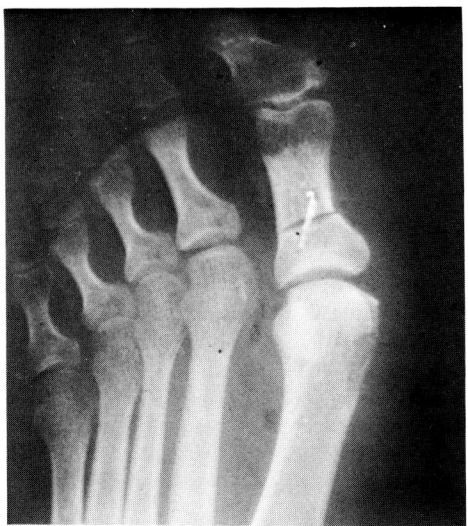

Fig. 7-9M. Pre-operative x-rays of patient shown in figs. 7-9A-L.

Fig. 7-9N. Post-operative x-ray. Note angle of wire.

BASIC BUNIONECTOMY WITH LATERAL SESAMOIDECTOMY (MCBRIDE TYPE BUNIONECTOMY)

Earl D. McBride described his technique for the correction of hallux valgus in 1928. Since that time, the term "McBride Bunionectomy" has been used and misused by generations of surgeons operating on the foot.

The salient points of the **McBride** operation are as follows:

1. The hyperostosis on the medial aspect of the metatarsal head is resected.
2. The lateral sesamoid is removed.
3. The head of adductor hallucis is transferred from its insertion on the base of the proximal phalanx, to the lateral aspect of the metatarsal head.

On paper, the idea of the adductor hallucis transfer would appear to be an excellent method of correcting the metatarsus primus varus. However, the **adductor** and **abductor hallucis** are essentially stabilizing muscles, they **do not adduct** or **abduct** as do their counter parts in the hand, adductor and abductor pollices. Their main function is to hold the proximal phalanx against the metatarsal head, thus **stabilizing** the hallux, during the toe-off portion of the gait cycle.

In reality, the adductor hallucis in hallux valgus is an **attenuated** muscle and, if transplanted to the metatarsal head, it cannot be expected to correct an **osteal deviation** such as metatarsus primus varus. For this reason, a **true** McBride bunionectomy is seldom, if ever, performed in modern foot surgery.

Habits die hard, however, and today surgeons still insist on using the term McBride bunionectomy for any hallux valgus surgery where the lateral sesamoid is resected.

Technique for Lateral Sesamoidectomy

The lateral sesamoid is removed in conjunction with hallux valgus surgery, when it is 50% or more in the intermetatarsal space as viewed on a dorsal-plantar weight bearing x-ray.

The removal of the lateral sesamoid is a **simple** task, if the surgeon is careful with its dissection and takes time to identify and use the important anatomical landmarks.

The Basic bunionectomy as outlined in the beginning of this chapter, is performed first. We then retract the wound lateralwards and go through the thin **gossamer-like** tissue which overlays the intermetatarsal space, exposing the first intermetatarsal space.

In figure 7-10A, we can see the important anatomy found in this area. The tendons of **extensor hallucis longus** and **brevis**; the **first dorsal interossei**; the lateral head of **flexor hallucis brevis**; the conjoined tendons of **adductor hallucis** which blend into an aponeurosis over the lateral sesamoid forming the **sesamoidal bulge**; and the **first anterior perforating artery** which descends into this area but is seldom seen during surgery.

The **sesamoidal bulge** is identified and a stab incision is made inbetween the sesamoid and the metatarsal head (fig. 7-10B). The incision is extended proximally and distally. A thumb and finger forceps is used to grasp the conjoined tendon of **adductor hallucis** (fig. 7-10C) and the sesamoid is **carefully** peeled from it.

The sesamoid has a **distal attachment** (into the base of the proxinal phalanx), a **proximal attachment** (the lateral head of Flexor Hallucis Brevis), and a **medial attachment** (the intersesamoidal ligament) which must be cut before the sesamoid can be resected.

Care is taken, when peeling the sesamoid from its attachment, to avoid cutting the **flexor hallucis longus** tendon which lies immediately under the sesamoid (fig. 7-10D).

A section of the **conjoined tendons** of Adductor Hallucis is then resected. This will insure complete detachment of the conjoined tendons into the base of the proximal phalanx and allow for the proper positioning (correction) of the hallux.

The hallux is then held in the corrected position and the capsule is sutured with 2-0 Dexon as shown in figure 7-6S. The deep and superficial tissues as well as the skin, are sutured with the material of choice.

Precautions

1. The McBride type bunionectomy is used for the correction of **moderate hallux valgus.**
2. The lateral sesamoid is removed in conjunction with hallux valgus surgery **only** if it is 50% or more in the intermetatarsal space as viewed on a dorsal-plantar weight bearing x-ray.

Lateral Sesamoidectomy

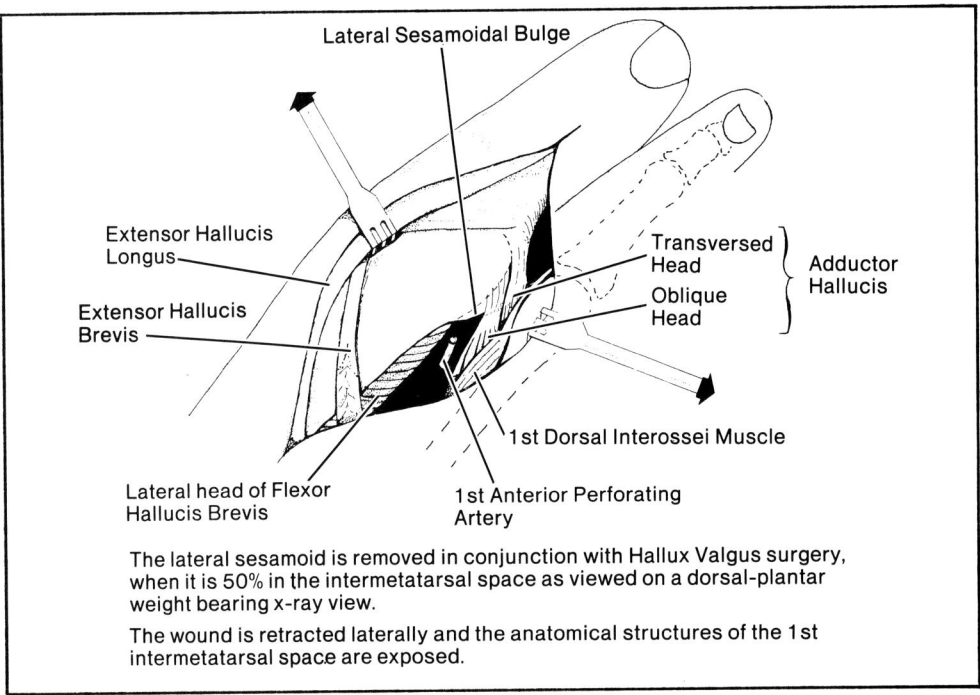

Fig. 7-10A

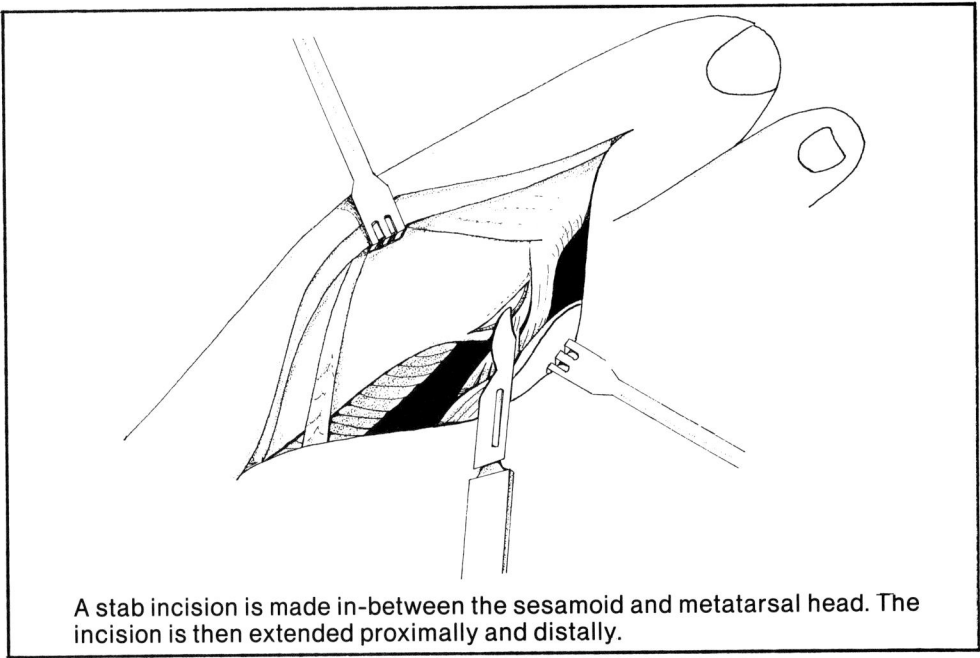

Fig. 7-10B

HALLUX VALGUS SURGERY

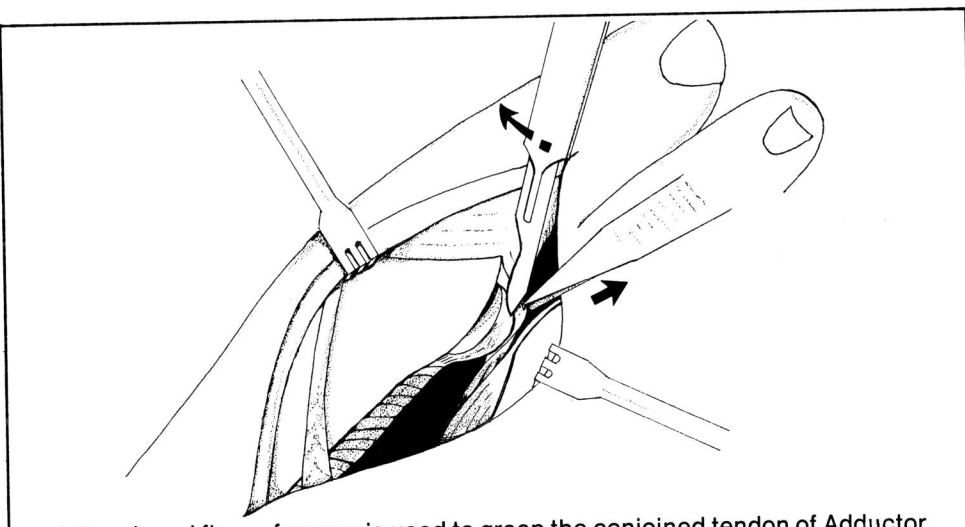

A thumb and finger forceps is used to grasp the conjoined tendon of Adductor Hallucis and the sesamoid is carefully peeled from it.

Remember that the sesamoid has a **distal attachment** (into the base of the proximal phalanx), a **proximal attachment** (the lateral head of Flexor Hallucis Brevis), and a **medial attachment** (the Intersesamoidal Ligament) which must be cut before the sesamoid can be resected.

Fig. 7-10D

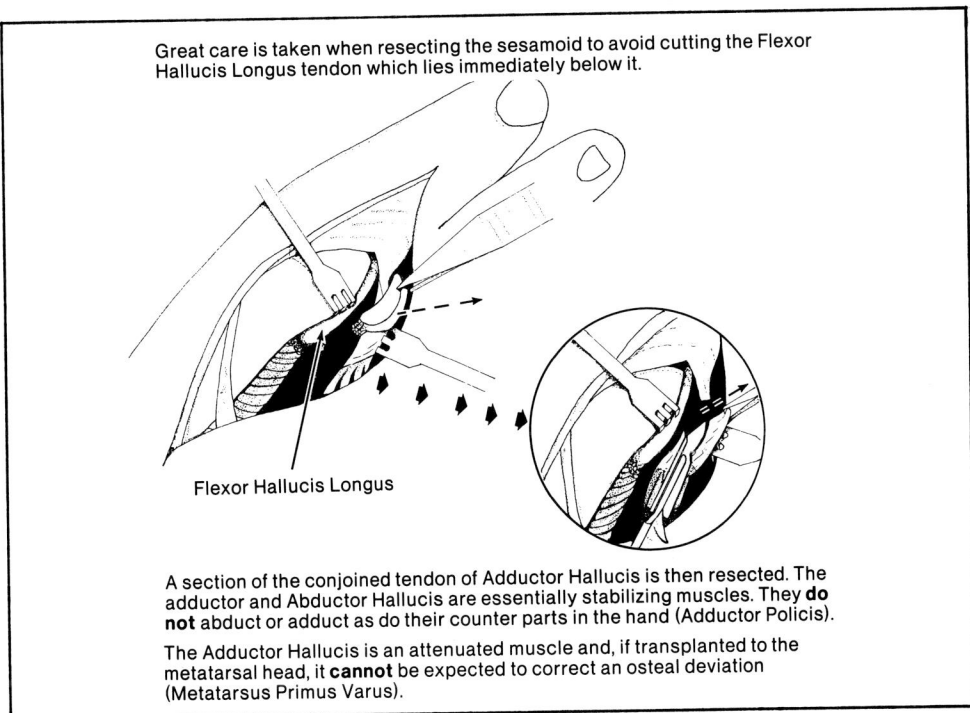

Great care is taken when resecting the sesamoid to avoid cutting the Flexor Hallucis Longus tendon which lies immediately below it.

Flexor Hallucis Longus

A section of the conjoined tendon of Adductor Hallucis is then resected. The adductor and Abductor Hallucis are essentially stabilizing muscles. They **do not** abduct or adduct as do their counter parts in the hand (Adductor Policis).

The Adductor Hallucis is an attenuated muscle and, if transplanted to the metatarsal head, it **cannot** be expected to correct an osteal deviation (Metatarsus Primus Varus).

Fig. 7-10C

THE REVERDIN OPERATION

The Reverdin Operation was first described by **J. L. Reverdin** in Switzerland, in 1881 . . . almost **100** years ago!

It was one of those little known operations that for years remained buried in the mountain of surgical procedures that have been written on hallux valgus.

It wasn't until the early 70's, when the new Genre' of power equipment and blades became available that the technique became popular.

Essentially, the procedure aims at the realignment of a laterally displaced articular fascet of the first metatarsal head by a **wedge shaped ostectomy.** One has to marvel at the ingenuity of Reverdin, who, in an age of poor instrumentation and even worse **anesthesia,** was able to become so **selective** in his hallux valgus surgery.

Today, the Reverdin operation — which incidentally was the **first osteotomy** described for hallux valgus surgery — is used in cases where the articular fascet of the metatarsal head is so **laterally displaced** that it would be futile to perform a Basic or McBride type bunionectomy.

In fact, if a **Basic** or **McBride** type bunionectomy were performed, one of two things could happen;

1. The hallux would inevitably slip back into valgus since **structure will follow function** and the metatarsal head cartilage is functioning in a lateral plane.
2. The hallux would be overcorrected, to overcome its tendency to slip back into a valgus position, and a **hallux varus** would result.

Surgical Criteria

The surgical criteria that we use at Franklin Boulevard Community Hospital, is as follows:

1. **The first metatarsal must not be too short.**

    The Reverdin Osteotomy only shortens the metatarsal by a couple of millimeters. However, on a very short first metatarsal, it could create a post-operative lesion under the second metatarsal head. In cases were a short first metatarsal is present, the **Distal Crescentic Osteotomy** is recommended.

2. **The inter-metatarsal angle must be taken into account.**

    The Reverdin Operation will sometimes decrease an inter-metatarsal angle. This happens because the articular fascet is realigned into a normal functioning position, thus releasing the **buttressing** affect of the proximal phalangeal base on the metatarsal head. If there is a metatarsus primus varus present, however, then the surgeon must correct it with an additional osteotomy.

3. **The deviation of the cartilage must be evaluated at the time of the operation.**

    Sometimes the radiographic findings of a laterally deviated articular fascet are not confirmed on the operating table, in which case the Reverdin operation **is not** indicated.

Technique

The Reverdin Operation is performed as follows:

The standard lineal incision of hallux valgus is used. A modified V-shaped Silver capsulotomy is performed on the medial aspect of the metatarsal-phalangeal-joint. As can be seen in our illustration (figure 7-11A), the apex of the V-capsule lies proximal on the metatarsal shaft. The V-flap is carefully underscored and retracted with a long suture of 3-0 Dexon.

The joint capsule is then carefully underscored, taking care to release the lateral collateral ligament, and the metatarsal head is exposed (figure 7-11B).

Note how the articular fascet is laterally displaced. The hyperthrophic bone is then resected from all around the head (figure 7-11C). Care is taken in resecting the medial eminence to leave the **crista,** the articulate fascet for the medial sesamoid, intact.

The wedge shaped osteotomy is then outlined (figure 7-11D). Note that the distal line is approximately 1 cm. from the tip of the cartilage. This cut is extremely important since **cartilage** has **no circulation** of its own and depends on the sub-chondral bone from its nutrition. If the cartilage is to remain viable, it must have enough sub-chondral bone.

The apex of the wedge is lateralwards, where a **hinge** will be left. The **hinge** will be thinned out to the consistency of cardboard paper (figure 7-11E).

The creation of this hinge will be the most important step of the operation — for two reasons:

First, the hinge will prevent displacement of the articular fragment. It will allow movement only from lateral to medial, thus creating a **very stable** osteotomy.

Secondly, by thinning out the hinge to the consistency of **cardboard paper,** there will be a resilliency, actually springiness to the bone. This springiness is necessary as it will allow for the **compression** which is so desirable in cancellous bone healing.

Once the hinge is thinned out to its proper thickness, the articulate fascet will be easily realigned into a normal position (figure 7-11F).

The compression on the osteotomy is maintained when the hallux is repositioned on the metatarsal head. The capsule is then sutured first, as shown in the insert in our illustration 7-11G, in the area where the capsular flap was taken from. The suturing of the capsular flap is next. The V-flap will maintain the proximal phalanx tight against the metatarsal, thus creating the compression which will enhance cancellous bone healing.

The mobile **V-flap** has the following advantages:

1. It will **derotate** any hallucial rotation present.
2. It **reinforces** the medial capsule.
3. It provides **pressure** coaptation, actually compression of the osteotomy site.

The capsule is closed with 2-0 Dexon. The deep and superficial fascia are closed in 4-0 Dexon. The wound is closed with the suture material of choice. Healing is **uneventful.**

Precautions

The surgeon should keep the following important points in mind when performing the Reverdin Operation:

1. Place your Osteotomy so that the distal cut is 1cm. from the articular tip, this will insure **cartilagenous viability.**
2. As with any other procedure, it is important that the **proper indications** are present.

Conclusion

The osteotomy line for the Reverdin operation lies distal to the sesamoids (see X-rays). In our **long** experience with the Reverdin operation, we **have not** had any incidence of sesamoidal irritation or joint movement limitation.

The Reverdin Operation has served us well for a good number of years. When performed as described here, it will yield consistently **good results.**

The Reverdin Operation

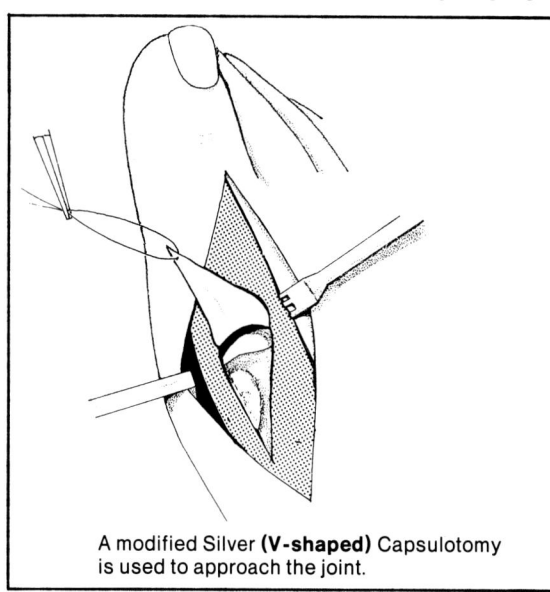

A modified Silver **(V-shaped)** Capsulotomy is used to approach the joint.

Fig. 7-11A

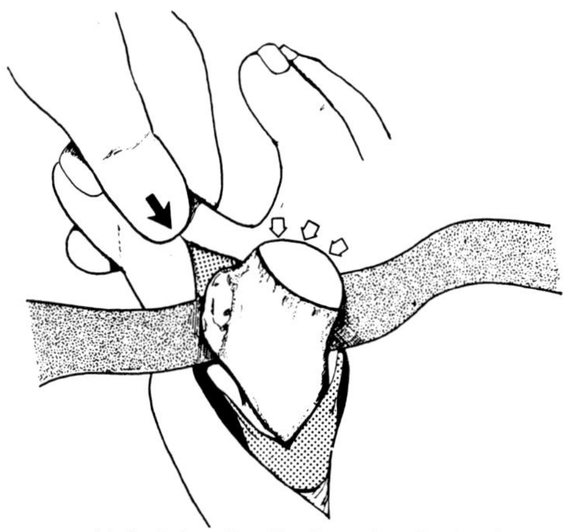

Note laterally displaced articular facet

Fig. 7-11B

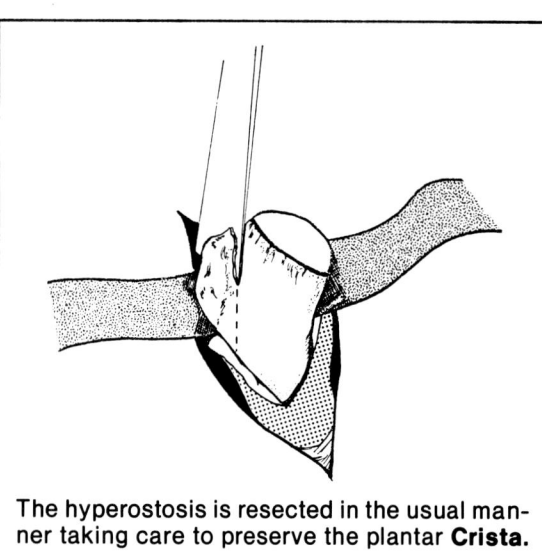

The hyperostosis is resected in the usual manner taking care to preserve the plantar **Crista.**

Fig. 7-11C

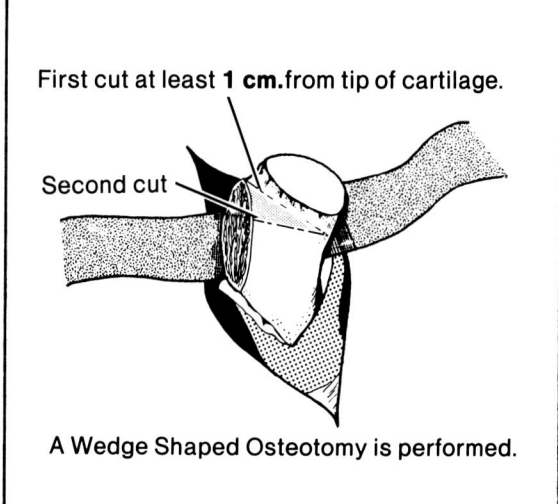

First cut at least **1 cm.** from tip of cartilage.

Second cut

A Wedge Shaped Osteotomy is performed.

Fig. 7-11D

HALLUX VALGUS SURGERY

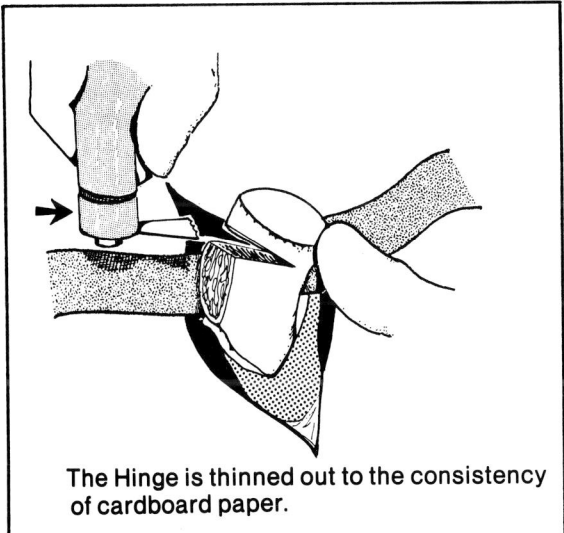

The Hinge is thinned out to the consistency of cardboard paper.

Fig. 7-11E

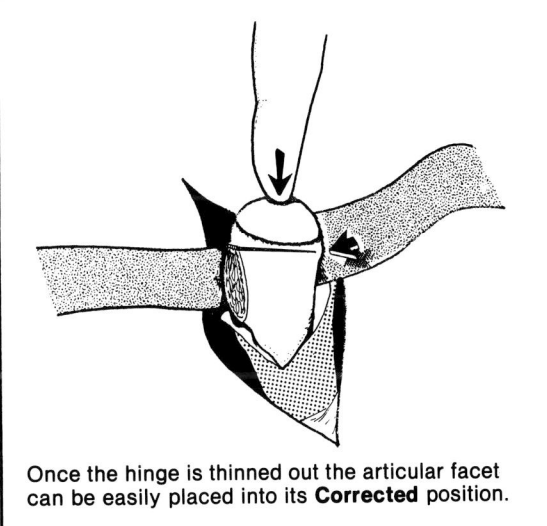

Once the hinge is thinned out the articular facet can be easily placed into its **Corrected** position.

Fig. 7-11F

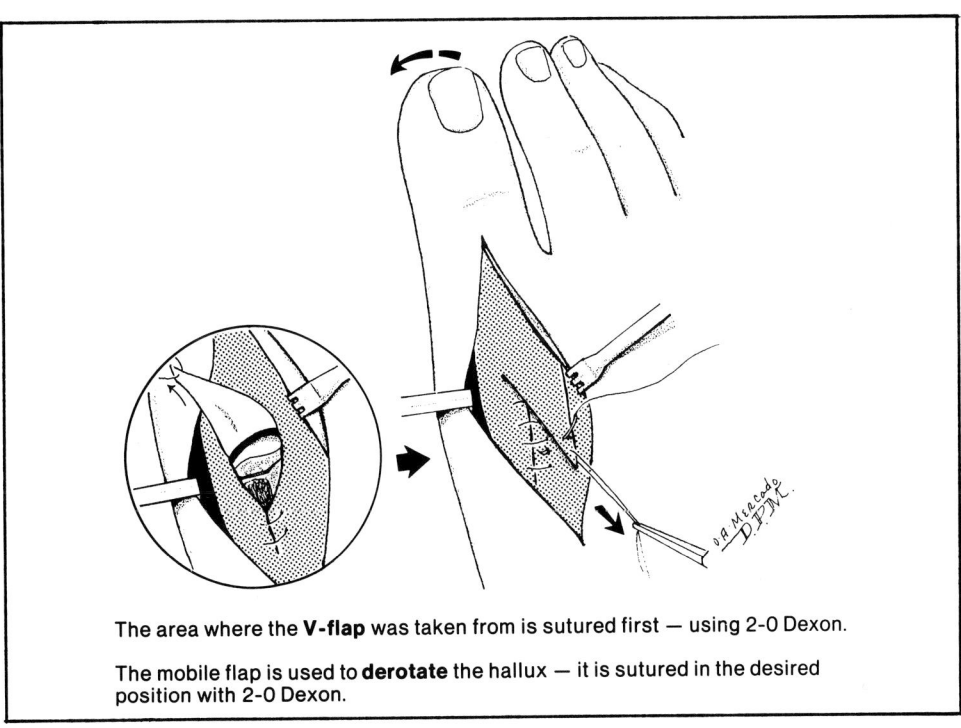

The area where the **V-flap** was taken from is sutured first — using 2-0 Dexon.

The mobile flap is used to **derotate** the hallux — it is sutured in the desired position with 2-0 Dexon.

Fig. 7-11G

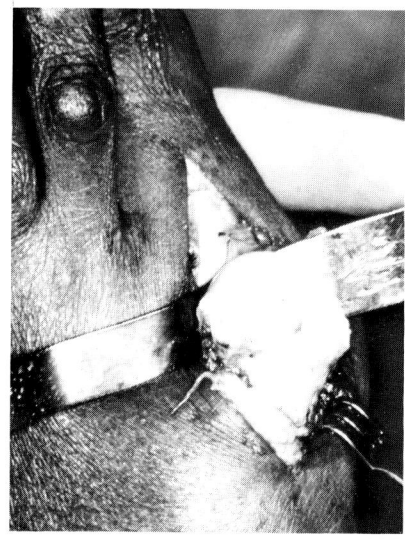

Fig. 7-12A. Note laterally displaced articular facet.

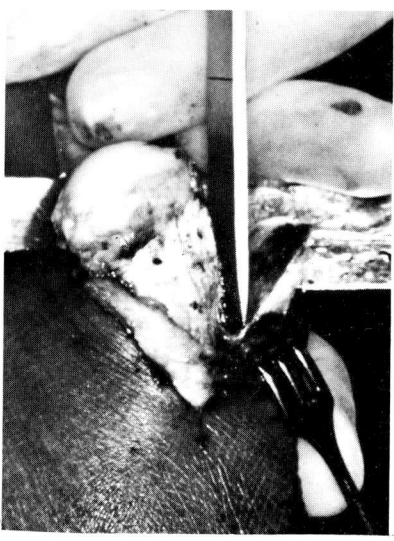

Fig. 7-12B. The hyperostosis is resected in the usual manner taking care to preserve the plantar **Crista.**

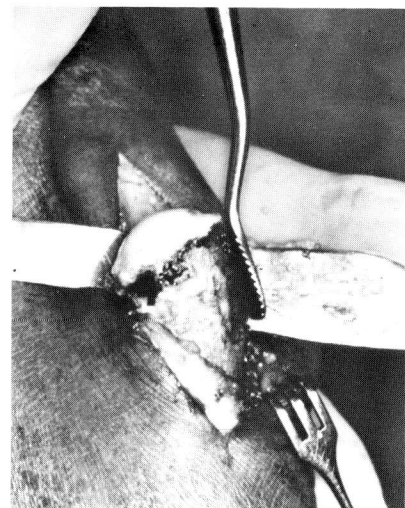

Fig. 7-12C. The bone is rasped smooth.

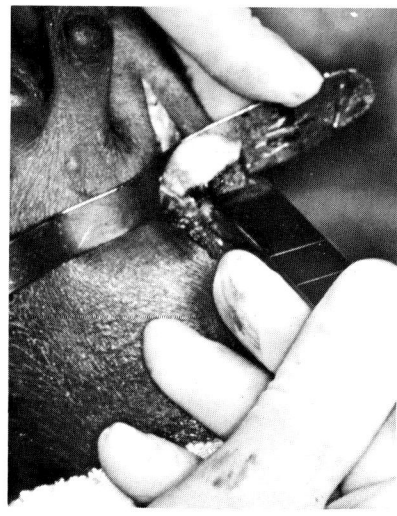

Fig. 7-12D. The osteotomy lines are carefully marked with an osteotome.

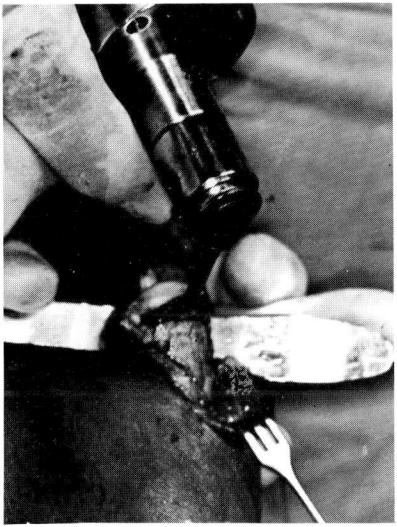
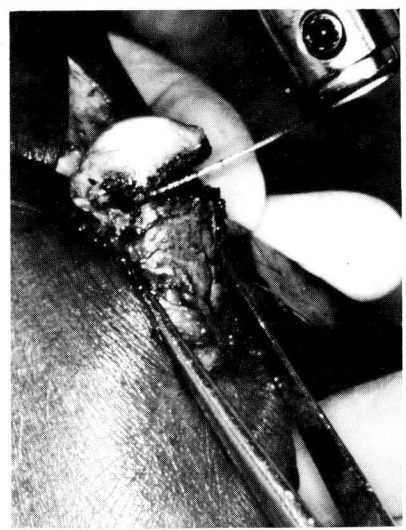

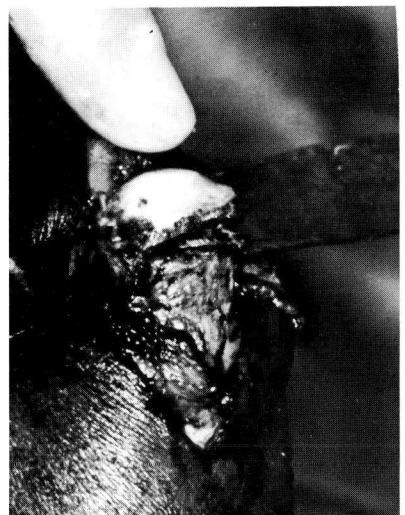
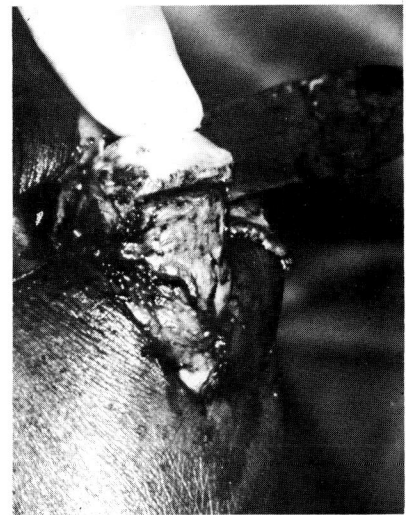

Fig. 7-12G. Once the hinge is thinned out the articular facet can be easily placed ...

Fig. 7-12H. ... into its **Corrected** position.

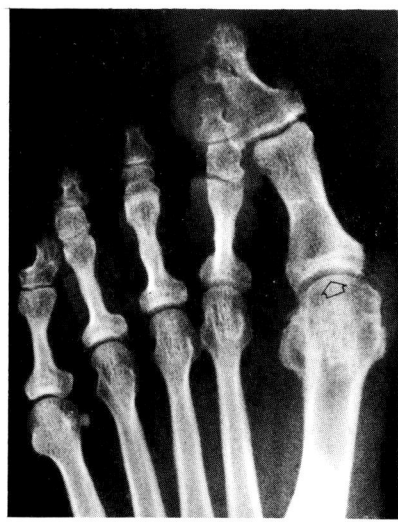 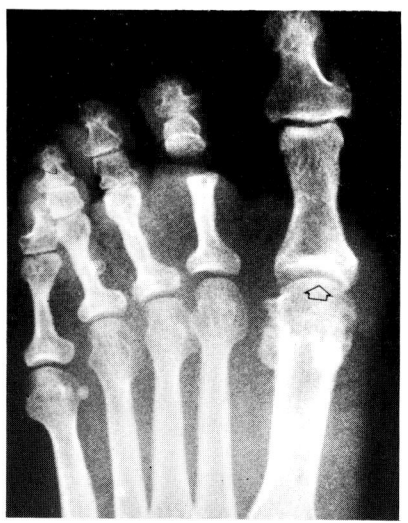

Fig. 7-13A. pre-operative x-ray of patient shown in figs. 7-12A-H. Arrow points to laterally deviated articular facet.

Fig. 7-13B. Two months after surgery, osteotomy line is almost invisible. Note that the osteotomy line lies distal to the sesamoids. Arrow points to realigned articular facet.

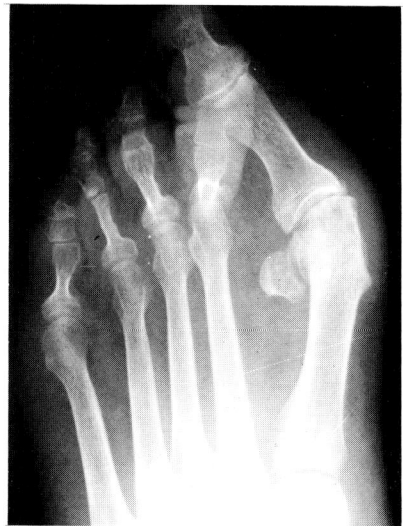 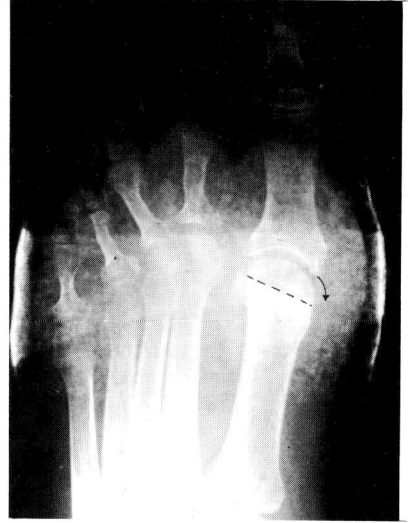

Fig. 7-14A. Pre-operative x-ray of patient who had a simple bunionectomy performed — when in fact what was indicated was a **Reverdin** operation.

Fig. 7-14B. Post-up x-ray. Revesion surgery was performed, using the Reverdin operation. The correction was excellent.

DISTAL CRESCENTIC OSTEOTOMY

The Distal Crescentic Osteotomy is a technique used in moderate hallux valgus when there is a laterally displaced articulate fascet on a **short** first metatarsal. In other words, the indications are the same as for the Reverdin operation, except it is performed on a short first ray (Fig. 7-15A). While the Reverdin operation only shortens the metatarsal a couple of millimeters or so, on a short metatarsal this can be enough to cause a **transfer lesion** on the second metatarsal head post-surgically.

Crescentic osteotomies are of recent vintage in the field of foot surgery. They came about in the early 1970's as the instrumentation, particularly the thin crescentic-shaped blade used, became available.

The advantage of the Distal Crescentic Osteotomy is that it allows repositioning of the laterally displaced articulate fascet without **significant** shortening of the first ray. Also, since the total head is repositioned on the metatarsal shaft, there is a reduction of the intermetatarsal angle. This I.M. angle reduction can be particularly useful in **hallux valgus juveniles** where a closing wedge osteotomy cannot be performed because of the **epiphyseal plate** present on the first metatarsal base.

Technique

Our approach to the first metatarsal phalangeal joint is the same as for any other hallux valgus procedure with the notable exception that the lateral collateral ligament is **not cut (fig. 7-15B).**

The hyperostosis on the medial and dorsal aspect of the metatarsal head is resected as previously described. As a rule, the lateral sesamoid is not removed in this procedure.

A **crescentic** blade is then used to perform the osteotomy. The cut extends from the anatomical neck area on the lateral aspect and curves slightly anteriorwards on the medial aspect (fig. 7-15C). The osteotomy transects the metatarsal head completely — **no** plantar hinge is left. The hallucial segment is then moved from lateral to medial — thus correcting the valgus position of the great toe (fig. 7-15D).

The head of the metatarsal is then fixated with Kirschner wire into its new position — remember to planti-flex the head ever so slightly, to prevent a second metatarsal intractable plantar keratosis (fig. 7-15E).

The K-wire is advanced until it comes out through the skin on the medial aspect of the foot. The K-wire driver is disengaged and attached again to the wire protruding through the skin. The wire is then slowly pulled until the wire is just beneath the cartilage of the metatarsal head (fig. 7-15F).

The wound is then closed in the usual manner. The wire is cut and bent so that it can be incorporated in the dressing. An above the ankle cast is applied for three weeks at which time it is removed along with the K-wire. Healing is usually uneventful.

Precautions

The following points are important for the surgeon to keep in mind when performing the Distal Crescentic Osteotomy:

1. Be sure of the indications for the procedure. A normal length first metatarsal does not need a Distal Crescentic Osteotomy, a Reverdin operation can be used for these cases. The only exception would be in hallux valgus juveniles, where the I.M. angle needs to be reduced.
2. **Do not cut** the lateral collateral ligament as it adds stability to the osteotomy site.
3. Fixate the osteotomy as outlined here, for best results.
4. Apply an above the ankle cast for at least three weeks to insure proper healing of the osteotomy site.

Conclusion

The Distal Crescentic Osteotomy, when performed as outlined here, will yield consistently good results.

Distal Crescentic Osteotomy

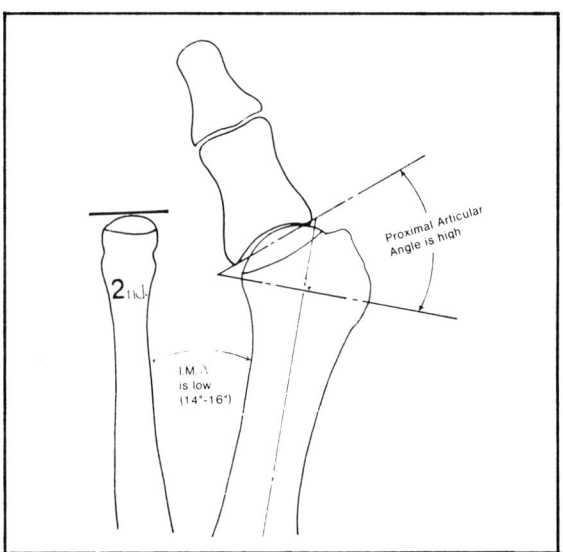

Fig. 7-15A

HALLUX VALGUS SURGERY

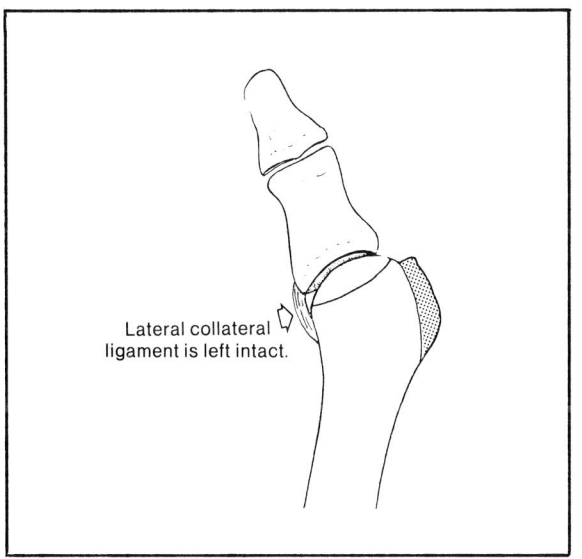

Lateral collateral ligament is left intact.

Fig. 7-15B

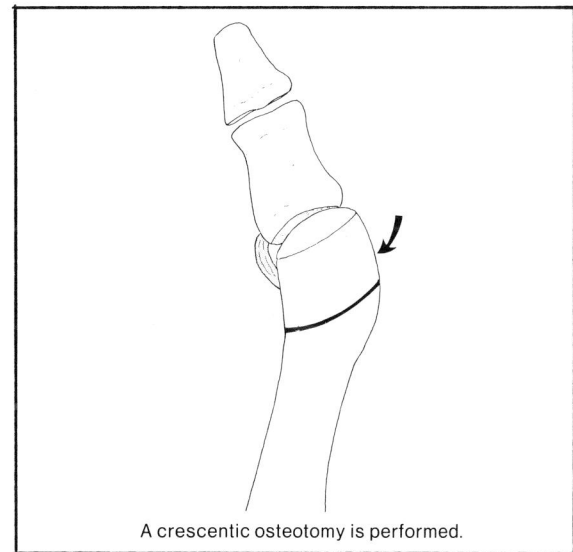

A crescentic osteotomy is performed.

Fig. 7-15C

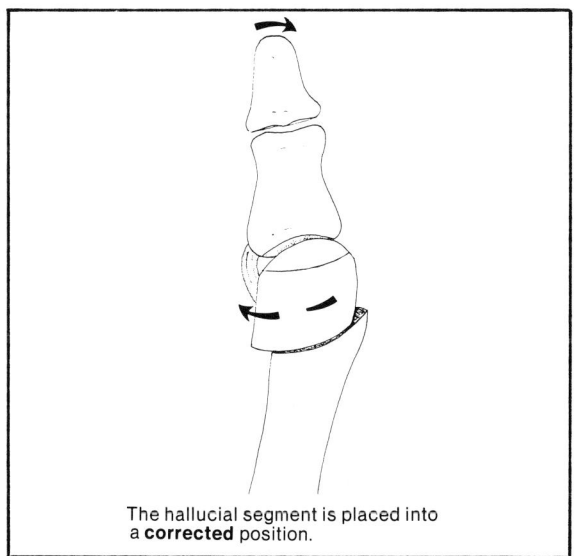

The hallucial segment is placed into a **corrected** position.

Fig. 7-15D

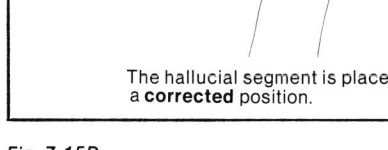

Note that head is plantiflexed slightly to prevent 2nd. meta. I.P.K.

A Kischner wire is used to fixate osteotomy. The wire will go through the head and shaft and into the skin on the medial aspect of the foot.

Fig. 7-15E

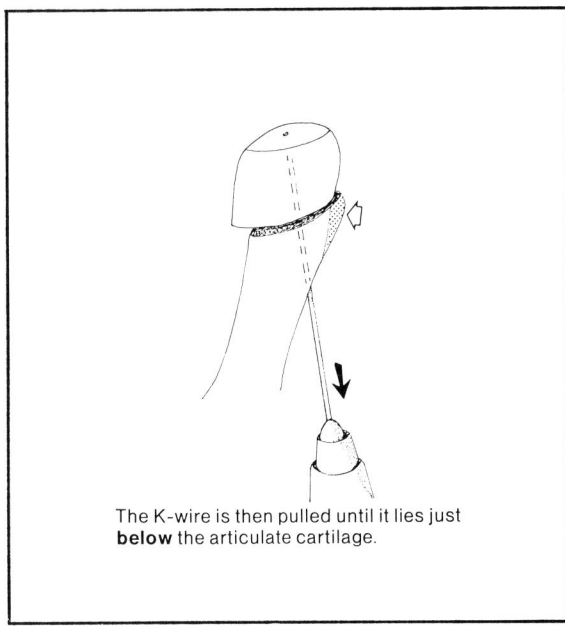

The K-wire is then pulled until it lies just **below** the articulate cartilage.

Fig. 7-15F

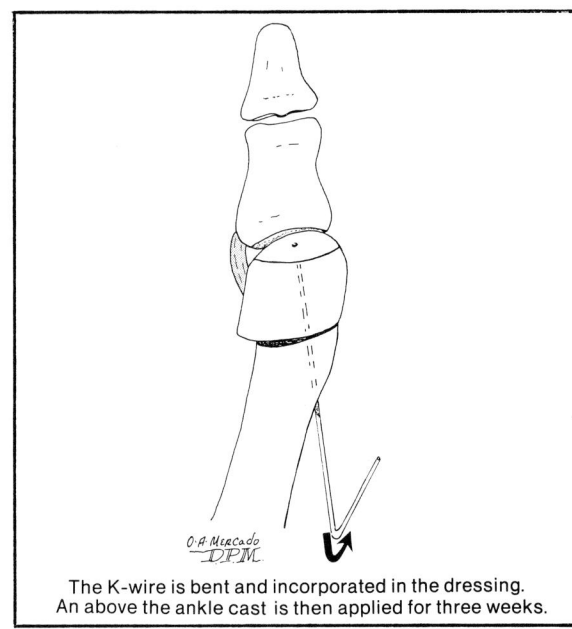

The K-wire is bent and incorporated in the dressing. An above the ankle cast is then applied for three weeks.

Fig. 7-15G

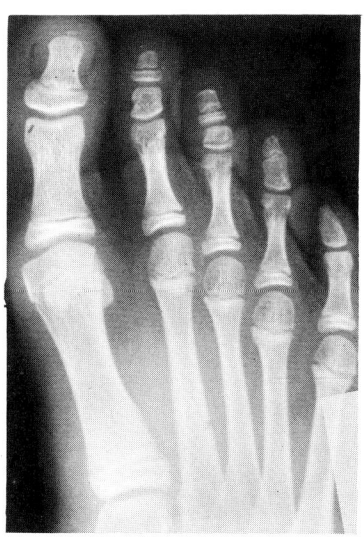

Fig. 7-16A. Pre-operative x-ray of thirteen year old girl with painful hallux valgus juveniles. Note epiphyseal plates.

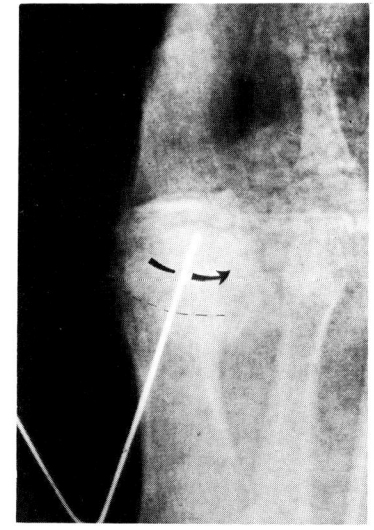

Fig. 7-16B. Post-operative x-ray. Distal Crescentic osteotomy was performed. Note location of K-wire used for fixation.

PROXIMAL CRESCENTIC OSTEOTOMY

The Proximal Crescentic osteotomy is perhaps my favorite Osteotomy to perform. It is indicated for the correction of **metatarsus primus varus** when the first metatarsal ray is **short.** If a closing wedge osteotomy were to be used on a short first metatarsal, a transfer lesion to the second metatarsal head could occur post-surgically. The Proximal Crescentic Osteotomy will correct the metatarsus primus varus without **significantly shortening** the first ray.

The Proximal Crescentic Osteotomy is my favorite osteotomy because, when performed correctly, it can truly be a **work of art.** Since it is a **difficult osteotomy** to perform and fixate, it has often been performed for the **wrong** indications thus leading to poor results. For these reasons, the osteotomy has fallen into disuse in many parts of the country.

I would like very much to stimulate the surgeons reading these lines to perform the osteotomy as described here. The results will be rewarding, to both the surgeon and the patient, and I am certain that the Proximal Crescentic Osteotomy will become an important addition to their hallux valgus surgery armamentarium.

Technique

After the hallux valgus problem has been corrected — using whatever technique is indicated — the incision is elongated proximally and dorsally over the first metatarsal-cuneiform joint (fig. 7-17A). The incision is carefully deepened and immediately the large vein of the **irregular dorsal venous network** will be seen.

The vein is carefully retracted with a **Penrose drain** — or umbilical cord tape — and the extensor digitorum longus is identified and retracted to expose the capsule and periosteum over the first metatarsal-cuneiform joint. (Fig. 7-17C).

A lineal incision is made on the dorsum of the first metatarsal base extending to the joint line. The capsule and periosteum are then carefully underscored — actually **peeled** — to either side of metatarsal base; this can easily be accomplished by using a thin periosteal elevator (Fig. 7-17D).

The capsule and periosteum are then retracted with the blunt end of a senn retractor. By retracting the capsule and periosteum in this manner, the **deep plantar artery** — which descends in between the bases of the first and second metatarsals — will be preserved when the osteotomy is performed.

We identify the first cuneiform joint line and measure at least one centimeter distal to it. A small, deep cut is then made into the bone — with a small power blade — creating what we like to call the **register mark** (Fig. 7-17F).

The register mark will allow us to **gauge** the amount of lateral movement that will take place on the distal metatarsal segment after the crescentic osteotomy is performed and the metatarsus primus varus is corrected.

A crescentic blade is chosen which will give the proper size cut. A few important points to remember about the crescentic blade are the following:

1. The blade is approximately one-third of a circle — in order to make the crescentic cut, the surgeon has to slowly oscillate the instrument back and forth while the blade is cutting.

2. Crescentic blades are expensive and very **fragile** — they cannot be forced or they will break.

3. Be sure to keep the blade at 90° to the bone.

4. Once the cut — actually the **groove** — is started, the blade will cut the bone without difficulty (Fig. 7-17G).

Our osteotomy is made immediately over the register mark. The apex of the crescentic cut lies proximally as seen in fig. 7-17G. We have tried placing the cut so that the apex of the crescent lies distally, but found this method to be more difficult since the cut would often go into the metatarsal base thus making movement of the distal metatarsal segment almost impossible.

The osteotomy **does not** go all the way through the bone — this is the **key** to the success of this procedure. The **plantar cortex** has to be feathered (thinned out) so as to allow movement of the metatarsal's distal shaft lateral wards without dorsal or plantar displacement (Fig. 7-17H).

As the plantar cortex is being thinned out, we try to move the distal segment of the metatarsal shaft with the blunt end of a senn retractor as shown in fig. 7-17I.

When the plantar cortex is thinned out enough, the metatarsal shaft will readily move into its corrected position (Fig. 7-17J).

The register mark will show how much movement has taken place — actually how far laterally the distal metatarsal shaft has moved. All that is required is a **couple** of millimeters between the register mark to obtain the desired reduction of the intermetatarsal angle.

The osteotomy is then fixated with a Kirschner wire. A few drops of decadron are infiltrated in the osteotomy site to cut down post-operative inflammation and pain. The periosteum and capsule are sutured with 3-0 Dexon. Sometimes a simple suture is used to pull the large vein away from the K-wire (fig. 7-17L).

The wound is then closed in the usual manner utilizing the suture material of choice (Fig. 7-17M).

The K-wire is carefully bent and incorporated in the dressing. An above the ankle cast is applied for three weeks — at that time the cast is removed along with the wire. Healing is usually uneventful.

Precautions

The Proximal Crescentic Osteotomy is a beautiful little technique to use in the correction of metatarsus primus varus on a short first metatarsal ray. The technique has fallen into disuse in the past, because it just **was not** performed correctly. The surgeon should keep the following points in mind:

1. The **register mark** is one of the most important steps of the operation. It has to be made deep enough so that when the crescentic osteotomy is performed, the surgeon will be able to see it easily.
2. Place the osteotomy at **least** 1 cm. from the joint line.
3. Keep the blade at **90°** to the bone.
4. **Do not** go all the way through the bone, this is **extremely important.** The plantar cortex has to be feathered (thinned out) to the consistency of thin cardboard paper. This will allow movement of the metatarsal shaft's distal end, from medial to lateral without dorsal or plantar displacement.
5. The **register mark** will gauge how far laterally the distal metatarsal shaft has moved. All that is required is a couple of millimeters between the register marks.
6. Fixate the osteotomy externally with a kirschner wire as outlined here.
7. Apply an above the ankle cast for at least 3 weeks.

Conclusion

I hope that we have cleared some of the mystery behind the Proximal Crescentic Osteotomy. The reader can rest **assured** that when performed as outlined here and for the proper indications, the osteotomy will yield consistently **good** results.

HALLUX VALGUS SURGERY

Proximal Crescentic Osteotomy

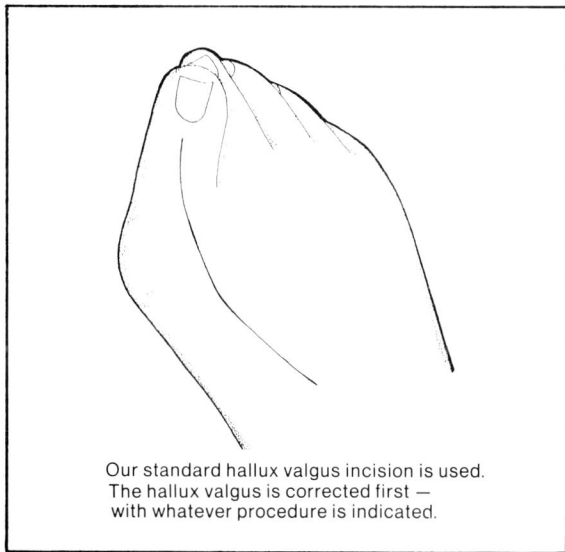

Our standard hallux valgus incision is used. The hallux valgus is corrected first — with whatever procedure is indicated.

Fig. 7-17A

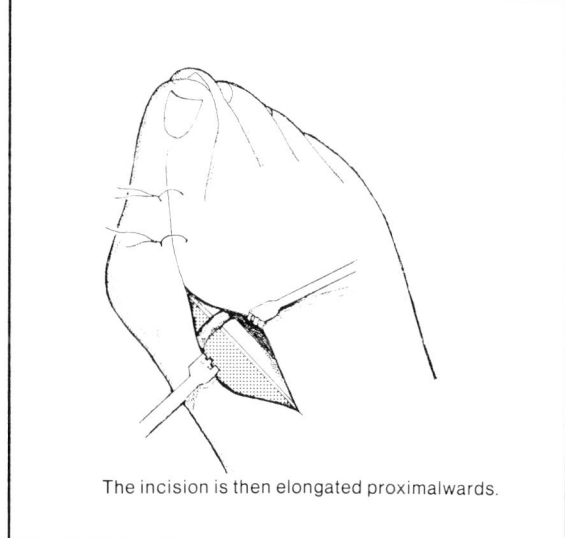

The incision is then elongated proximalwards.

Fig. 7-17B

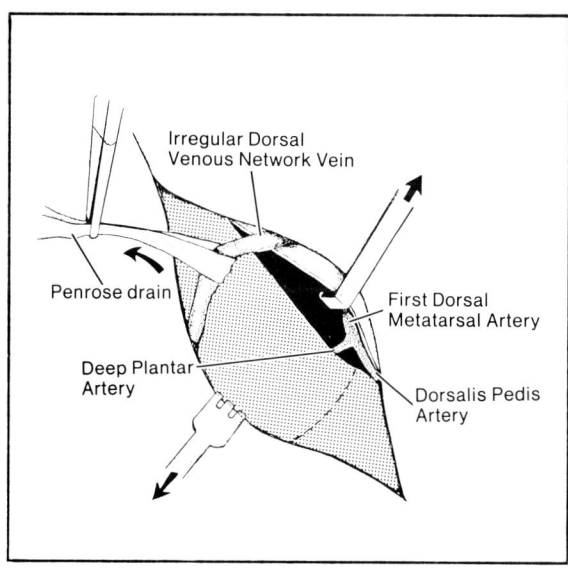

Penrose drain — Irregular Dorsal Venous Network Vein — First Dorsal Metatarsal Artery — Deep Plantar Artery — Dorsalis Pedis Artery

Fig. 7-17C

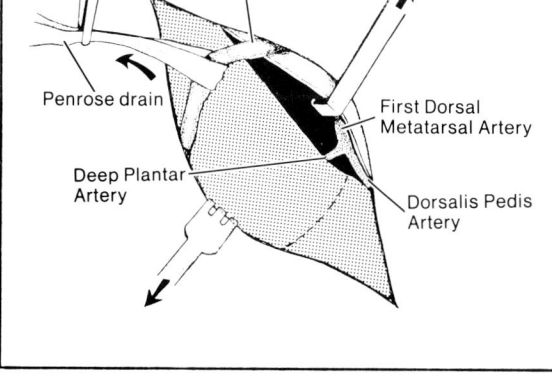

A periosteal elevator is used to retract (peel) periosteum from bone.

Fig. 7-17D

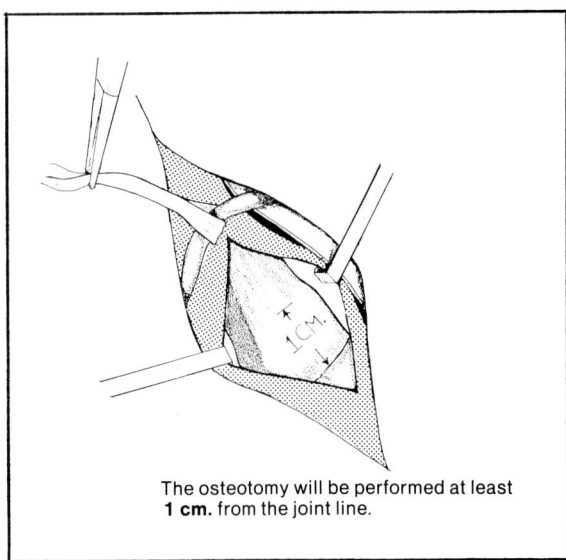

Fig. 7-17E

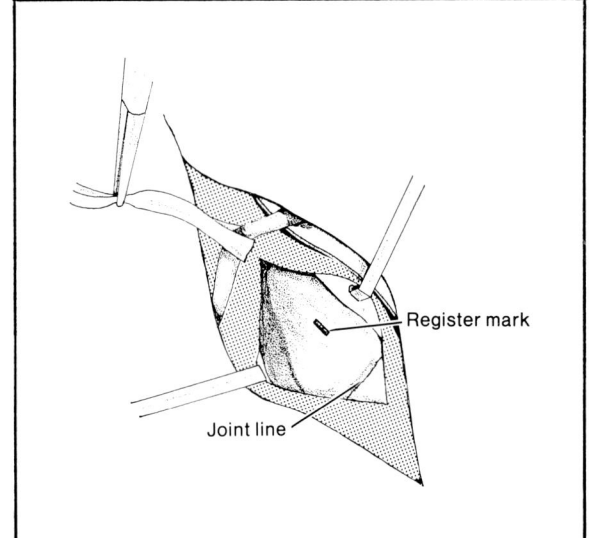

Fig. 7-17F

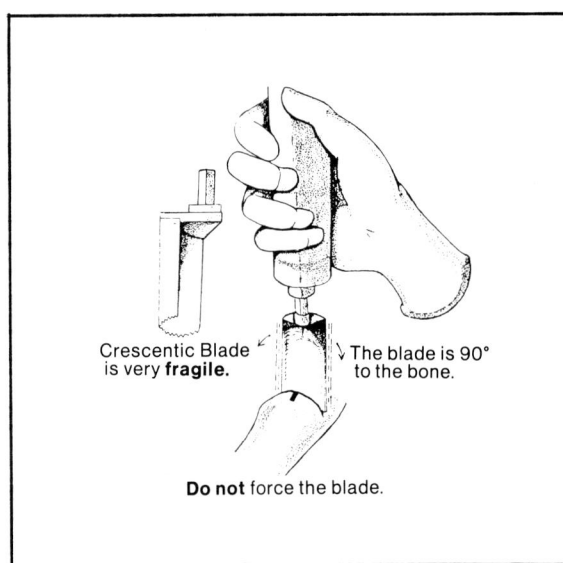

Fig. 7-11G

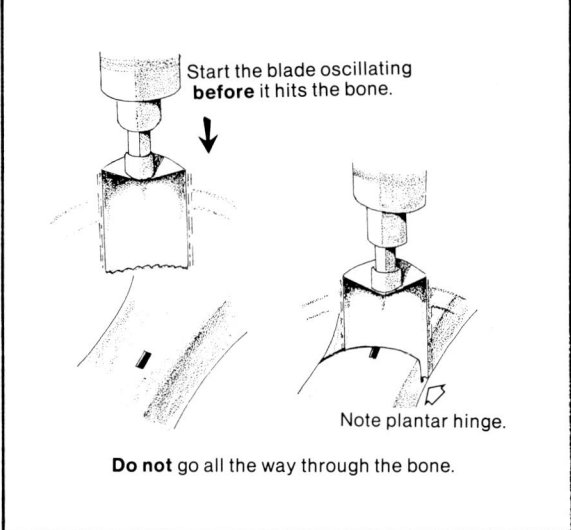

Fig. 7-17H

HALLUX VALGUS SURGERY

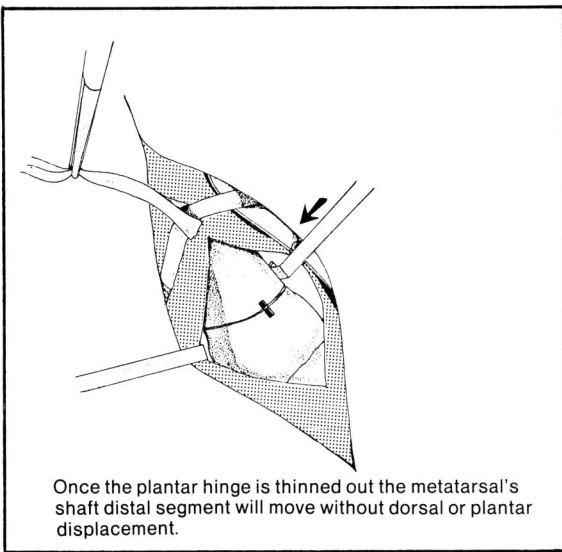

Once the plantar hinge is thinned out the metatarsal's shaft distal segment will move without dorsal or plantar displacement.

Fig. 7-17I

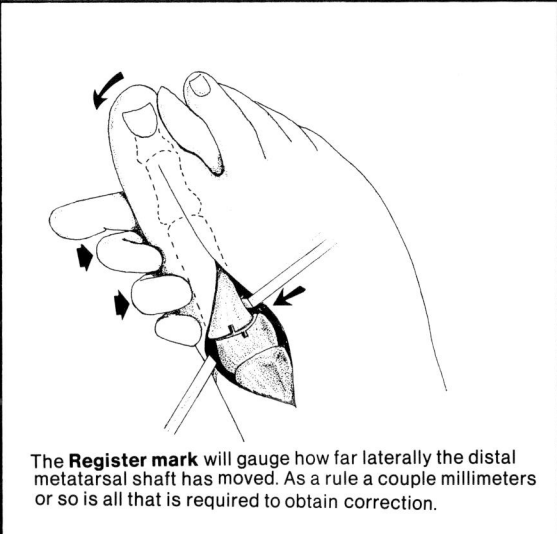

The **Register mark** will gauge how far laterally the distal metatarsal shaft has moved. As a rule a couple millimeters or so is all that is required to obtain correction.

Fig. 7-17J

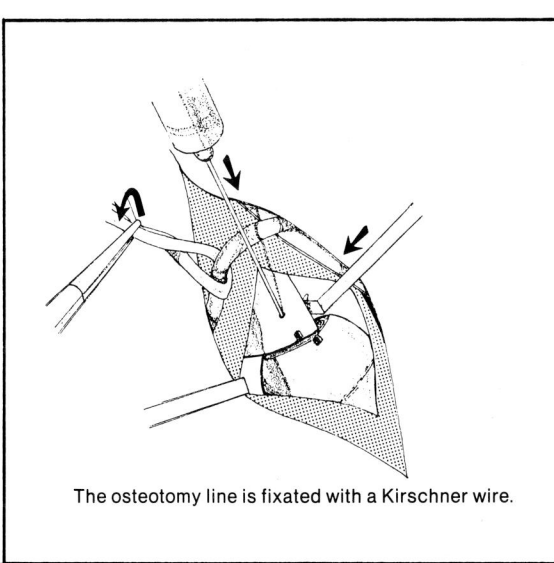

The osteotomy line is fixated with a Kirschner wire.

Fig. 7-17K

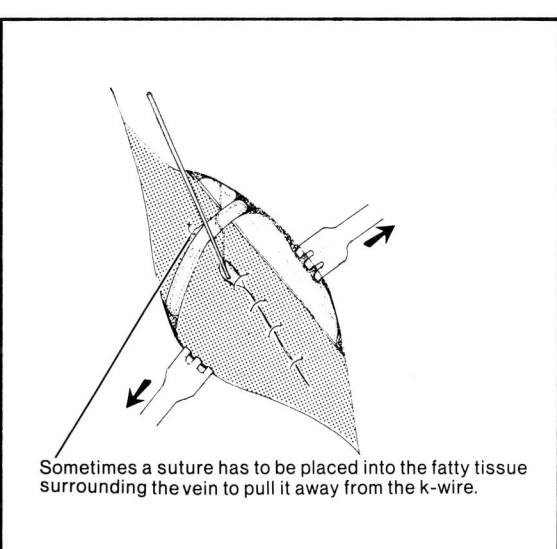

Sometimes a suture has to be placed into the fatty tissue surrounding the vein to pull it away from the k-wire.

Fig. 7-17L

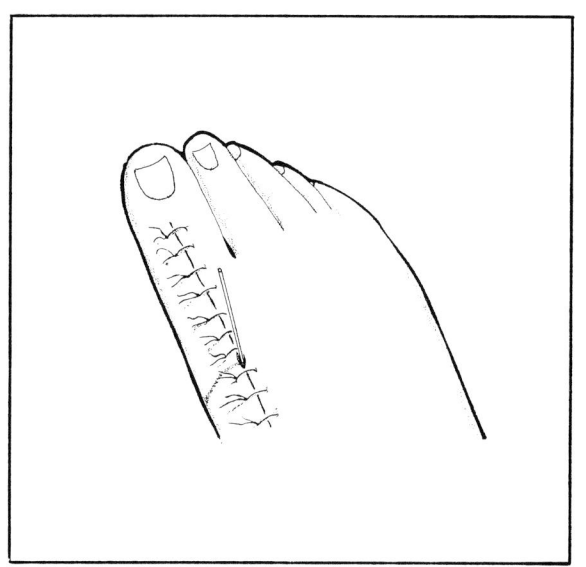

Fig. 7-17M

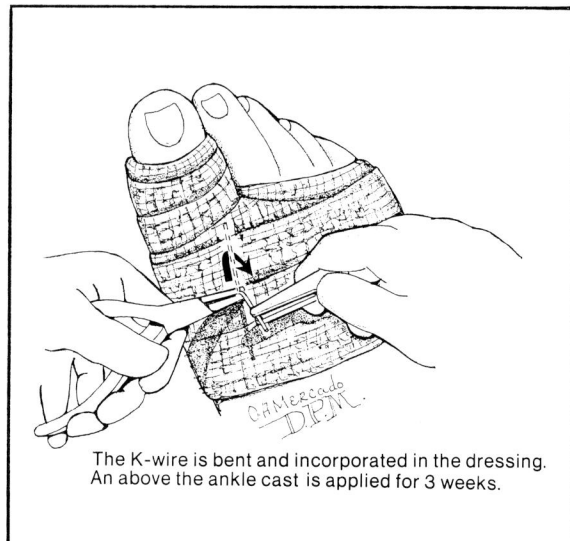

The K-wire is bent and incorporated in the dressing. An above the ankle cast is applied for 3 weeks.

Fig. 7-17N

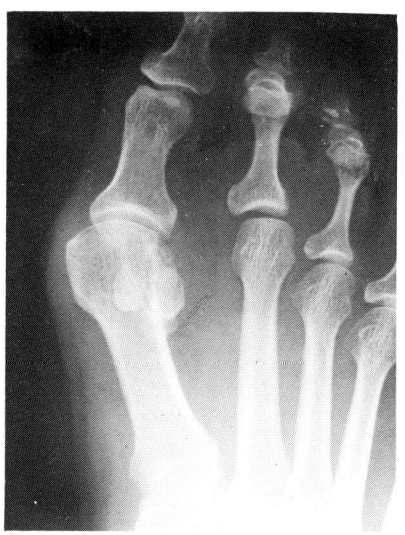

Fig. 7-18A. Pre-operative x-ray.

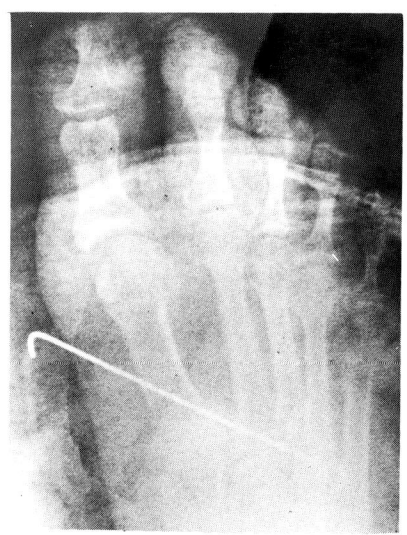

Fig. 7-18B. Proximal Crescentic Osteotomy has been performed. Since plantar hinge is used — all that is required for fixation is a single K-wire.

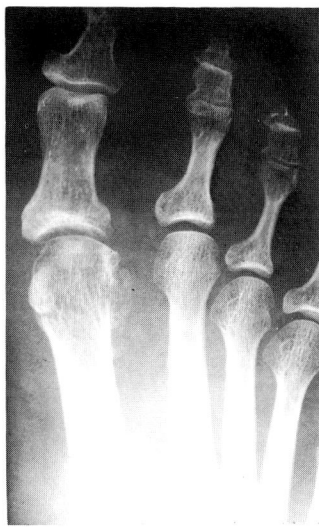

Fig. 7-18C. Three months after surgery shows excellent alignment.

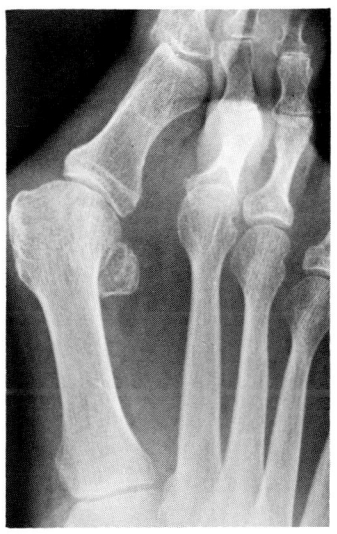

Fig. 7-19A. Pre-operative x-ray. Note metatarsus primus varus with short first ray. Also note stable first metatarsal — cuneiform joint.

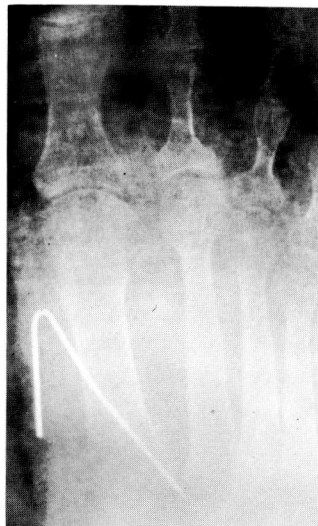

Fig. 7-19B. Post-operative x-ray. Note location of single K-wire used for fixation.

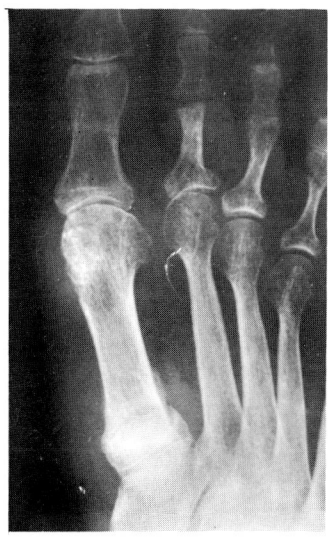

Fig. 7-19C. Three months after surgery — good correction has been achieved.

Closing Wedge Osteotomy

The Closing Wedge Osteotomy is perhaps the most common procedure used for the correction of metatarsus primus varus. The technique is easy to perform and, because of its medial hinge, exceedingly **stable.**

It is indicated for the correction of metatarsus primus varus, when the first metatarsal ray is of normal length. When the first metatarsal is short, a crescentic osteotomy should be performed to avoid a possible transfer lesion under the second metatarsal head area.

Technique

The hallux valgus problem is first corrected utilizing the technique indicated. The standard hallux valgus incision is then elongated proximally and dorsally.

The capsule and periosteum around the base of the first metatarsal are exposed and retracted in the same manner as the proximal crescentic osteotomy (fig. 7-17 B, C, D and E).

The joint line of the first metatarsal-cuneiform is identified. We then measure **at least** 1cm. (usually 1.2cm.) distal to the joint line and make a small mark with a number 15 blade (fig. 7-20A).

The shape of the wedge is carefully outlined by striking an osteotome against the bone. The wedge is placed so that its apex lies medialwards. **Remember,** it is **not** necessary to remove a great deal of bone. It is best to be on the **conservative** side — if a bigger wedge is required it is a simple matter to remove more bone (fig. 7-20B).

The wedge of bone is then resected taking care to keep both cuts angled at 90° to the bone to insure **adequate coaptation** when the osteotomy is closed (Fig. 7-20C).

The medial end of the osteotomy is carefully thinned out to the consistency of cardboard paper to create a **hinge.** This hinge is extremely important as it will only allow movement of the metatarsal shaft from medial to lateral — without dorsal or plantar displacement — thus creating a **very stable** osteotomy (fig. 7-20D).

The metatarsal shaft is then placed into its corrected position (fig. 7-20E and F). The osteotomy line is fixated with a Kirschner wire. (Fig. 7-29G). The capsule and periosteum are sutured with 3-0 Dexon after a few drops of Decadron have been infiltrated into the osteotomy site.

The wound is closed in the usual manner with the suture material of choice. The Kirschner wire is bent and incorporated in the dressing. An above the ankle cast is applied (Fig. 7-20H). The cast and wire are removed in three weeks. Healing is usually uneventful.

Conclusion

The Closing Wedge Osteotomy is easy to perform and extremely stable. However, the surgeon should keep the following points in mind to insure a trouble free osteotomy:

1. The Closing Wedge Osteotomy should **only** be used when the first metatarsal is of **normal** length (it can also be used on long metatarsals).
2. A short first metatarsal requires a crescentic osteotomy to avoid a possible transfer lesion to the second metatarsal.
3. It is **important** to create a medial hinge — to prevent dorsal or plantar displacement.
4. Fixation (K-wire is my preference) and casting are essential to insure adequate coaptation and healing of the osteotomy.

HALLUX VALGUS SURGERY

Closing Wedge Osteotomy

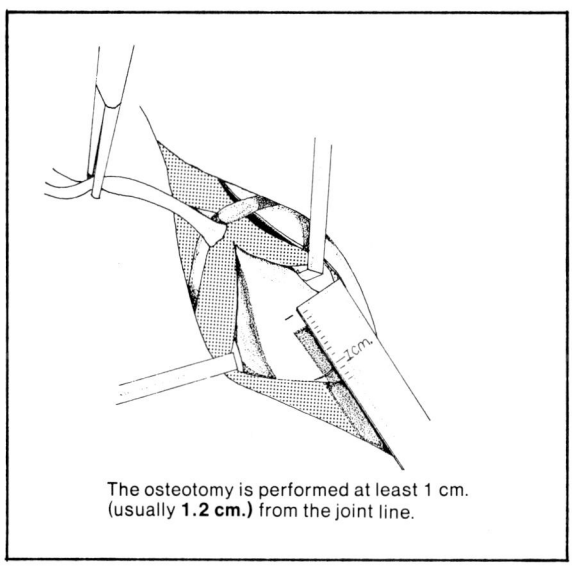

The osteotomy is performed at least 1 cm. (usually **1.2 cm.**) from the joint line.

Fig. 7-20A

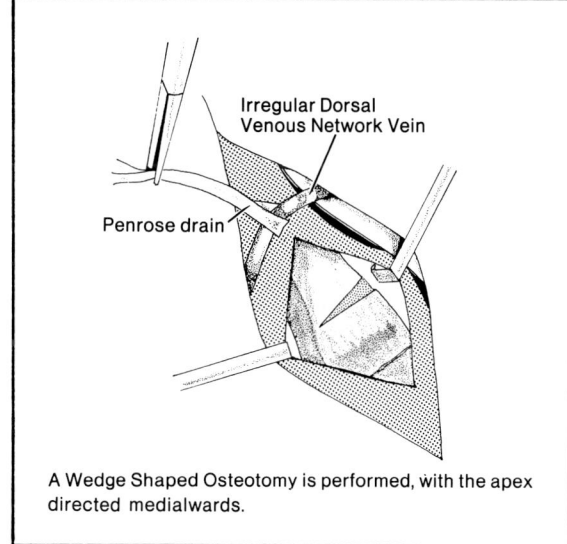

A Wedge Shaped Osteotomy is performed, with the apex directed medialwards.

Fig. 7-20B

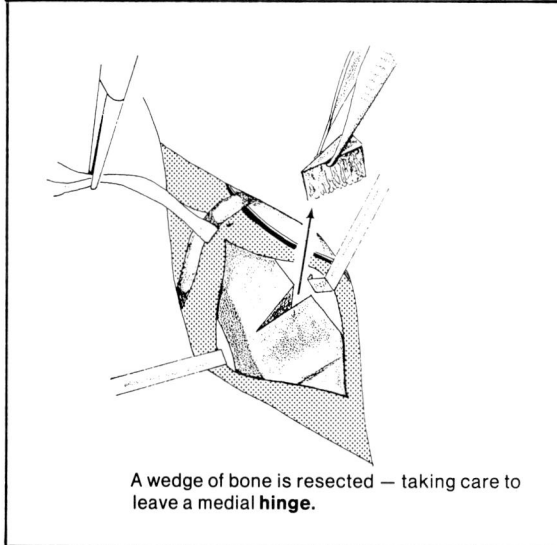

A wedge of bone is resected — taking care to leave a medial **hinge.**

Fig. 7-20C

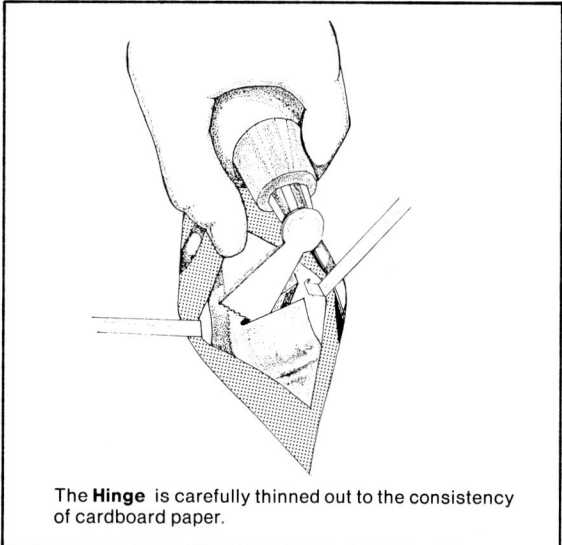

The **Hinge** is carefully thinned out to the consistency of cardboard paper.

Fig. 7-20D

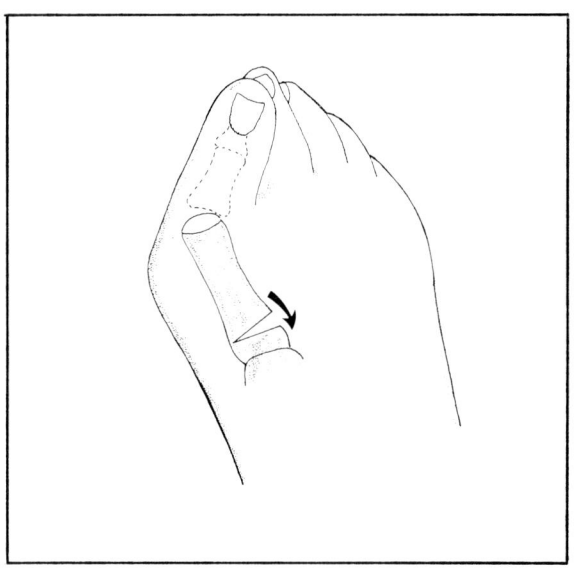

Fig. 7-20E

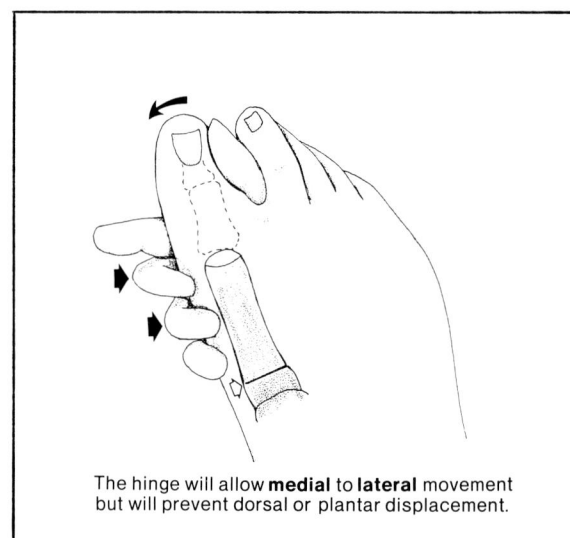

The hinge will allow **medial** to **lateral** movement but will prevent dorsal or plantar displacement.

Fig. 7-20F

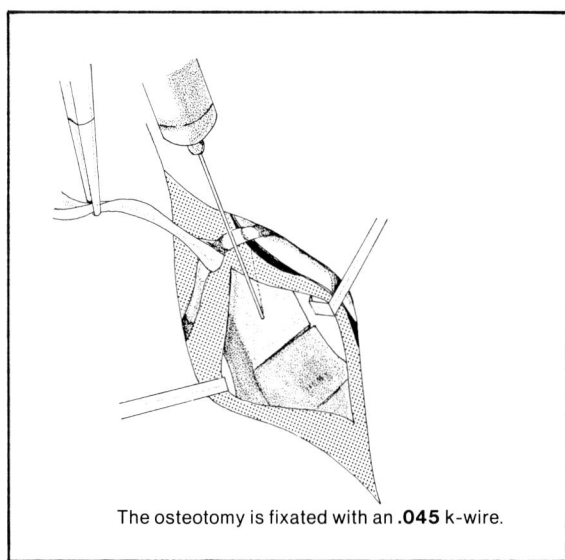

The osteotomy is fixated with an **.045** k-wire.

Fig. 7-20G

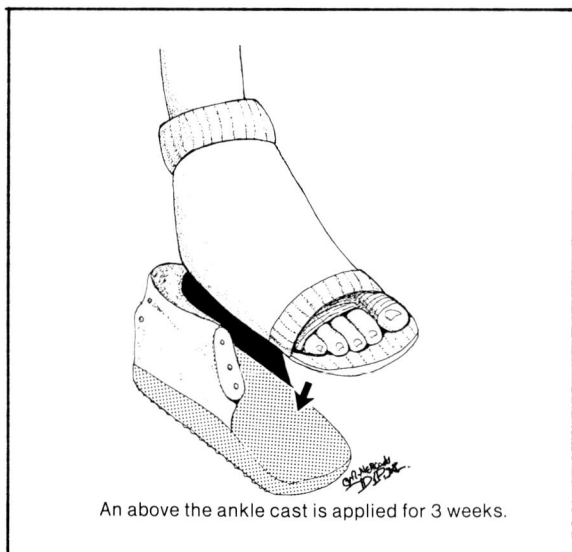

An above the ankle cast is applied for 3 weeks.

Fig. 7-20H

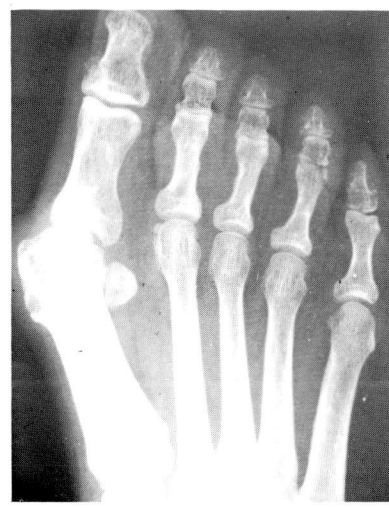 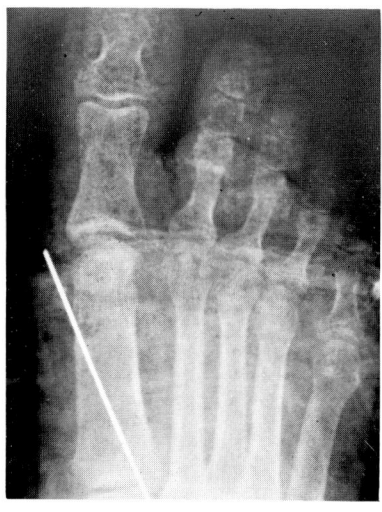

Fig. 7-21A. Pre-operative x-ray. Note **deviated** shaft causing metatarsus primus varus — compare with Fig. 7-3C (page 190).

Fig. 7-21B. Post-operative x-ray. Osteotomy line coaptation is so tight — that it is almost invisible.

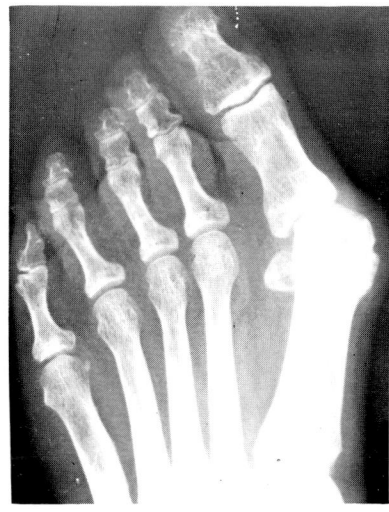 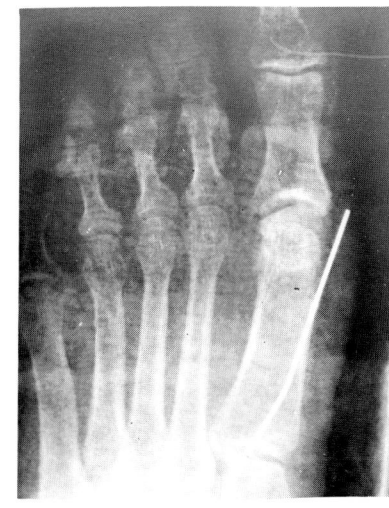

Fig. 7-21C. Pre-operative x-ray.

Fig. 7-22B. Post-operative x-ray.

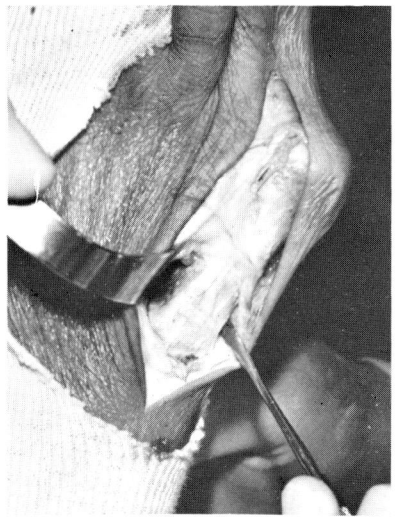

Fig. 7-23A. A periosteal elevator is used to retract (peel) the periosteum from bone.

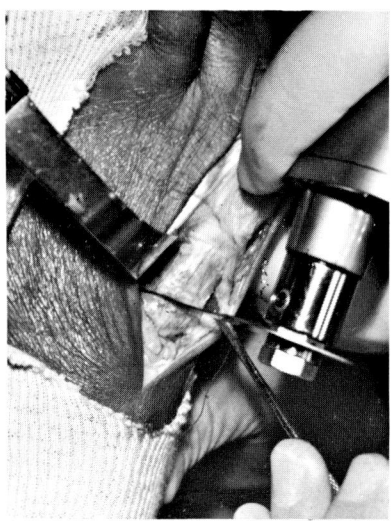

Fig. 7-23B. After careful measurements are taken — at least 1 cm. from joint line — the shape of the wedge is outlined and the osteotomy is performed. Note angle of blade in our first cut.

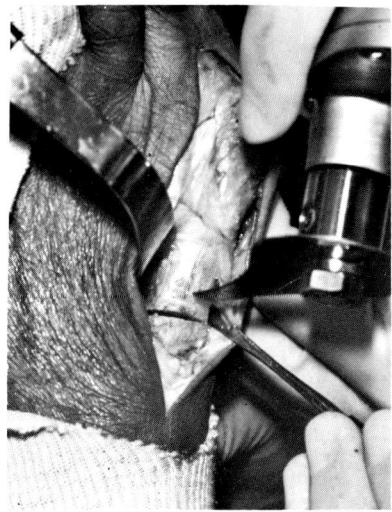

Fig. 7-23C. For the second cut the angle of the blade has changed (although it is still 90° to the bone) to create the wedge. Also note that blade is moving before coming in contact with the bone.

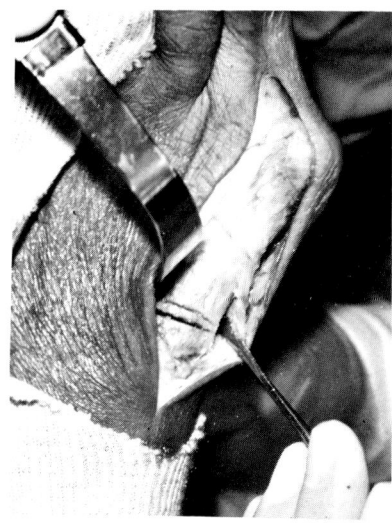

Fig. 7-23D. The apex of the wedge lies medialwards. Remember, it is **not** necessary to remove a great deal of bone.

HALLUX VALGUS SURGERY

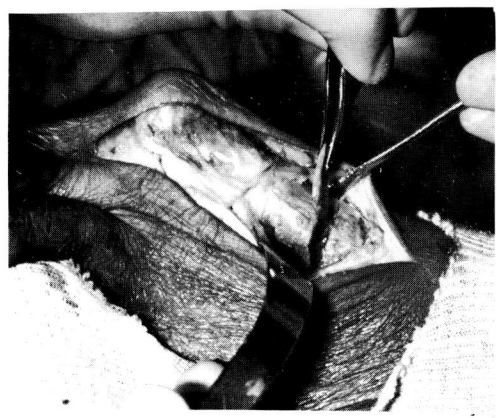

Fig. 7-23E. The wedge of bone is then resected.

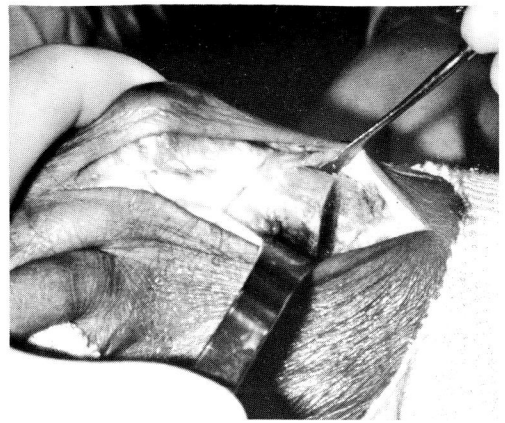

Fig. 7-23F. The medial end of the osteotomy is carefully thinned out to the consistency of cardboard paper to create a **hinge.**

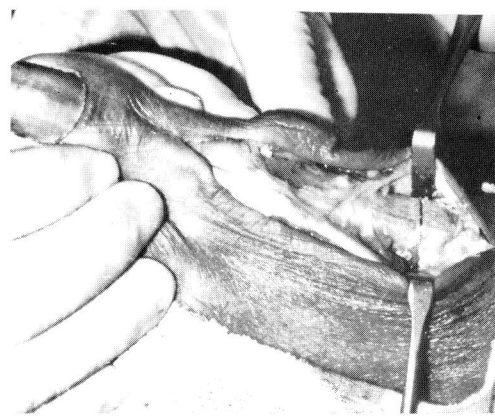

Fig. 7-23G. The metatarsal shaft is then placed into its corrected position ...

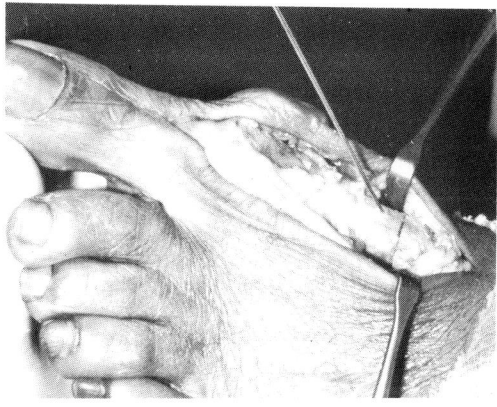

Fig. 7-23H. ... and fixated with a K-wire.

The Lapidus Operation

Paul W. Lapidus, first described his operation for the correction of metatarsus primus varus in 1934. Since that time he has been the most ardent advocate of cuneometatarsal fusion in hallux valgus surgery.

The Lapidus operation never became popular with foot surgeons, and of late it has been more in style to osteotomize the first metatarsal base to correct metatarsus primus varus.

Perhaps the main reason for the lack of popularity for the operation has been its improper use. Part of the blame must go to Lapidus, himself, who — like most early surgeons writing on hallux valgus — persisted in advocating the use of his technique for **all** hallux valgus problems. Of late, Lapidus, has been more conservative in his application of his technique. Unfortunately, many surgeons are still performing fusion of the cuneometatarsal joint when perhaps another simpler operation would have sufficed.

Indications for the Lapidus Operation

The Lapidus operation is an excellent technique for the reduction of metatarsus primus varus. When performed properly, it will markedly reduce the width of the forefoot and stabilize the first metatarsal ray segment.

The surgeon should keep the following points in mind when evaluating a patient for the Lapidus operation:

1. The Lapidus operation **will not** correct the valgus of the hallux, this has to be accomplished by another procedure (Basic bunionectomy, Reverdin, etc.). It will only correct the metatarsus primus varus deformity.
2. The Lapidus operation should only be performed when the intermetatarsal angle is 15° or more.
4. The technique **can** be performed on the elderly patients (sixth and seventh decade) as long as they are in good health, have no medical contraindications and their circulation is patent.
5. **Casting** post-operative (above the ankle cast) for three weeks is essential in order to achieve adequate fusion.
6. In our experience, external fixation with Kirschner wire, which is removed in three weeks at the time that the cast is removed, has proven to be the best method of maintaining the osteotomy site.
7. The technique can be performed bilaterally, however the patients must understand that they will have difficulties ambulating with the casts.
8. The patient with acute osteoporosis is **not** a good candidate for the technique.

Technique

The technique that we have used at Franklin Boulevard Community Hospital for a good number of years is as follows:

First, we correct the hallux valgus problem with whatever technique is indicated (Basic bunionectomy, Reverdin, etc.). The incision is then elongated dorsally and lateralwards over the first cuneometatarsal joint (see fig. 7-24A). The wound is deepened, the **extensor hallucis longus** is retracted laterally and the capsular ligament is exposed.

Anatomically speaking, we have the **dorsalis pedis artery** which terminates in two branches. The **first dorsal metatarsal artery** and the **deep plantar artery** which descends in between the bases of the first and second metatarsals (fig. 7-24B). By underscoring the capsule and periosteum from the joint line, the deep plantar will be adequately protected when the osteotomy is performed.

The cuneometatarsal joint, incidentally, is quite **unique.** Unlike the bases of the other metatarsals, which are flat or triangular in shape, the first metatarsal-cuneiform joint is kidney bean shaped and concavo-convex. The cuneiform being convex and the base of the metatarsal concave.

Once the wound is retracted to expose the capsular ligament, the capsule and periosteum are carefully underscored and retracted and the joint is exposed. We first resect the articular fascet of the cuneiform. It is not necessary to resect a **formidable** amount of bone. A slight wedge of bone is taken (see fig. 7-24C) with the base of the wedge laying laterally.

Once the cuneiform fascet has been resected, you will be surprised at the depth of the joint. The cuneometatarsal joint is approximately **2.5-3.5cm. deep,** so don't make your cut too shallow, as this will result in improper fusion.

After the cuneiform fascet is cut, the metatarsal base is easily visualized when the metatarsal shaft is plantiflexed. Visualization is even more enhanced when Seeburger Retractors are used to elevate the base (see fig. 7-24D).

Again with the power saw, the articular fascet is carefully cut. **Do not** cut more than the articular fascet, that is all that's required (see fig. 7-24E). Incidentally, since the base is concave, it is necessary to start your cut a couple of millimeters behind the joint line to ascertain the removal of the articular fascet in-toto.

The wound is thoroughly washed with saline solution, then the metatarsal ray is positioned into its proper alignment — in other words, the metatarsus primus varus is reduced (see fig. 7-24F). It is **important** when positioning the metatarsal into its corrected altitude, not to have plantar or dorsal movement as this may result in improper fusion or even a sub-luxation of the hallux valgus (fig. 7-24I).

Once the metatarsal is aligned properly, a thin Kirschner wire is driven through the cuneometatarsal joint to hold the correction in place (see fig. 7-24G).

The joint capsule is carefully closed with 2-0 Dexon and the first metatarsal-phalangeal-capsule is closed, also using 2-0 Dexon. The deep and superficial fascias are closed with 4-0 Dexon and the wound is approximated with the suture material of choice (see fig. 7-24H).

The cast and kirschner wire are removed in three weeks. The K-wire is easily removed in the office, without anesthesia. The post-operative recovery period is usually uneventful. The patient is encouraged to walk the second day post-op.

As in the findings of Charnley, the British orthopedist, clinical fusion occurs in 21 days. However, it takes months to have a complete fusion.

It is not unusual to have a patient complain after a couple of months of pain on the cuneometatarsal joint. This is usually a **traumatic arthritic flare-up,** and can be readily treated with short term cortico-steroid therapy.

Conclusion

When the Lapidus operation is performed as described here, and for the proper indications, it will yield consistently **good results.**

The important points for the surgeon to keep in mind are:

1. The Lapidus operation is used in a deviated first cuneometatarsal joint with an intermetatarsal angle of **15° or more.**
2. Take only a **very thin** wedge from the cuneiform and the articular fascet of the metatarsal base.
3. Move the metatarsal in one plane **only,** medial to lateral. Movement in other planes, dorsal or plantar, can result in improper fusion; sub-luxation of the hallux or even a transfer lesion to the second metatarsal head (fig. 7-24I).
4. Maintain a **cast** for at least three weeks.

The Lapidus Operation

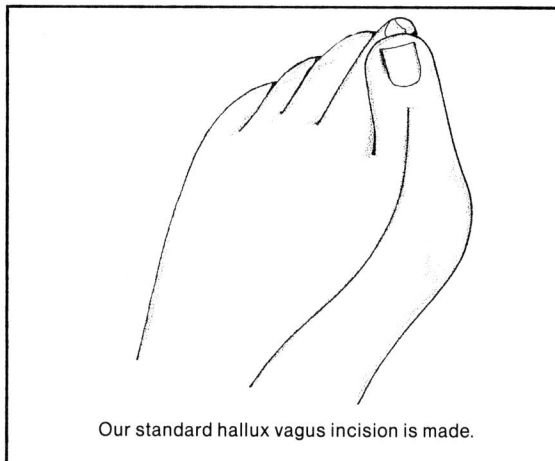

Our standard hallux vagus incision is made.

Fig. 7-24A

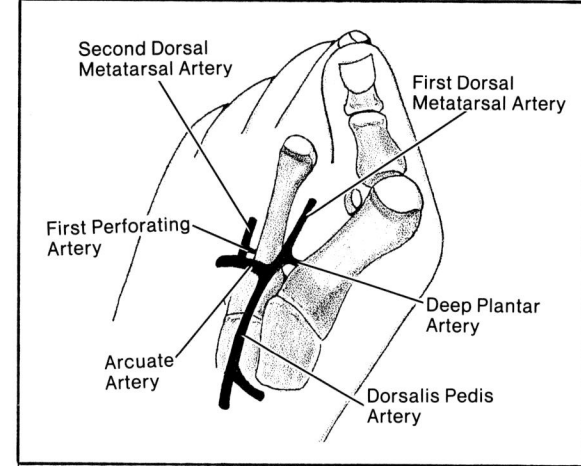

Fig. 7-24B

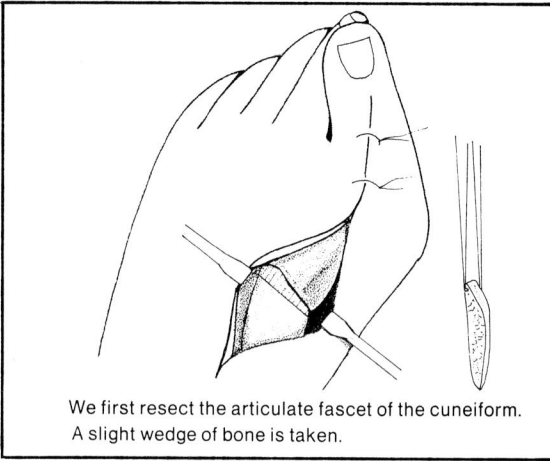

We first resect the articulate fascet of the cuneiform. A slight wedge of bone is taken.

Fig. 7-24D

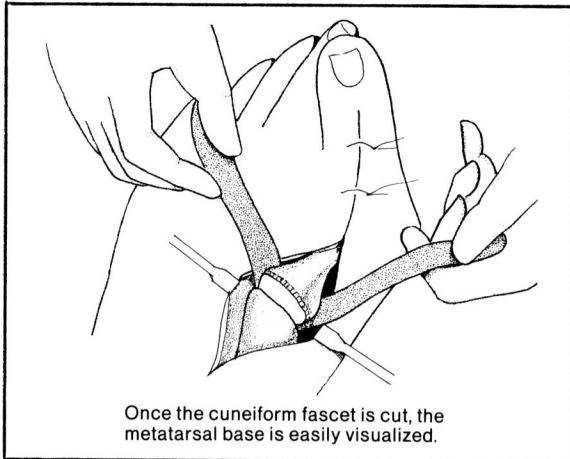

Once the cuneiform fascet is cut, the metatarsal base is easily visualized.

Fig. 7-24C

HALLUX VALGUS SURGERY

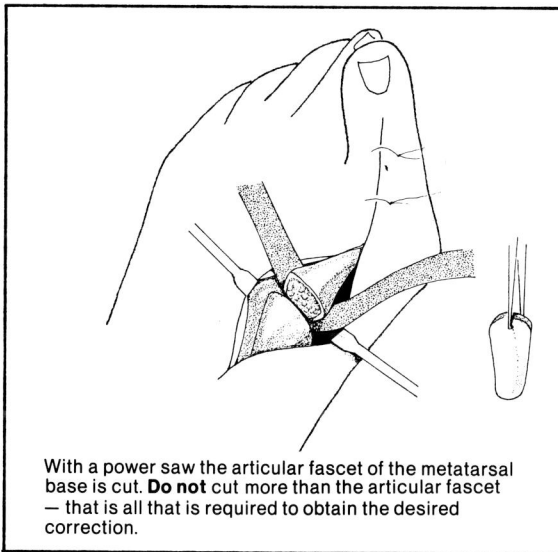

With a power saw the articular fascet of the metatarsal base is cut. **Do not** cut more than the articular fascet — that is all that is required to obtain the desired correction.

Fig. 7-24E

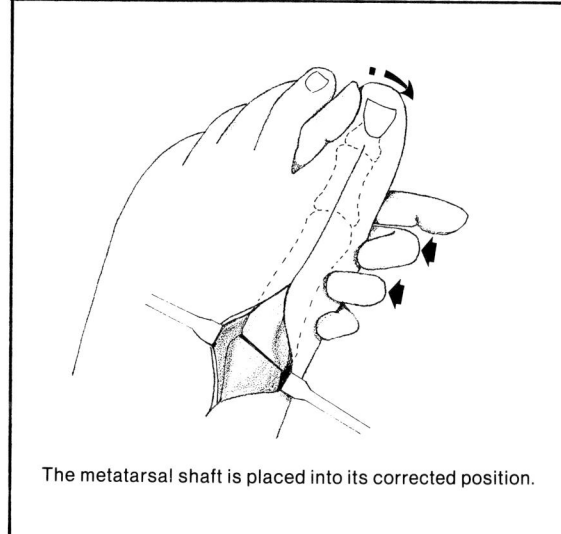

The metatarsal shaft is placed into its corrected position.

Fig. 7-24F

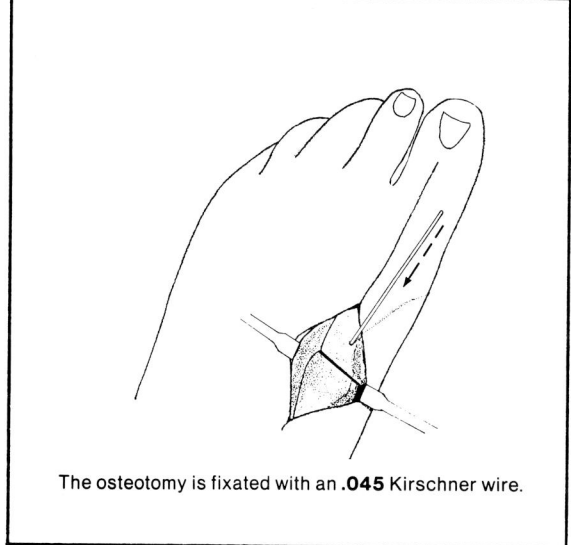

The osteotomy is fixated with an **.045** Kirschner wire.

Fig. 7-24G

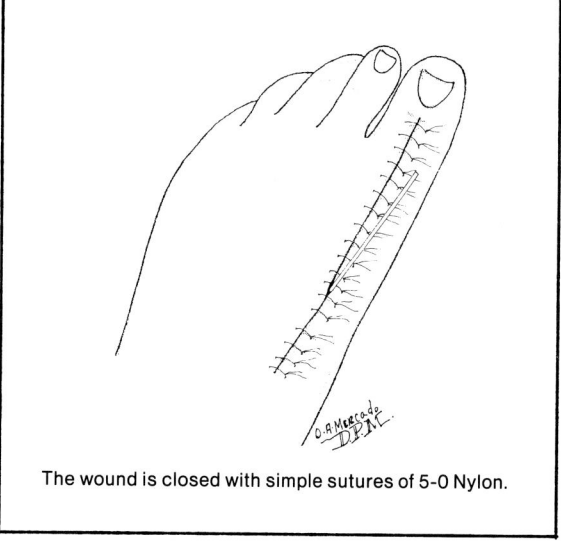

The wound is closed with simple sutures of 5-0 Nylon.

Fig. 7-24H

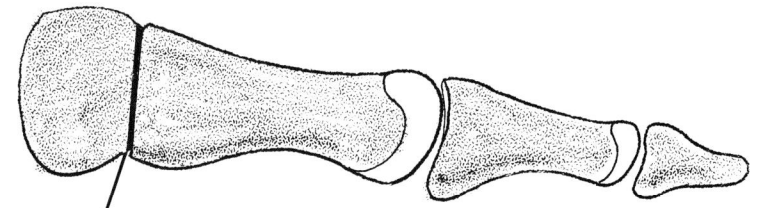

Properly angled osteotomy is easy to fixate and will **heal** uneventfully.

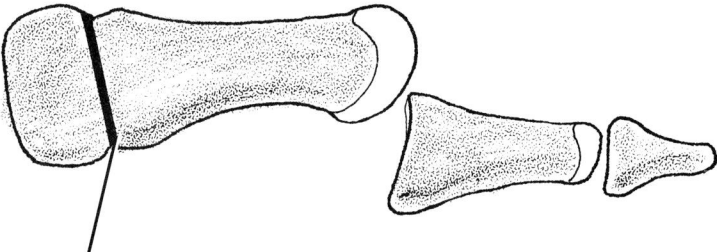

This osteotomy was angulated causing dorsi-flexion and plantar dislocation.

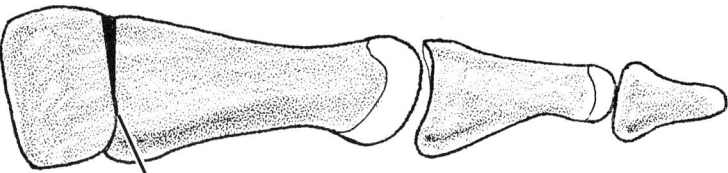

This osteotomy **did not** go plantarwards enough — thus causing an improperly healed osteotomy site.

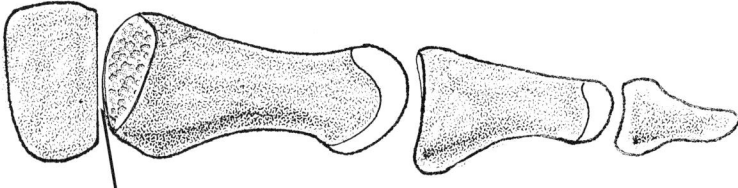

Too much bone was taken — resulting in a mal-healed osteotomy.

Fig. 7-241

HALLUX VALGUS SURGERY

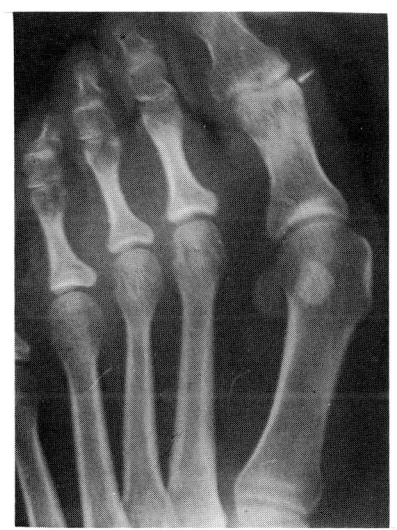

Fig. 7-25A. Pre-operative x-ray

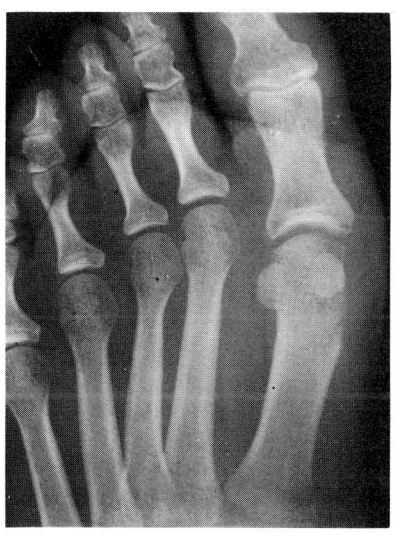

Fig. 7-25B. Six-months after surgery. Note fusion of first metatarsal-cuneiform joint.

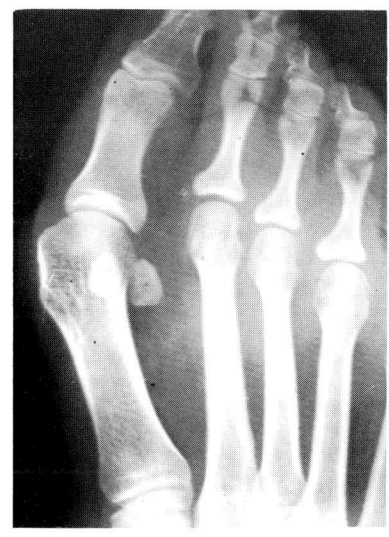

Fig. 7-26A. Pre-operative x-ray.

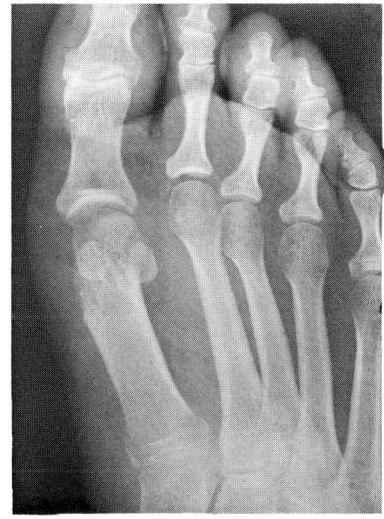

Fig. 7-26B. Post-operative x-ray. Note alignment of sesamoids and first ray.

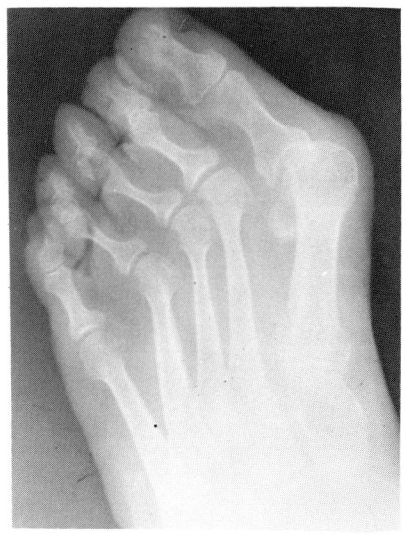

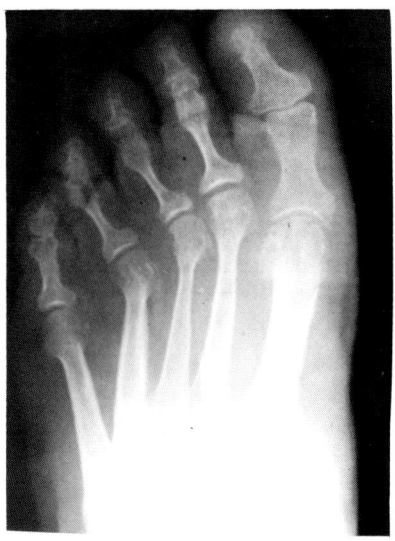

Fig. 7-27A. Pre-operative x-ray. Note acute lateral deviation of hallux and lesser three toes.

Fig. 7-27B. One year post-op. A Lapidus Operation was performed, nothing was done to the lesser toes. Since the first ray was **stabilized**, the toes can now function normally — *structure follows function.*

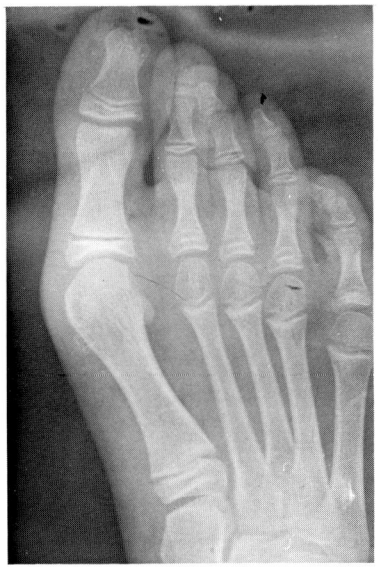

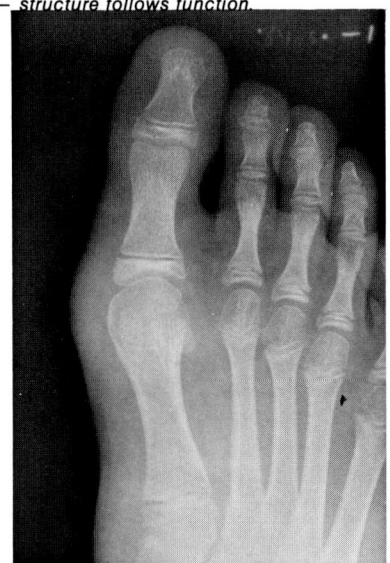

Fig. 7-28A. Pre-operative x-ray of twelve year old girl. Note deviated first metatarsal-cuneiform joint (see Fig. 7-3B).

Fig. 7-28B. A modified Lapidus was performed, a wedge was taken from the cuneiform — nothing was done to the base of the metatarsal.

HALLUX VALGUS SURGERY

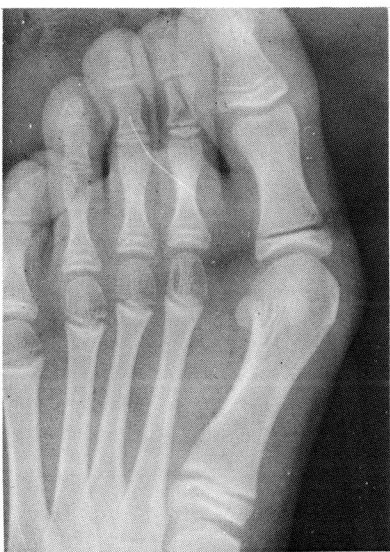 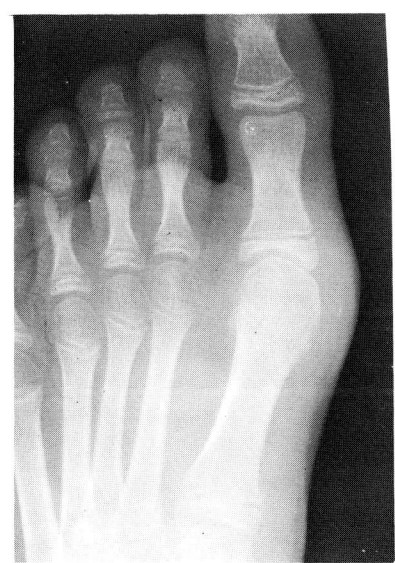

Fig. 7-29A. Pre-operative x-ray, note epiphyseal plates.

Fig. 7-29B. Post-operative x-ray. A wedge was taken from the anterior aspect of the cuneiform. The cartilage on the base of the metatarsal was left intact. Correction was excellent.

Silicone Rubber Implants

Silicone rubber implants for surgery of the great toe were introduced in 1965 by **Dr. Alfred B. Swanson.** After many years of research — with a great variety of materials — Dr. Swanson created a flexible implant to replace the base of the proximal phalanx. This implant has been extremely useful and, when used for the proper indications, will stand up under long-term use.

Dow-Corning Corporation, who manufacturers the implant, has conducted **mechanical stress tests** in a specially designed machine which simulates the action of the first metatarsal phalangeal joint. During testing, the implant was able to withstand the **stress** of **250,000,000** movements — the equivalent of walking around the earth **101 Times.**

Today, there are two types of silicone rubber implants used for the metatarsal phalangeal joints. The **hemi-implant,** used to replace the base of the proximal phalanx; and the **total joint implant,** used to replace the complete metatarsal phalangeal joint.

Precautions

There are some important points that should be covered before we go into the actual surgical technique. First, it is important that the patient be properly **educated** as to what the **implant will do** and what **it cannot do.**

In this television age of Marcus Welby and The Six Million Dollar Man, it is easy enough for a patient to have **unrealistic expectations** from surgery — specially when we use the terms **joint implant** or **joint replacement.**

In my practice, I refer to the implant as a **spacer.** I tell the patient that we **cannot** create a joint that will be as good as a **normal** one. We can, however, by replacing the arthritic portions of the bone with a special rubber-like spacer, create a **pain free joint** which will have a **good range of motion.**

I am careful to point out that the big toe will stay slightly elevated on weight bearing and **will not** be able to **purchase** as well as the other toes. Also, I **frankly** tell the patient that in the literature there have been incidents where the spacer had to be removed, resulting in a shorter hyper-mobile toe. However, I also point out that in my experience I have had to remove only **two spacers.** One was in a patient who accidentally dropped a large can on his toe, fracturing the implant; and another in a patient who, after the surgery, formed an exostosis on the metatarsal head which rubbed against the implant — resulting in an inclusion cyst forming around the small fragments rubbed off from the implant. In both cases, we were able to **successfully** replace the defective implants with new ones.

Indications for the Hemi Implant

1. **Hallux Rigidus,** where the articulate cartilage of the proximal phalanx is so destroyed that it cannot be remodeled.

2. **Rheumatoid Arthritic** changes within the metatarsal phalangeal joint. In advance cases, a total implant joint is used.

3. **Revision Surgery** for unstable or painful joints following Keller procedures or resection of proximal bases which have led to accordion type toes.

4. **Freiberg Infraction,** when the base of the proximal phalanx cannot be remodeled.

5. **Hallux Valgus,** where the phalangeal base cartilage is destroyed; or in cases with an extremely long proximal phalanx.

Technique for Hemi-Implant

The surgical technique utilized is essentially the same for all indications. For our purposes here, we will illustrate a typical **Hallux Rigidus** case.

As we can see in our illustration in fig. 7-30A, a **normal** first metatarsal phalangeal joint can be readily dorsi-flexed with little trouble and **no pain.** In a patient where a Hallux Rigidus is present, the articular facets have undergone arthritic changes resulting in **articular lipping** (Fig. 7-30B). This lipping will cause a great deal of pain and prevent **dorsi-flexion** of the joint.

Our approach to the joint is by a standard hallux valgus incision (fig. 7-30C). The wound is deepened and the metatarsal head is exposed in the usual manner. Our illustration (Fig. 7-30D) reveals a typical arthritic metatarsal head — note the great amount of arthritic lipping and **cartilagenous changes** found.

The hypertrophic eminence is resected (Fig. 7-30E). Care is taken to aim our osteotome so as to **preserve** the medial articular facet (the crista) for the medial sesamoid.

The hypertrophic dorsal lipping is also carefully removed (Fig. 7-30F). Our aim is to remodel the metatarsal head so as to create a more **normal** looking and functioning metatarsal head.

The base of the proximal phalanx is exposed and carefully examined (fig. 7-30G). If the cartilage on the base is viable, then we just merely remove the hypertrophic lipping around the base and then carefully close the wound in the usual manner (Fig. 7-30H).

If, however, the articular cartilage is **destroyed** (Fig. 7-30I), we then replace the base of the phalanx with a Silastic® Implant.

In order to successfully replace the base with the implant, the bone has to be cut in a very **exacting manner.** As shown at the top of our fig. 7-30J, the amount of the phalangeal base removed must be equal or slightly larger than the **collar** of the replacing implant. Also, when the osteotomy is performed, the blade must be at 90° to the bone so that a straight cut is achieved — this will allow the implant to be inserted at the **proper angle** once the medullary canal is reamed out.

The illustration in Fig. 7-30K, shows what can happen when the surgeon makes the cut at less than 90° — the osteotomy is angulated. When the medullary canal is reamed out, the implant will go in **improperly** and will not function adequately.

The singularly **most important** step in the successful application of a Silastic® Implant is the proper preparation of the medullary canal for the acceptance of the **implant stem.** We first find the opening to the medullary canal with a very thin periosteal elevator. Next, using a small drill bit, we carefully fashion a **cave-like canal** which conforms to the shape of implant stem — flat on the bottom and sides, and dome-shaped dorsally (Fig. 7-30L). The canal is reamed out deep enough to accept most of the implant stem. As a rule, the stem is too long and a small piece has to be cut off from the tip.

While the medullary canal is being reamed out, its size and depth is tested with a Silastic® sizer. The proper implant size is chosen by trying the different sizes until we find the one that fits well. In fig. 7-30M, we see a lateral view of the metatarsal head. The top implant is too large; the middle one is too small, the bottom implant is the proper size.

On a dorsal-plantar view (Fig. 7-30N) we again try to pick the proper size for the metatarsal head — the implant on the right hand side is the perfect size. Incidentally, the most common size that we use is a **No. 2** implant.

Once the medullary canal has been fashioned into the right size and depth, a few drops of a cortico-steriod solution (Decadron) are instilled into the canal. This will cut down the inflammatory reaction, caused by the implant, and lessen post-operative pain (Fig 7-30O).

The surgeon asks for the proper size implant and the nurse places it in a cup filled with **saline solution.** Using blunt ended forceps, the implant is held and the desired amount from the tip of the stem is cut — as the stem is usually too long.

It is **important** to note that the implant is only handled with instruments. Silicone rubber, because of **static electricity,** can attract dust and lint which can create a great deal of inflammation post-operatively.

The implant is then carefully inserted into the reamed out medullary canal (fig. 7-30P). The wound is closed in the usual manner. Healing is usually uneventful.

Conclusion:

Silicone rubber implants have been heaven sent for the arthritic patients. When properly used, they can reward the surgeon with some of his most gratifying cases. To insure consistently good results the surgeon should:

1. Make sure that the patient has been **properly educated** as to what the implant can do and what it cannot do.
2. Warn the patient that sometimes the implants have to be **removed.**
3. Follow the **proper indications** for the use of the implant.
4. Take **meticulous care** when cutting the bone and in preparing the medullary canal for the insertion of the implant stem.
5. Use a few drops of a **corticosteroid** in the medullary canal before inserting the implant — this will keep postoperative inflammation down to a minimum.
6. Handle the implant **only** with instruments to avoid dust and lint adhering to it.
7. Do not use an implant when a **simpler** procedure will suffice.

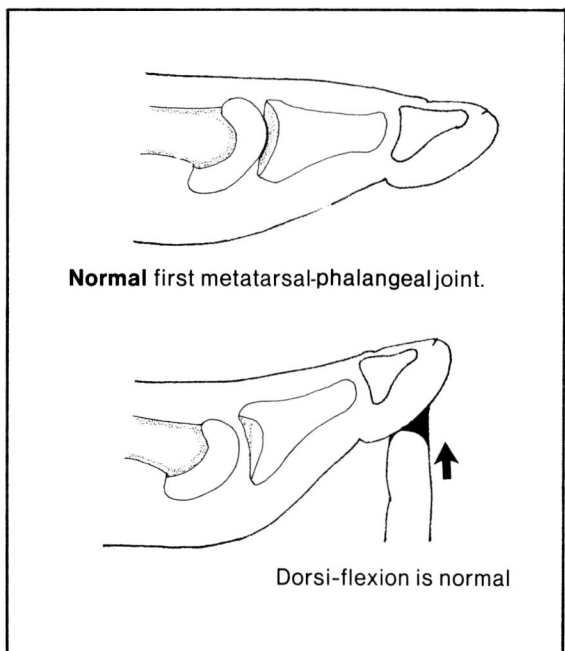

Fig. 7-30A

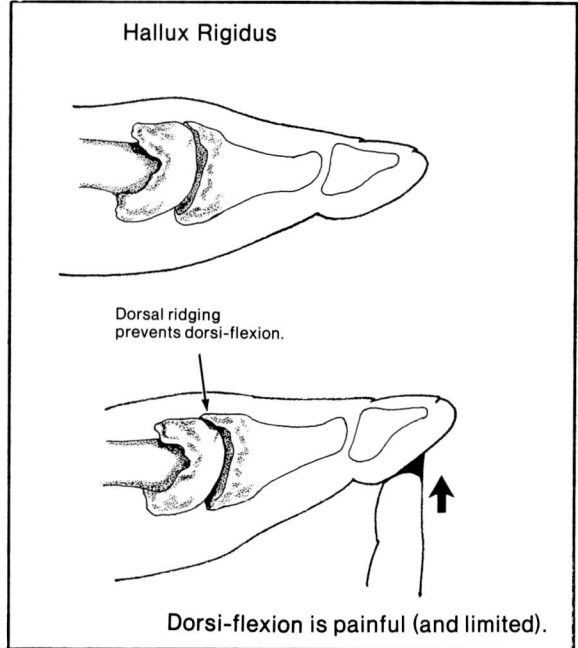

Fig. 7-30B

HALLUX VALGUS SURGERY

Technique for Hemi-Implant

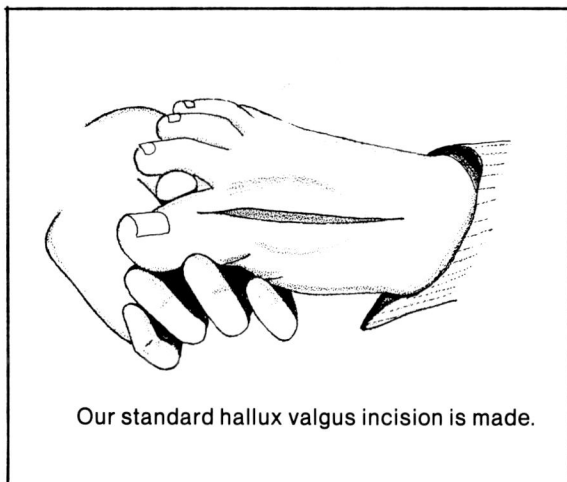

Our standard hallux valgus incision is made.

Fig. 7-30C

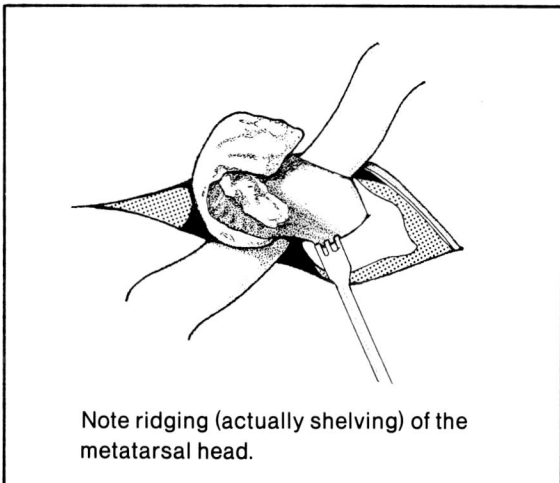

Note ridging (actually shelving) of the metatarsal head.

Fig. 7-30D

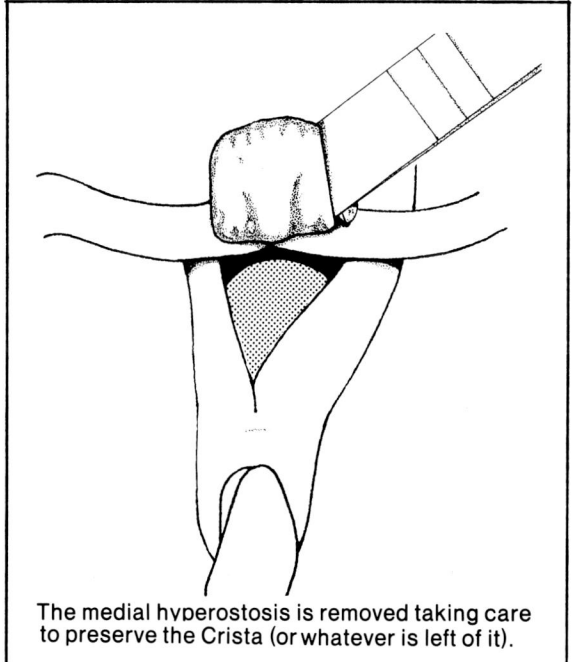

The medial hyperostosis is removed taking care to preserve the Crista (or whatever is left of it).

Fig. 7-30E

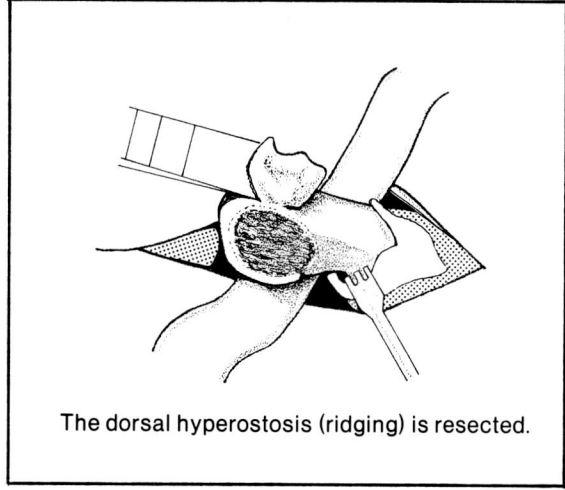

The dorsal hyperostosis (ridging) is resected.

Fig. 7-30F

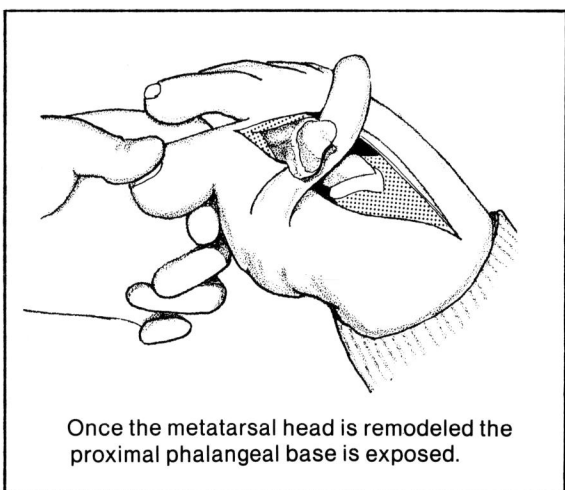

Once the metatarsal head is remodeled the proximal phalangeal base is exposed.

Fig. 7-30G

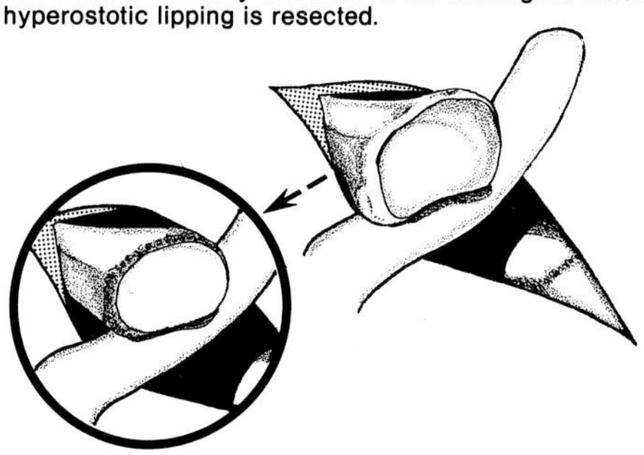

The head is carefully examined if the cartilage is **viable** — then the hyperostotic lipping is resected.

The base is remodeled — a **silastic®** implant **is not** needed.

Fig. 7-30H

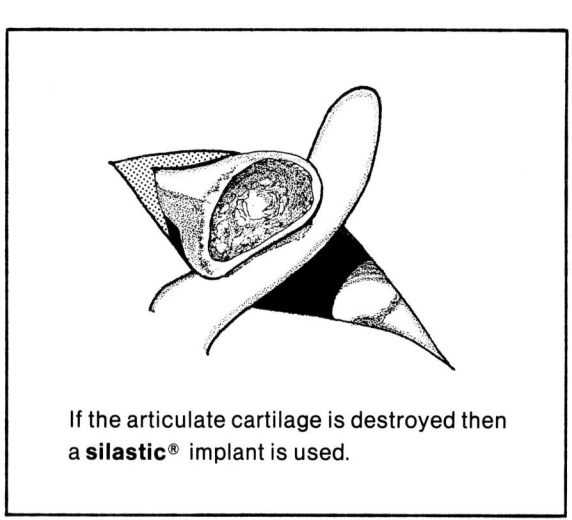

If the articulate cartilage is destroyed then a **silastic®** implant is used.

Fig. 7-30I

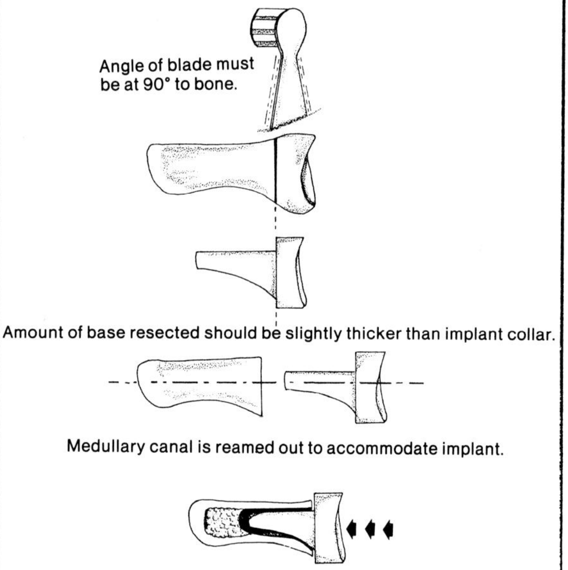

Angle of blade must be at 90° to bone.

Amount of base resected should be slightly thicker than implant collar.

Medullary canal is reamed out to accommodate implant.

Properly fitting implant will insure a long-lasting trouble-free implant.

Fig. 7-30J

HALLUX VALGUS SURGERY

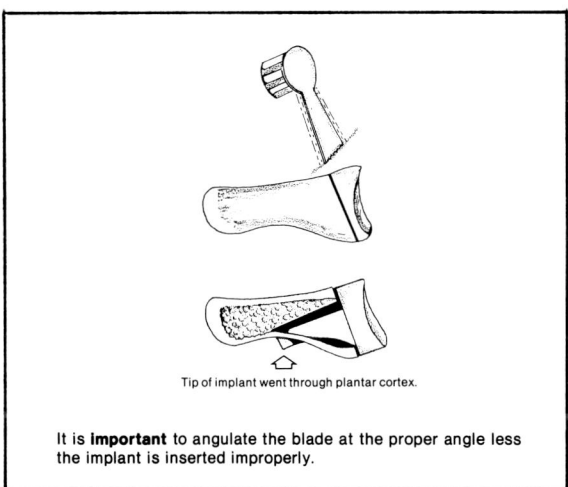

It is **important** to angulate the blade at the proper angle less the implant is inserted improperly.

Fig. 7-30K

The most **important** step of the operation is the preparation of the medullary canal — so that the implant fits well.

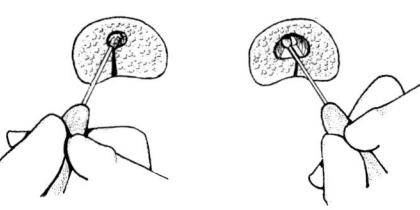

First, the medullary canal is identified — then using a small drill bit the canal is remodeled to resemble the shape of the implant stem.

Fig. 7-30L

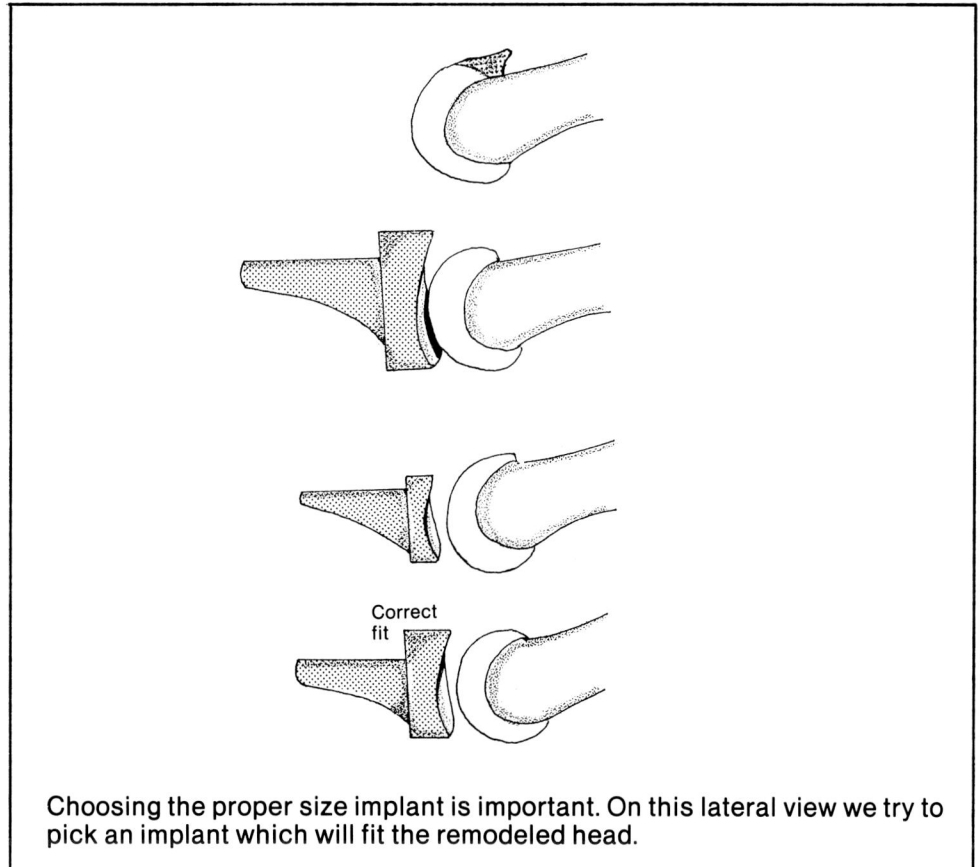

Choosing the proper size implant is important. On this lateral view we try to pick an implant which will fit the remodeled head.

Fig. 7-30M

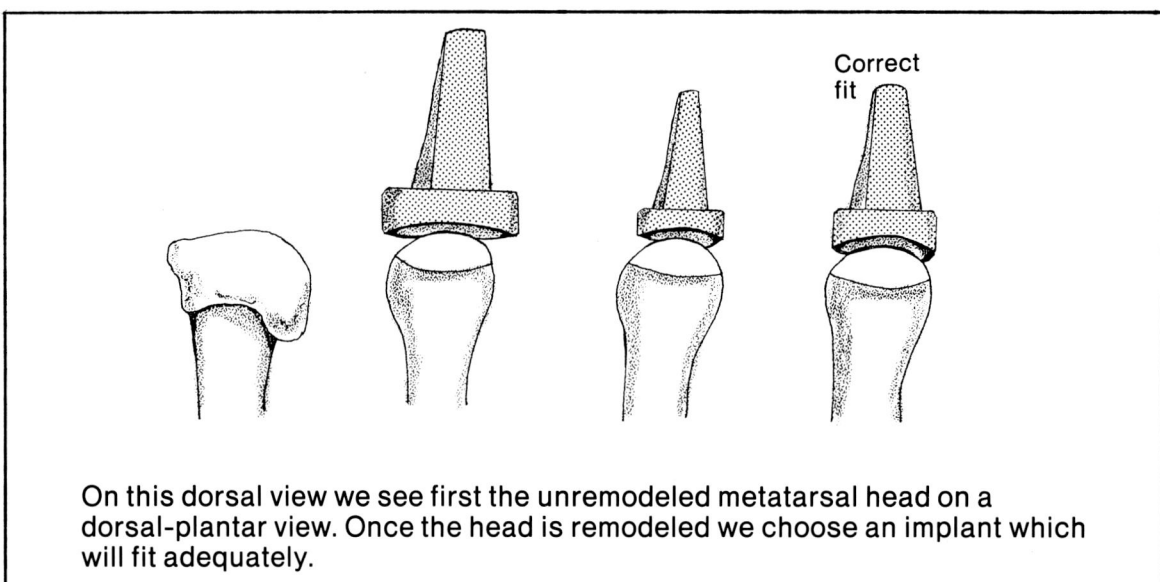

On this dorsal view we see first the unremodeled metatarsal head on a dorsal-plantar view. Once the head is remodeled we choose an implant which will fit adequately.

Fig. 7-30N

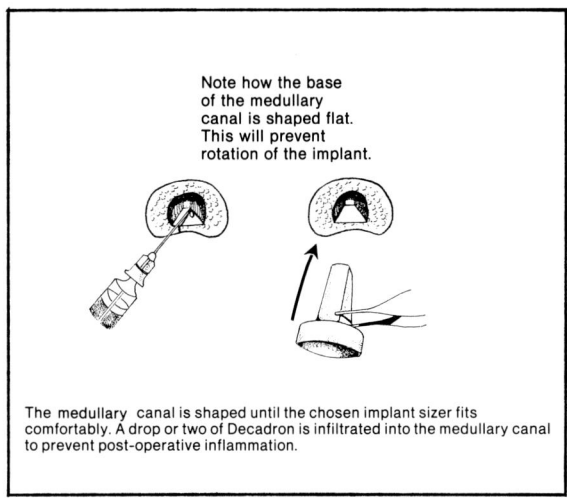

Note how the base of the medullary canal is shaped flat. This will prevent rotation of the implant.

The medullary canal is shaped until the chosen implant sizer fits comfortably. A drop or two of Decadron is infiltrated into the medullary canal to prevent post-operative inflammation.

Fig. 7-30O

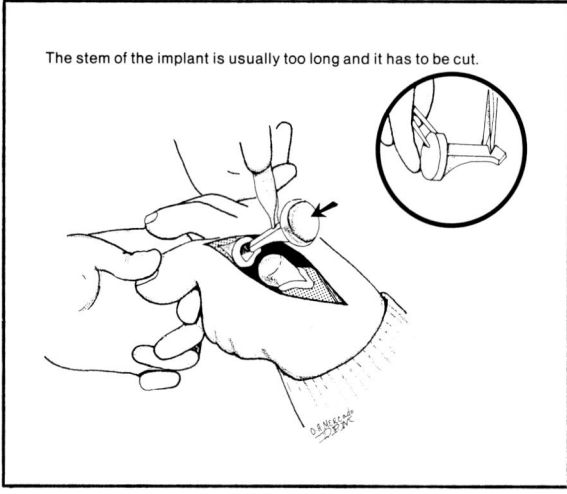

The stem of the implant is usually too long and it has to be cut.

Fig. 7-30P

HALLUX VALGUS SURGERY

Technique for Hemi-Implant

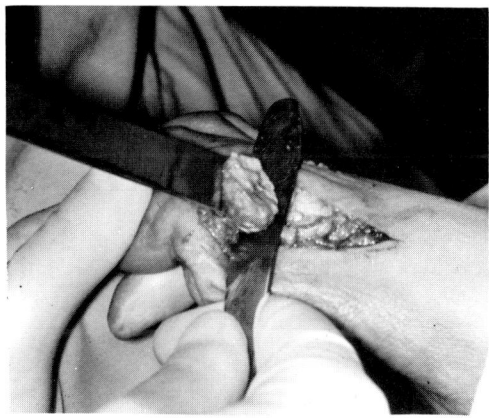

Fig. 7-31A. The base of the proximal phalanx is exposed and examined. Here we see that the cartilage is destroyed. The amount of bone to be removed is marked with an osteotome ...

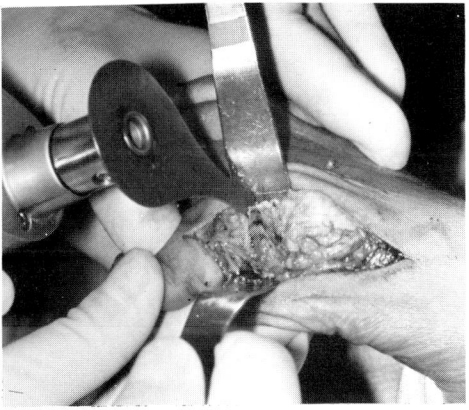

Fig. 7-31B. ... and removed with power equipment. Note that angle of blade is 90° to the bone.

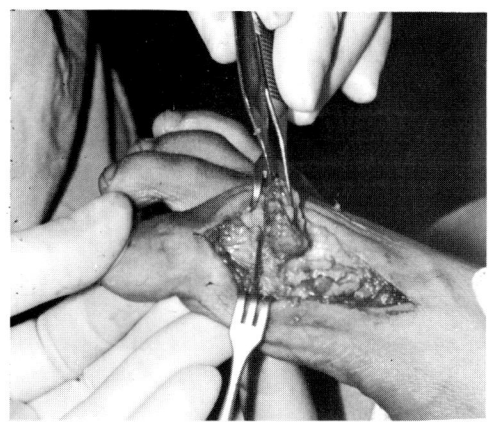

Fig. 7-31C. The base is resected.

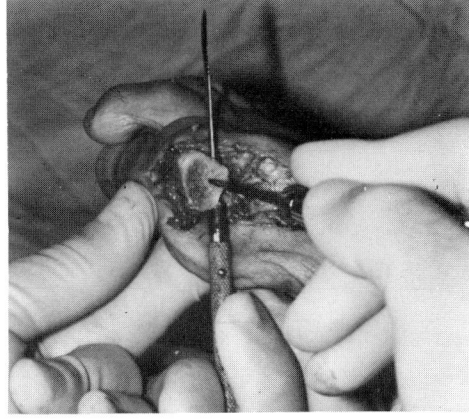

Fig. 7-31D. The most **important** step of the operation is the preparation of the medullary canal.

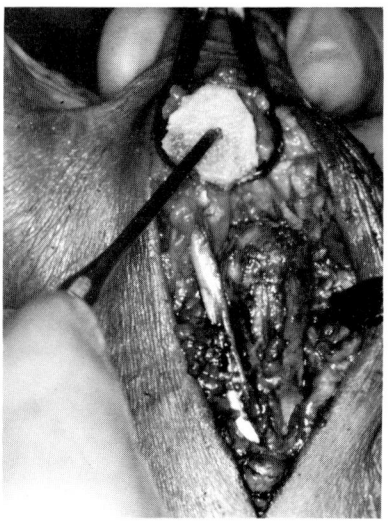

Fig. 7-31E. First we find the opening to the medullary using a thin periosteal elevator.

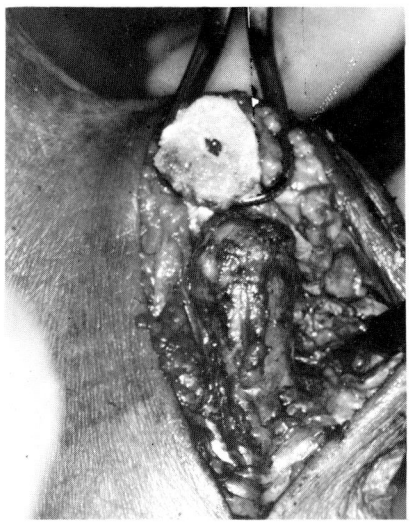

Fig. 7-31F. The meduallary canal is marked.

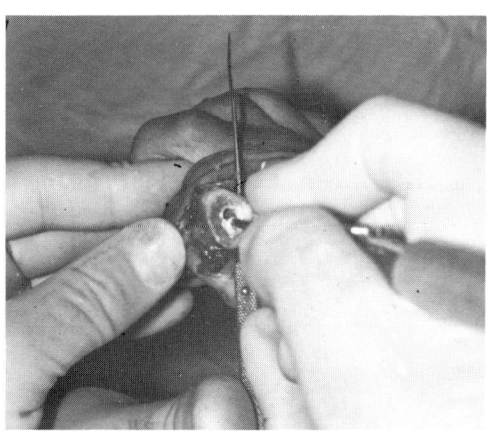

Fig. 7-31G. Using a **small** drill bit, we carefully fashion a cave-like canal.

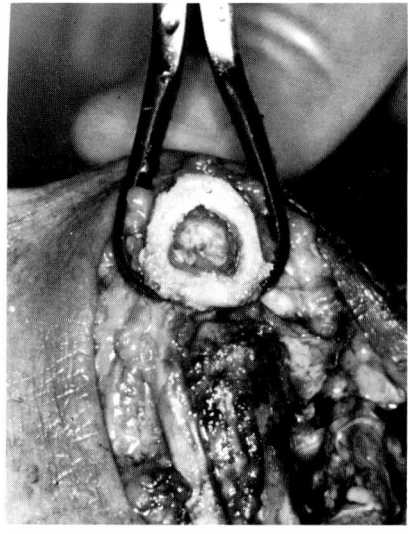

Fig. 7-31H. Note how the base of the medullary canal is shaped flat. This will prevent rotation of the implant.

HALLUX VALGUS SURGERY

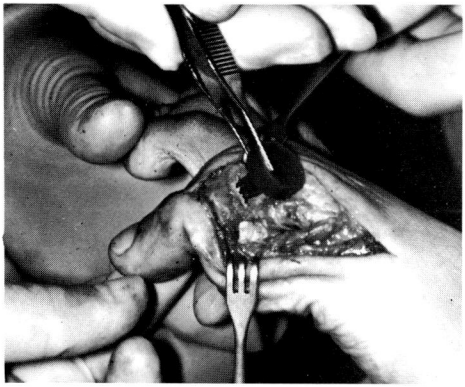

Fig. 7-31I. The medullary canal is shaped until the chosen implant sizer fits comfortably. Here a sizer is being used to gauge size of canal.

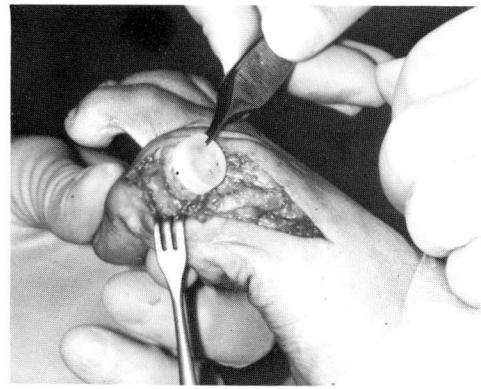

Fig. 7-31J. When the medullary canal is ready, the proper Silastic® implant is then inserted.

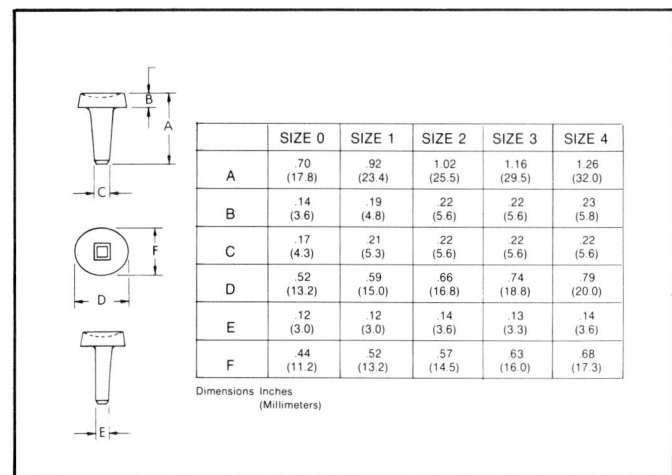

	SIZE 0	SIZE 1	SIZE 2	SIZE 3	SIZE 4
A	.70 (17.8)	.92 (23.4)	1.02 (25.5)	1.16 (29.5)	1.26 (32.0)
B	.14 (3.6)	.19 (4.8)	.22 (5.6)	.22 (5.6)	.23 (5.8)
C	.17 (4.3)	.21 (5.3)	.22 (5.6)	.22 (5.6)	.22 (5.6)
D	.52 (13.2)	.59 (15.0)	.66 (16.8)	.74 (18.8)	.79 (20.0)
E	.12 (3.0)	.12 (3.0)	.14 (3.6)	.13 (3.3)	.14 (3.6)
F	.44 (11.2)	.52 (13.2)	.57 (14.5)	.63 (16.0)	.68 (17.3)

Dimensions Inches (Millimeters)

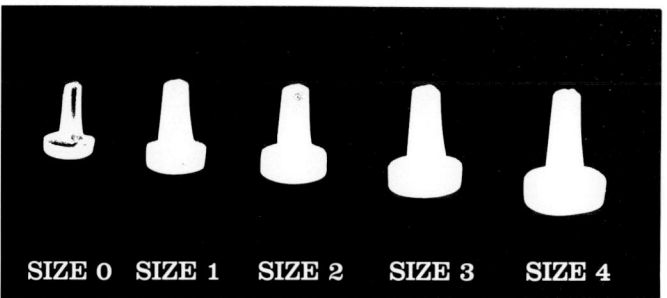

© Copyright 1972 and 1975, Dow Corning Corporation. All Rights Reserved.
SILASTIC® is a registered trademark of Dow Corning Corporation.

* A. B. Swanson, M.D., F.A.C.S., Grand Rapids, Michigan

Fig. 7-32. Used with permission from Dow Corning Corporation.

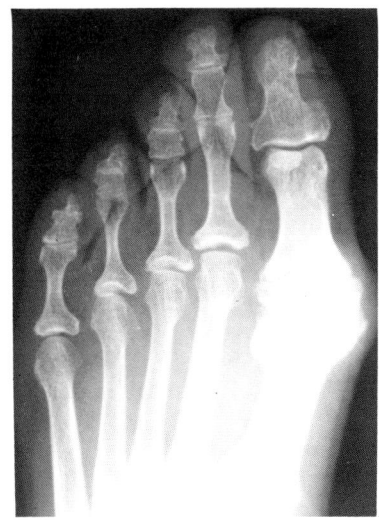
Fig. 7-33A. Dorsal-plantar x-ray view of hallux rigidus.

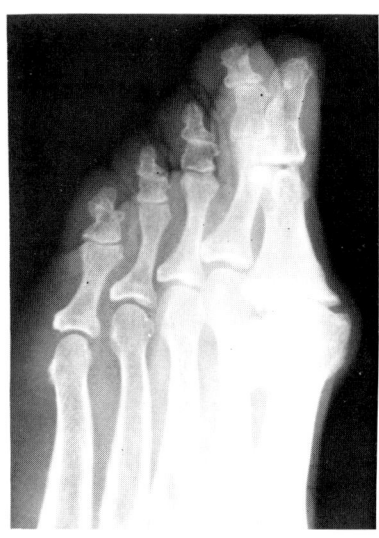
Fig. 7-33B. Oblique x-ray view of hallux rigidus.

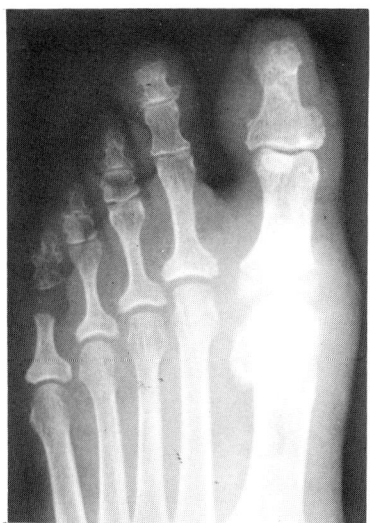
Fig. 7-33C. Post-operative dorsal-plantar view. Hallux rigidus has been corrected with a Silastic® implant.

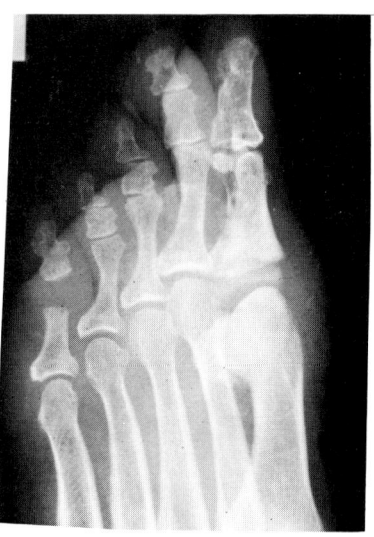
Fig. 7-33D. Post-operative oblique view. Shows excellent insertion of Silastic® implant.

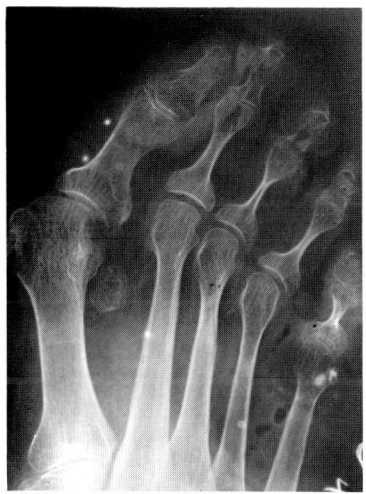 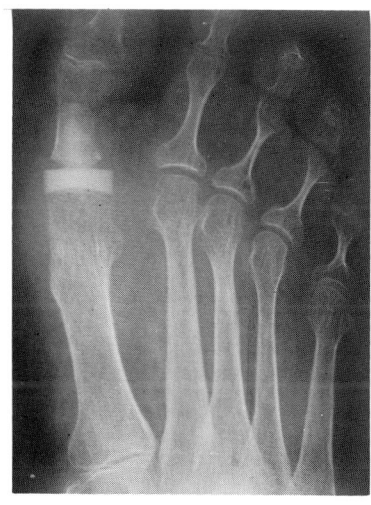

Fig. 7-34A. Pre-operative x-ray of 65 year old nun. Note lateral deviation of all toes.

Fig. 7-34B. Post-operative x-ray (one year later). This patient was operated almost eight years ago — she has been able to continue her active life as a business manager for a large hospital.

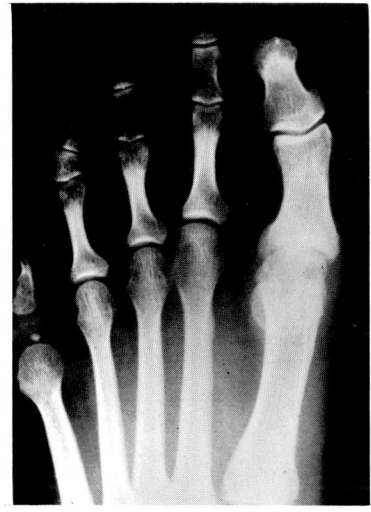 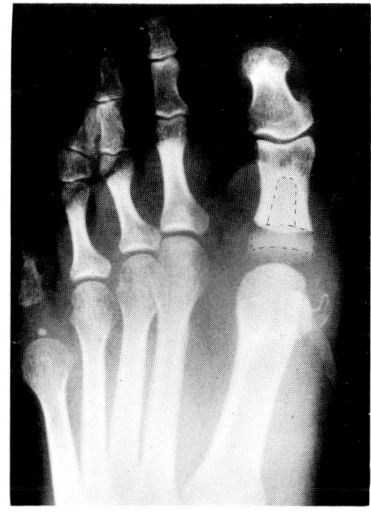

Fig. 7-35A. This twenty-one year old female patient was operated at age nineteen for a hallux rigidus but condition progressed.

Fig. 7-35B. Surgery was performed and a Silastic® implant was used. The patient has had implant in for six years with excellent results.

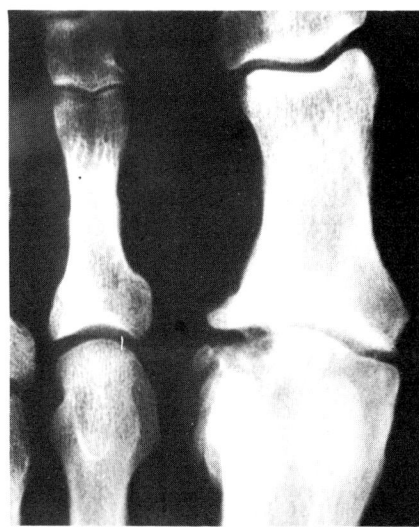

Fig. 7-36A. Pre-operative x-ray reveals hallux rigidus with associated lateral deviation of interphalangeal joint (hallux valgus interphallangeus).

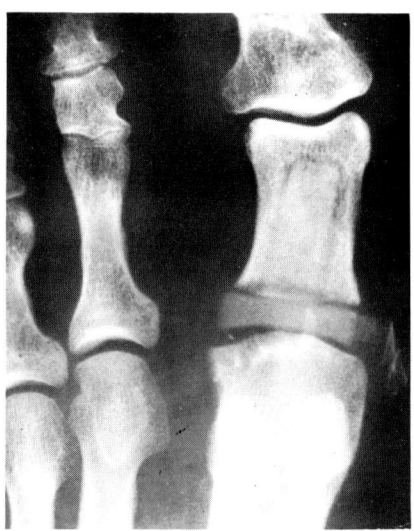

Fig. 7-36B. Post-operative x-ray. Note that base was cut at an angle to correct the lateral deviation of the interphalangeal joint.

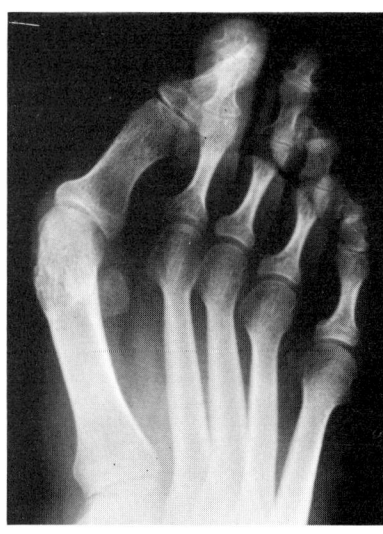

Fig. 7-37A. Pre-operative x-ray. Patient had unsuccessful hallux valgus surgery.

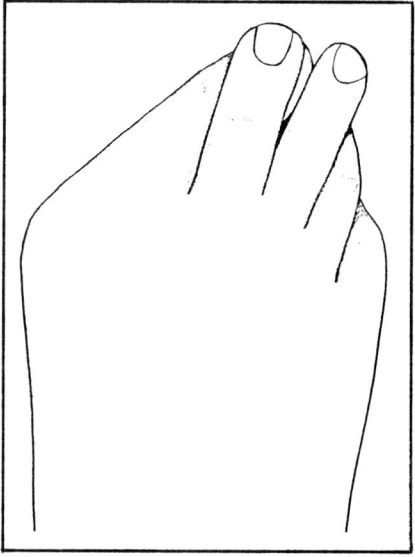

Fig. 7-37B. Line drawing of patient's foot in Fig. 7-37A.

HALLUX VALGUS SURGERY

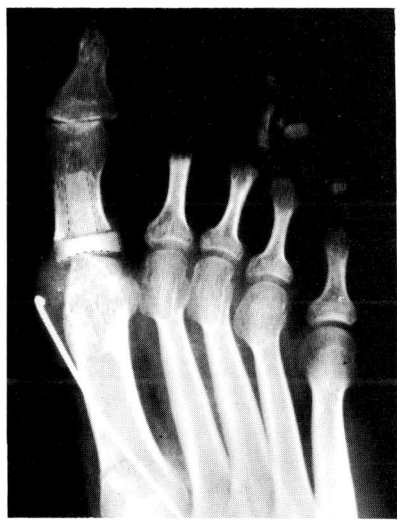
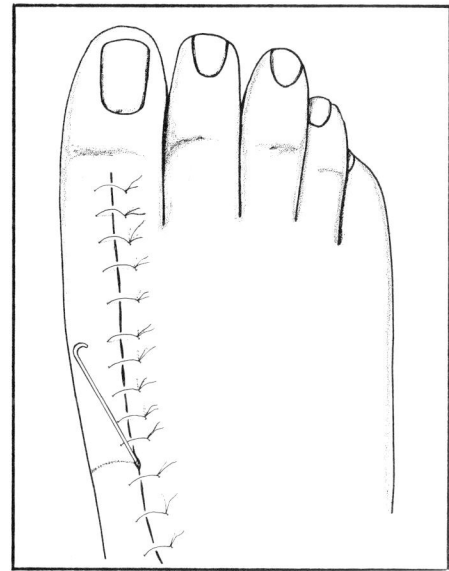

Fig. 7-37C. Post-operative x-ray. A Silastic® implant was used as well as a Closing Wedge Osteotomy.

Fig. 7-37D. Line drawing of patient's foot in Fig. 7-37C.

Total Joint Implant

Total joint implants were released for general use late in 1977. There are two companies which manufacture these ingenious prostheses, **Dow-Corning** and **Cutter Biomedical.**

The Dow-Corning implant is called the Silastic® Flexible Hinge Toe Implant H.P. (Fig. 7-38). The Cutter Biomedical implant is manufactured under the name of Cutter Hinged Great Toe (Fig. 7-39).

For years the need for a total joint replacement prosthesis had been in the minds of many surgeons and some of them tried gallant — if unsucessful — efforts. Two such individual should be mentioned here, lest an injustice of historical reporting be committed. **Dr. Russell Seeburger,** the late and tremendously talented surgeon from Michigan, was using metal implants in the late 1950's for metatarsal phalangeal joint replacements. **Dr. L.S. Weil,** also, manufactured a total joint replacement for the first metatarsal phalangeal joint in the early 1970's.

Today, it appears that silicone rubber is the material of choice for total joint replacement in the foot.

Precautions

While our clinical experience with the hemi-implants is now almost a decade old, total joint protheses are of **recent vintage.** We just do not have the **long term** experience in the use of these implants.

For this **important** reason, the surgeon should use the total joint implant **only** in cases where the joint is **painful** and **severely destroyed** and **cannot** be repaired with a more **conservative** procedure.

Technique

Both the Cutter and Silastic® great toe implants are inserted in the same fashion. Our illustration in fig. 7-40A shows the relative size and configuration of the Cutter prosthesis.

The joint is approached in the same manner as for the hemi-implant (fig. 7-40B). The head of the metatarsal is exposed as is the base of the proximal phalanx. We then estimate the amount of bone that is to be resected (fig. 7-40C). Remember, the bones **must** be cut at 90° to insure proper implant fit.

The head of the metatarsal is resected first. It is only necessary to take the anterior cartilagenous portion of the bone. The base of the proximal phalanx is then removed in the same manner as for a hemi-implant.

The medullary canals of the metatarsals and phalangeal shafts are then prepared to accept the stems of the prosthesis. The medullary canals are fashioned into the proper shape of the stems and herein lies the difference between the Silastic® and the Cutter implants.

In the case of the **Silastic® implant,** the medullary canals are fashioned (as illustrated in figs. 7-30L and 7-30O) into a **cave-like canal** which conforms to the shape of the stems (fig. 7-41)

For the **Cutter implant,** the medullary canals are reamed out into a **round hole** which will accept the polyester mesh sleeve covered stems (Fig. 7-40C).

The sizer set is used to find the proper size prosthesis. It is **not** necessary to cut the stems. The metatarsal stem (the longer of the two) is inserted first (Fig. 7-40D). The hallux is planti-flexed and the distal stem is **bent** and carefully inserted into the reamed out proximal phalangeal medullary canal (Fig. 7-40E).

The prosthesis is **only** handled with blunt instruments. Note that the Silastic® implant is inserted with the hinged portion of the implant facing up.

A few drops of a cortico steroid solution are infiltrated into the medullary canal to reduce post-surgical pain and inflammation. The prosthesis is kept in a sterile solution — a **prophylactic antibiotic solution** can be used — until it is implanted. The wound is then carefully closed in the usual manner.

Conclusion

There is a great temptation to utilize the total joint implant as a method of obtaining a straight toe following hallux valgus surgery. However, the surgeon should fight off this temptation as the procedure calls for the **removal** of the joint. If the joint removed is **"bad"** then the prosthesis will improve joint motion and alleviate pain; if, however, a **"good"** joint is needlessly destroyed, then the procedure is **doomed** to failure.

A few points that the surgeon will do well to keep in mind are:

1. Use **meticulous care** in the preparation of the bone and medullary canals.
2. Handle the prosthesis **only** with blunt instruments.
3. Choose the **proper size** implant.
4. I must admit that of the two protheses mentioned here, my **preference** is for the Silastic® implant.
5. Choose and **educate** your patients properly.

HALLUX VALGUS SURGERY

SILASTIC® Flexible Hinge Toe Implant H.P.
BRAND
(Swanson Design*)

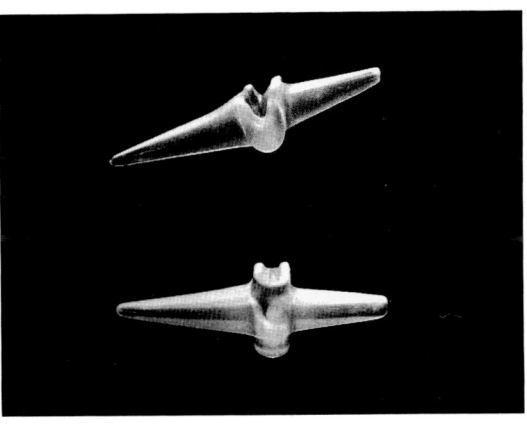

Typical Dimensions

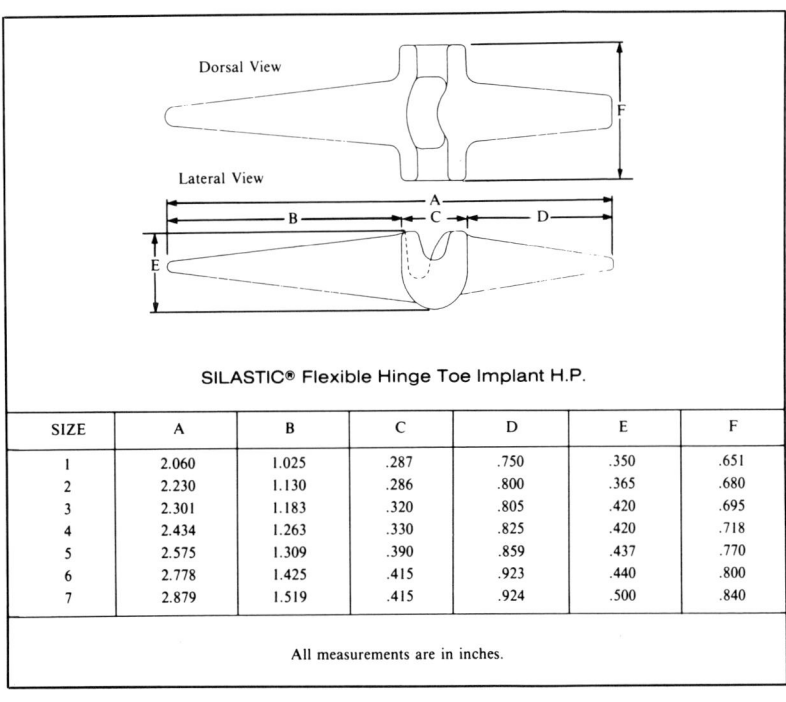

SILASTIC® Flexible Hinge Toe Implant H.P.

SIZE	A	B	C	D	E	F
1	2.060	1.025	.287	.750	.350	.651
2	2.230	1.130	.286	.800	.365	.680
3	2.301	1.183	.320	.805	.420	.695
4	2.434	1.263	.330	.825	.420	.718
5	2.575	1.309	.390	.859	.437	.770
6	2.778	1.425	.415	.923	.440	.800
7	2.879	1.519	.415	.924	.500	.840

All measurements are in inches.

Fig. 7-38. Used with permission from Dowing Corning Corporation.

CUTTER HINGED GREAT TOE

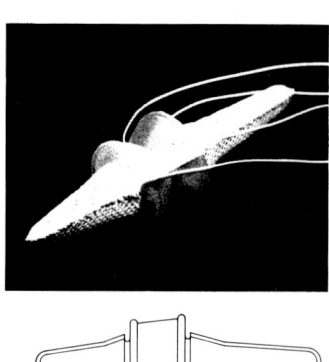

CATALOG NUMBER	SIZE
GT-10	Small
GT-20	Medium
GT-30	Large

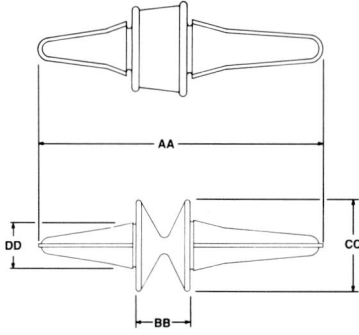

CATALOG NUMBER	SIZE	AA	BB	CC	DD
GT-10	SMALL	1.780/45.2	.358/9.1	.580/14.7	.280/7.11
GT-20	MEDIUM	2.120/53.8	.420/10.7	.680/17.3	.340/8.64
GT-30	LARGE	2.55/64.7	.494/12.55	.800/20.3	.400/19.3

ENGLISH/METRIC

Great Toe Sizer

CATALOG NUMBER	SIZE
GT-105	Small
GT-205	Medium
GT-305	Large

(SIZERS ARE FABRICATED OF RED SILICONE.)

The Hamer Soft Tissue Retractor

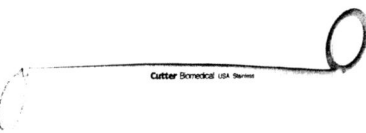

CATALOG NUMBER
FR-70

Stabilization Suture Passer

CATALOG NUMBER
SP-70

Cutter Biomedical

Fig. 7-39. Used with permission from Cutter Biomedical.

HALLUX VALGUS SURGERY

Technique for Total Implant

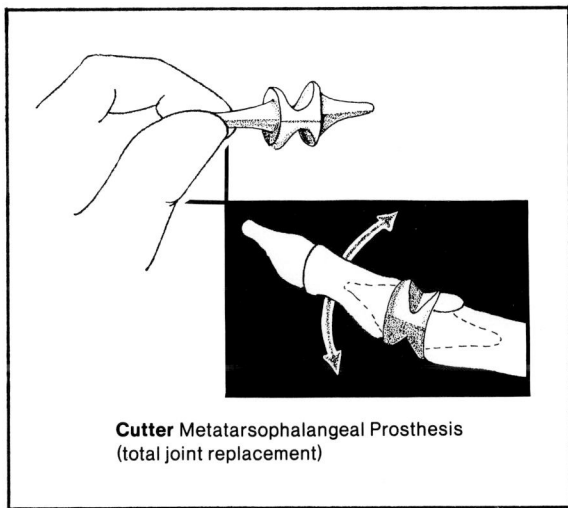

Cutter Metatarsophalangeal Prosthesis (total joint replacement)

Fig. 7-40A

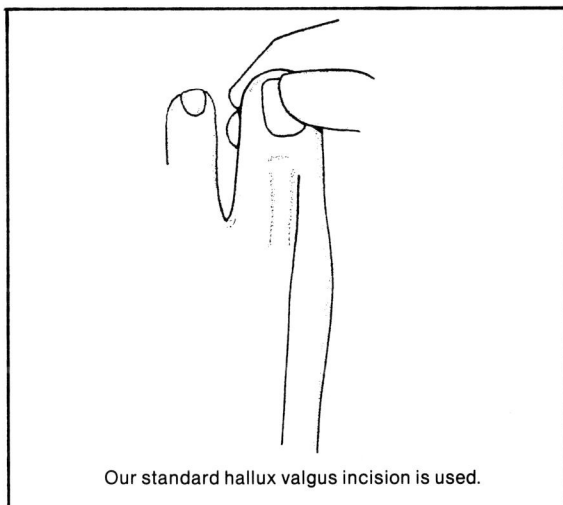

Our standard hallux valgus incision is used.

Fig. 7-40B

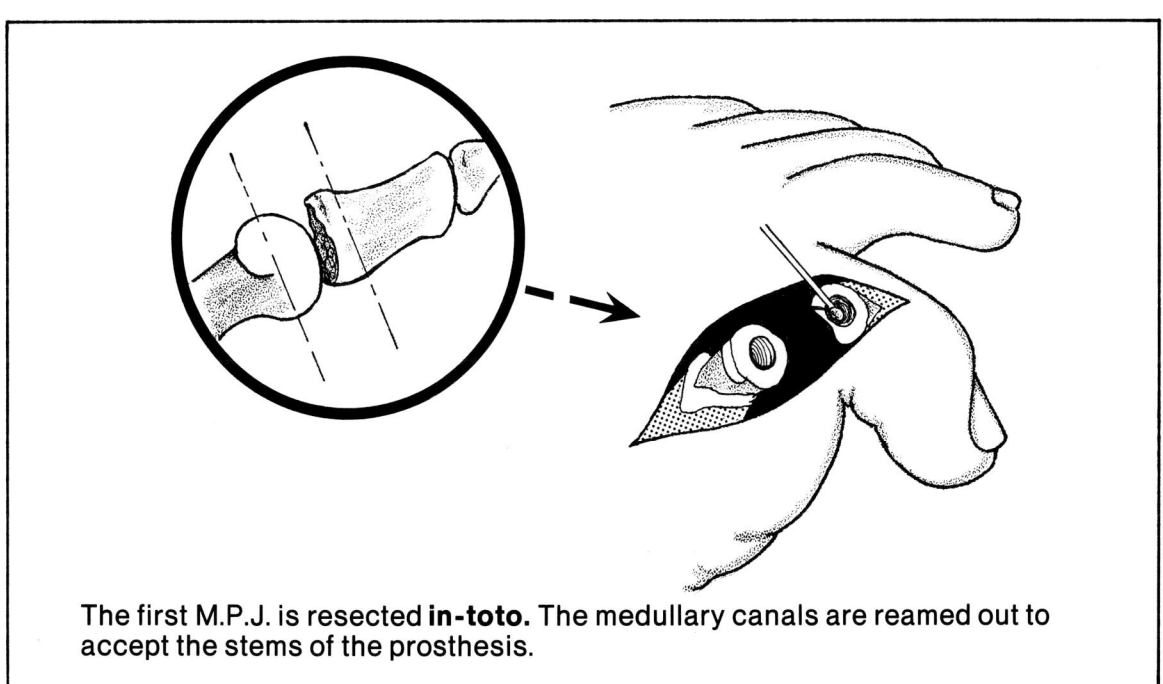

The first M.P.J. is resected **in-toto.** The medullary canals are reamed out to accept the stems of the prosthesis.

Fig. 7-40C

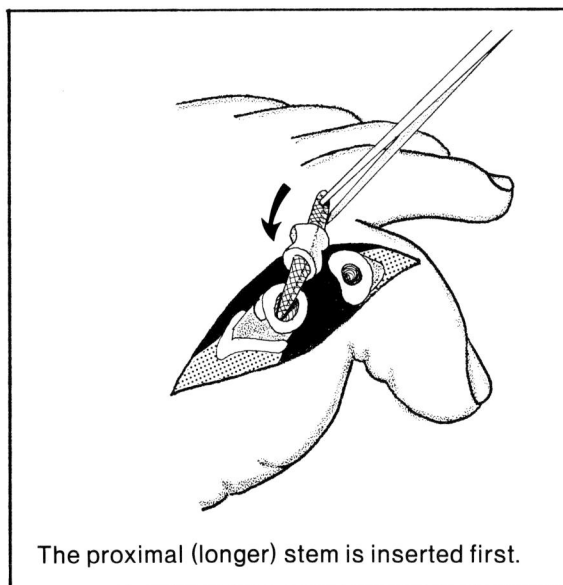

Fig. 7-40D

The proximal (longer) stem is inserted first.

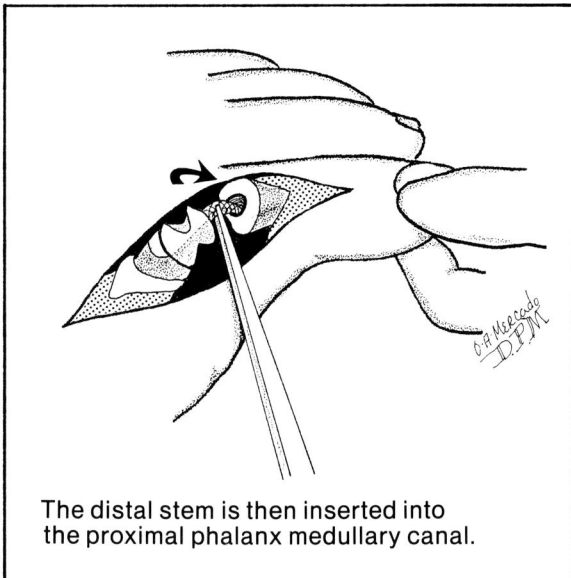

Fig. 7-40E

The distal stem is then inserted into the proximal phalanx medullary canal.

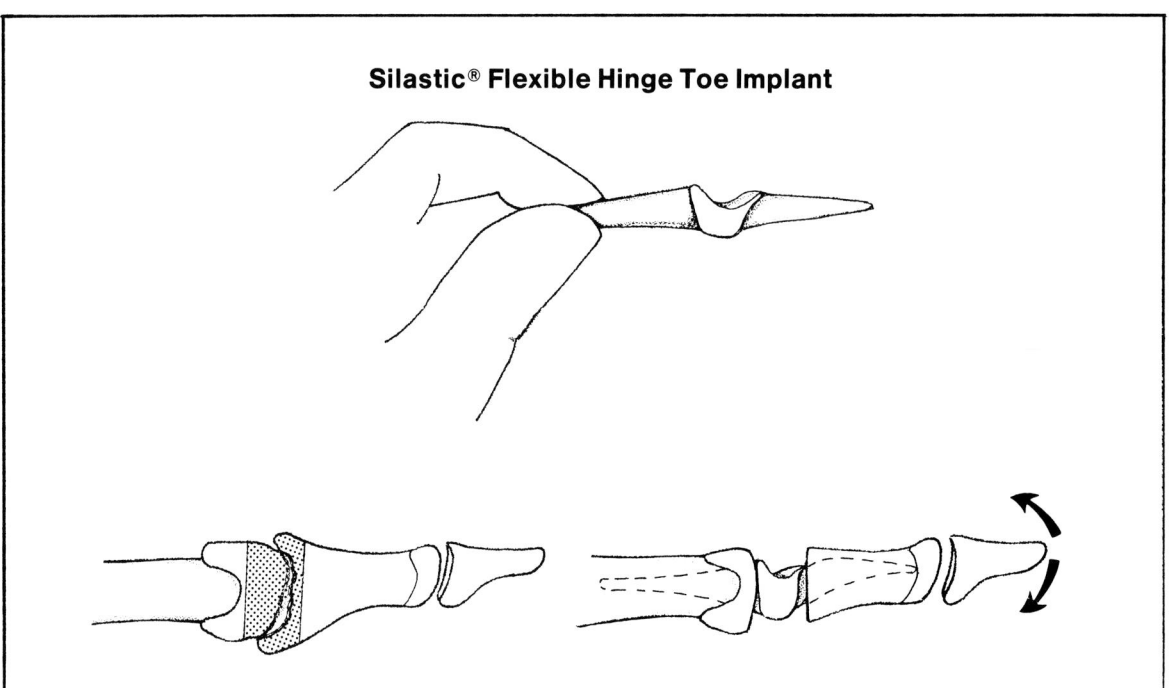

Silastic® Flexible Hinge Toe Implant

Fig. 7-41

HALLUX VALGUS SURGERY

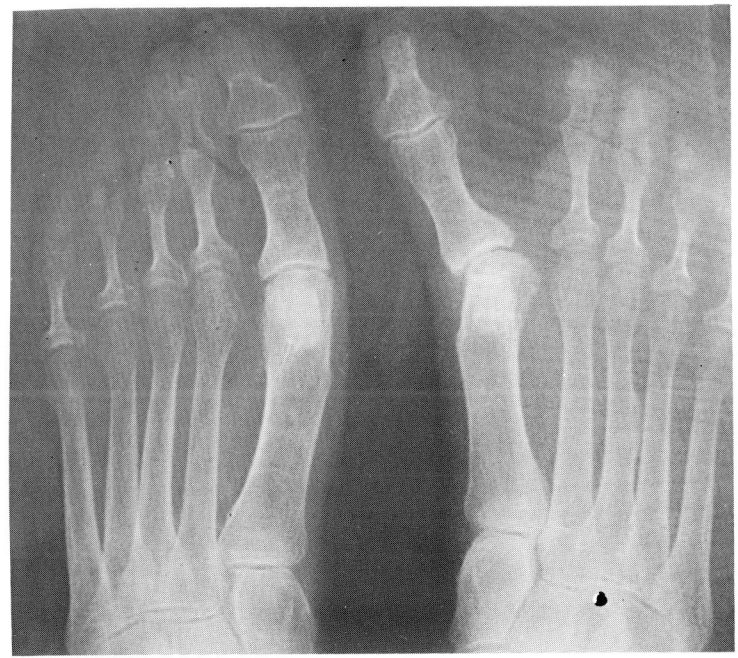

Fig. 7-24A. Pre-operative x-ray of hallux varus right foot.

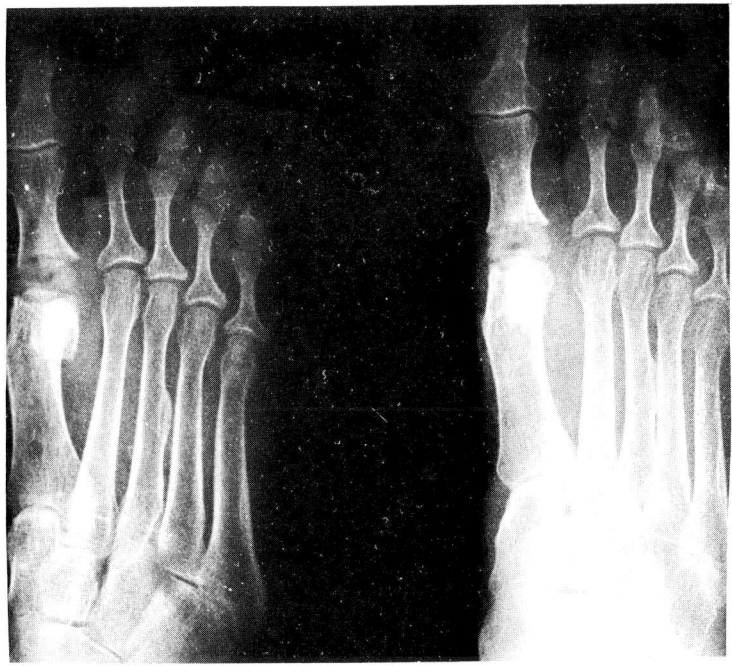

Fig. 7-24B. Post-surgical x-ray. Hallux varus was reduced with the use of a Silastic® Flexible Hinge Toe Implant.

Bibliography

Anesthesia — Chapter 1

Andriani, John: Labat's Regional Anesthesia — Techniques and Clinical Applications. W.B. Saunders Company, Philadelphia and London, 1969.

DeMoon, Patrick A. and Mercado, O.A.: Manual of Hospital Podiatry. National Academy of Hospital Podiatry, Chicago, 1975.

Dripps, R.D., Eckenhoff, J.E. and Vandam, L.D.: Introduction to Anesthesia: The Principles of Safe Practice, W.B. Saunders Company, Philadelphia, 1972.

Foldes, F., Davidson, G., Duncalf, D. and Kuwabara, S.: The intravenous toxicity of local anesthetic agents in man, Clin. Pharmacol. Ther., 6:328, 1965.

Goodman, L.S. and Gilman, A.: The Pharmacological Basis of Therapeutics, Ed. 5, MacMillian Company, New York, 1975.

Hollunger, G.: On the metabolism of lidocaine II. The biotransformation of lidocaine. Acta Pharmacol. Toxicol.

Kaplan, Earl G. Lectures to Surgical Residents at Civic Hospital, Detroit 1961.

Knox, P.R., North, W.C. and Stephen, C.R.: Pharmacological and clinical observation with mepivacaine, Anesthesiology, 22:987,1961.

Krantz, J.C. and Carr, C.J.: Pharmacological Principles of Medical Practice, The William and Wilkins Company, Baltimore, 1964.

Lee, J.A.: A Synopsis of Anesthesia, William and Wilkins, Baltimore, 1973.

Mercado, O.A.: The Fundamentals of Local Anesthesia. Current Podiatry, May 1972.

Moore, D.C.: Regional Block, Ed. 4, Charles C. Thomas, Springfield, Ill. 1975.

Pizzolato, P. and Mannheimer, W.: Histopathologic Effects of Local Anesthetic Drugs, Charles C. Thomas, Springfield, Ill.

Sanner, Fern,: Chief of Anesthesia, Franklin Boulevard Community Hospital. Personal Communication, 1978.

Sanner, Fern, and Lawton, James H.: Intravenous Regional Anesthesia in the Lower Leg and Foot, J.A.P.A., Vol. 64 No. 6, June 1974.

Scarlet, J.J., Walter, J.H., Bachmann, R.J.: Digital blood perfusion following injections of plain lidocaine and lidocaine with epinephrine, J.A.P.A., 68:339, 1987.

Weinstock, R.: Local infilltration anesthesia. 5th Annual Surgical Symposium, California College of Podiatric Medicine, San Francisco, 1975.

Wylie, W.D.: A Practice of Anesthesia. Year Book Medical Publishers, Inc., Chicago, 1972.

Young, Agatha: The Men Who Made Surgery. Hillman Books, New York, N.Y. 1961.

Nail Surgery — Chapter 2

Bartlett, R.W.: A conservative operation for cure of so-called ingrown toenail, J.A.M.A. 108:1257, 1937.

Bean, W.B.: Nail growth: a twenty-year study, Arch. Intern. Med., 111:476, 1963.

Bose, B.: A technique for excision of nail fold for ingrowing toenail, Surg. Gynec. Obstet., 132:511, 1971.

Burns, S.A., Ketai, R.S., Ketai, N.H.: Onychocryptosis: a brief review, J.A.P.A. 67:780, 1977.

DuVries, H.L.: Hypertrophy of Ungualabia, Chiropody Rec 16:11, 1933.

DuVries, H.L.: Ingrown nail, Chiropody Rec., 27:155, 164, 1944.

Emmert, C.: Operations for ingrown toenail, Arch. Klin. Chir., 11:268, 1869.

Freund, P.: Onychomycosis, diagnosis and treatment, J.A.P.A., 62:395, 1972.

Frost, L.: Root resection for incurvated nail, J. Nat. Ass. Chirop., 40:19, 1950.

Frost, L.: A definite surgical treatment for some lateral nail problems., J. Nat. Ass. Chirop., 47:10, 493, 1956.

Frost, L.: Atraumatic nail avulsion with a novel ungual elevator, J.A.P.A., 48:51,1958.

Graham, H.F.: Ingrown toe nail, Amer. J. Surg., 6:411, 1929.

Gray, H. and Goss, C. (Editors): Gray's Anatomy Ed. 28, Lea and Febiger, Philadelphia, 1970.

Harris, L.: A variation in the treatment concept of onychomycosis, J.A.P.A., 66:700, 1976.

Howard: Ingrown toenail, its surgical treatment. N.Y. Med. Surg. J., 57:579, 1893.

Kaplan, E.G.: Elimination of onychauxis by surgery, J.A.P.A., 50:111, 1960.

Keyes, E.L.: The surgical treatment of ingrown toenails, J.A.P.A., 102:1458, 1934.

Kilberg, A.J.: Surgical treatment of onychocryptosis. Clin. J. Chirop. Pod. Pedic. Surg., 7:222, 1935.

Krausz, C.E.: Nail survey: 28th October 1942 to 3rd April 1970, Brit. J. Chirop., 35:117, 1970.

Lloyd-Davies, R.W. and Brill, G.C.: The aetiology and out patient management of ingrowing toenails, Brit. J. Surg., 50:592, 1963.

Mercado, O.A.: The Anatomical Landmark of the Nail Matrix. Presented as a Scientific Exhibit at the First Annual Illinois Podiatry Conferrence, Chicago, Illinois, Feb. 1969.

Mercado, O.A.: The Kaplan Nail. Current Podiatry. April, 1972.

Ney, G.C.: An operation for ingrowing toenails, J.A.P.A., 80:374, 1923.

Nyman, S.: The phenol-alcohol technique for toenail incision, J. New Jersey Chiropodists Soc., 5:4, 1956.

Owens, R.E.: Surgical Correction for onychauxis, J.A.P.A., 52:591, 1962.

Pardo-Costello, V.: Diseases of the Nails, ed. 3, Springfield, Ill., 1960, Charles C. Thomas.

Polokoff, M.: Ingrown toenail and hypertrophied nail lip surgery by electrolysis, J.A.P.A., 51:805, 1961.

Samitz, M. and Dana, A.: Cutaneous Lesions of the Lower Extremities, J.B. Lippincott Co., Philadelphia, 1971.

Steinberg, M.D.: A simplified technique for surgery of ingrowing toenails, Surgery, 36:1132, 1954.

Suppan, R.J.: Podiatric Surgery, Rev. Ed., Ohio College of Podiatric Medicine, Cleveland, 1968.

Suppan, R.J., and Ristchlin, J.D.: A non-debilitating surgical procedure for ingrown toenail, J.A.P.A., 52:900, 1962.

Weisfeld, M.: Illustrated technique for the complete removal of nail matrix and hyponychium without skin incisions (Suppan Nail Technique No. 2), J.A.P.A., 65:481, 1975.

White, C.J. and Laipply, T.C.: Diseases of the Nails: 792 cases, Ind. Med. Surg., 27:325, 1958.

Winograd, A.M.: Modification in technique of operation for ingrown toenail,J.A.M.A., 92:299, 1929.

Winograd, A.M.: The surgical treatment of ingrown toenail, J.A.M.A., 102:1458, 1934.

Winograd,A.: Results in operations for ingrown toenails III. Med. J., 70:197, 1936.

Yale, J.F.: Phenol-alcohol technique for correction of infected ingrown toenail, J.A.P.A., 64:46, 1974.

Soft Tissue Surgery — Chapter 3

Anderson, I.: The treatment of plantar warts. Br. J. Derm. ,75 :725,1972.

Anderson, R. : The treatment of intractable plantar warts. Plast. Reconstr. Surg. ,19 :384,1957.

Baker,L. D. and Kuhn, H. H. : Morton's metatarsalgia; localized degenerative fibrosis with neuromatous proliferation of the fourth plantar nerve. So. Med. J. ,37 :123, 1944.

Barber, K. W. et al: Benign extraneural soft tissues tumors of the extremeties causing compression of nerves. JBJS, 44A: 98,1962.

Berlin, S. J. etal: Skin Tumors of the Foot: Diagnosis and Treatment. Futura Publ. Co.,N. Y. 1974.

Berlin, S. J., Donick, I. I., Block, L. D., and Costa, A. J. : Nerve tumors of the foot: diagnosis and treatment.JAPA, 65 :157, 1975.

Betts, L. O. : Morton's metatarsalgia: neuritis of fourth digital nerve. Med. J. Aust. , 1: 514, 1940.

Bickel,W. H. and Dockerty, M. A. : Plantar neuromas, Morton's toe. Surg. Gyn. and Obst. , 84: 111, 1947.

Blair, V. P. , Brown, J. B. and Byars, L. T. : Plantar warts, flaps and grafts. JAMA, 108:24, 1937.

Cox, H. T. : The Cleavage Lines Of The Skin. Brit. J. Surg, 29 :234, 1941.

Duncan, T. L. and Wright, J. L. : Plantar interdigital neuroma. So. Med. J. , 51 :49, 1958.

DuVries, H. L. : New approach to the treatment of intractable verruca plantaris (plantar wart).JAMA,152: 1202, 1953.

Editorial: Treatment of plantar warts. New Eng. J. Med. , 248 :659, 1953.

Falknor, G. W. : Needling- a new technique in verruca therapy, JAPA, 59: 51, 1969.

Gross, S. W. et al: Peripheral nerve tumors. Nuerol. , 7 :711, 1957.

Guthrie, L. G. : On a form of painful toe. Lancet, 1: 628, 1892.

Haggart,G. E. : The conservative and surgical treatment of plantar warts. Surg. Clin. N. Amer. , 14 :1211 ,1934.

Hauser, E. D. : Interdigital neuroma of the foot. Surg. Gyn. and Obst. , 133 :265 ,1971.

Inman, V. T. , editor: DuVries, Surgery of the Foot, 3 rd ed. , C. V. Mosby Co. St. Louis, 1973.

Journal of the American Podiatry Association- special issue devoted to podiatric oncology. S. J. Berlin, editor, Vol. 66 -No. 7, 1976.

Kelikian, R. : Hallux Valgus, Allied Deformities of the foot and metatarsalgia. W. B. Saunders; Co. , Philadelphia, 1965.

Lewis, D. and Hart, D. : Tumors of peripheral nerves. Ann.1930.

Lieberman, H. : An empirical treatment for mosaic verruca JAPA, 50 :737, 1960.

Luciano, C. S. : Verruca plantaris- a compendium of its understanding and treatment. JAPA, 67 :858, 1977.

McElvenny, R. T. : The etiology and surgical treatment of intractable pain about the fourth metatarsal-phalangeal joint. JBJS, 34 :490 1956.

McGregor ,I. A. : Fundamental Techniques of Plastic Surgery and their Surgical Applications, 5th ed. , William and Wilkins Co. , Baltimore, 1972.

Morton, T. S. K. : Metatarsalgia (Morton's painful affection of the foot) with an account of six cases cured by operation. Ann. Surg. , 17: 680, 1893.

Peacock, E. E. , Jr. , Madden, J. W. and Tier, W. C. : Biologic basis for the treatment of keloids and hypertrophic scars. So. Med. J. , 63: 755, 1970.

Peacock, E. E. , Jr. and Van Winkle, W. Jr. : Wound Repair. W. B. Saunders, Philadelphia, 1976.

Reed, R. W. : Verruca plantaris; a review of the problem. J. Foot Surgery, 15: 24, 1976.

Rodin, B. M. et al: Digital traumatic neuroma. A case report. JAPA, 63: 445 1973.

Woods-Jones, F. : Structure and Function as seen in the Foot. Baltimore, Williams and Wilkins, 1944.

Yale, I: Podiatric Medicine, William and Wilkins Co. Baltimore, 1974.

Digital Surgery — Chapter 4

Borg, I.: Operation for correction of hammer toe. Acta Chir Scan., 100:619, 1950.

Buggiani, F.P., Biggs, E.: Mallet toe. JAPA, 66:321, 1976.

Cahill, B.R. and Conner, D.E.: A long-term follow-up on proximal phalangectomy for hammer toes. Clin. Ortho., 86:191, 1972.

Creer, W.S.: Treatment of hammer toe. JBJS 21:977, 1939.

DuVries, H.L.: Deformities of the proximal phalangeal joint. The Chiropody Record, Vol. 16, No. 12:5, 1933.

Ely, L.W.: Hammertoe. Surg. Clin. N.A., 6:433, 1926.

Forrester-Brown, M.F.: Tendon transplantation for clawing of the great toe. JBJS, 20:56, 1938.

Fowler, A.W.: The surgery of fixed claw toes. JBJS, 39B:585, 1957.

Giannestras, N.J.: Foot disorders; Medical and Surgical Management, Lea and Febiger, Philadelphia, 1973.

Glassman, F., Wolin, I. and Sideman, S.: Phalangectomy for toe deformities. Surg. Clin. N.A., 29:275, 1949.

Green, D.R., Ruch, J.A. and Butlin, W.E.: Polydactylism repair. JAPA, 66:302, 1976.

Haber, L., Winthrop, L. and Weiner, S.S.: Biomechanical findings in a random survey of 5th toe abnormalities. JAPA, 65:206, 1975.

Higgs, S.L.: "Hammer-toe" Med. Press, 131:473, 1931.

Kelikian, H.: Hallux Valgus, Allied Deformities of the Forefoot and Metatarsalgic. W.B. Saunders Co., Philadelphia, 1965.

Kitting, R.W. and McGlamry, E.D.: Repair of hammer toe fifth. JAPA, 63:321, 1973.

Knecht, J.G.: Pathomechanical deformities of the lesser toes. JAPA 64:941, 1974.

Lantzouris, L.A.: Congenital subluxation of the fifth toe and its correction by a periosteo-capsulo-plasty and tendon transplantation. JBJS, 22:147, 1940

Lapidus, P.W.: Operation for correction of hammer toe. JBJS, 21:977, 1939.

Lapidus, P.W.: Transplantation of the extensor tendon for correction of overlapping fifth toe. JBJS, 24:555, 1942.

Macken, O.P.: Procedure for correction of distal digital contractures. J. Foot Surgery, 11:141, 1972.

McGlamry, E.D.: Forefoot reconstruction: a case study. JAPA, 63:231, 1973.

McGlamry, E.D., Kitting, R.W.: Repair of hammer toe, right Fourth. JAPA, 64:435, 1974.

Mercado, O.A.: The Receding Fifth Toe: The Pedal Fallacy. Current Podiatry, Vol. 12 No. 11, 1963.

Parrish, T.: Dynamic correction of claw toes. Ortho. Clin. N.A., 41:1, 1973.

Perrone, M.A.: Podiatric Nail and Bone Surgery With a Rotary Airmotor. The Weber Dental Manufacturing Co., Canton, 1972.

Rice, J.R.D.: Digital arthroplasty by power surgery with minimal incision. JAPA 67:811, 1977.

Roven, M.D.: Phalangeal set - semi closed reduction of malaligned digits. JAPA, 60:80, 1970.

Sarrafian, S.K. and Topouzian, L.K.: Anatomy and physiology of the extensor apparatus of the toes. JBJS, 51A:699, 1969.

Selig, S.: Hammer toe: a new procedure for its correction, Surg. Gyn. and Obst., 72:101, 1941.

Sgarlato, T.E.: Transplantation of the flexor digitorum longus muscle tendon in hammer toe. JAPA, 60:383, 1970.

Sorto, L.A.: Surgical correction of hammer toes: a five year post-operative study. JAPA, 64:930, 1974.

Soule, R.E.: Operation for the cure of hammertoe. N.Y. Med. J., p. 649, 1910.

Subotnick, S.I.: Digital deformities: etiology and treatment. JAPA, 65:543, 1975.

Tartack, I., Glick, M.: Congenital-bilateral cock-up toe deformity — a case report. JAPA, 66:95, 1976.

Taylor, R.G.: An operative procedure for the treatment of hammer-toe and claw-toe. JBJS, 22:608, 1940.

Taylor, R.G.: The treatment of claw-toes by multiple transfers of flexor into extensor tendons. JBJS, 33:539, 1951.

Trethowan, H.W.: The treatment of hammer toes. Lancet, 1:1257 & 1312, 1925.

Wilson, J.N.: V-Y correction for various deformity of the fifth toe. Brit. J. Surg., 41:133, 1953.

Woodhams, L.E.: A three-year follow-up study of hammer digit syndrome of the hallux. JAPA 64:955, 1974.

Young, C.S.: An operation for the correction of hammer toe and claw toe. JBJS, 20:715, 1938.

Principles of Bone Surgery — Chapter 5

Charnley, John: Compression Arthrodesis. E. & S. Livingstone Ltd. Edinburgh and London, 1953.

DePalma, A.F., Mckeever, C.D. and Subin, D.K.: Process of repair of articular cartilage, demonstrated by histology and autoradiology with tritiated thymidine. Clin. Orthop., 48:229, 1966.

Eggers, G.W.N., Schindler, T.O. and Pomerat, C.M.: The influence of the contact-compression factor on osteogenesis in surgical fractures. JBJS, 31A:693, 1949.

Eggers, G.W.N.: Clinical significance of contact-compression factor in bone surgery. Arch. Surg., 62:467, 1951.

Epker, B.N. and Frost H.M.: Correlation of bone resorption and formation with the physical behavior of loaded bone. J. Dent. Res., 44:33, 1965.

Friedenberg, Z.B. and French, G.T.: The effects of known compression forces on fracture healing. Surg. Gyn. and Obst., 94:743, 1952.

Fuller, J.A., Ghadially, F.N.: Ultrastructural observations on surgically produced partial-thickness defects in articular cartilage. Clin. Orthop., 86:193, 1972.

Ghadially, F.N., Ailsby, R.L., Oryschak, A.F.: Scanning electron microscopy of superficial defects in articular cartilage. Ann. Rheum. Dis., 33:327, 1971.

Ghadially, F.N., Fuller, J.A., and Kirkaldy-Will, W.H.: Ultrastructure of full thickness defects in articular cartilage. Arch. Pathol., 92:356, 1974.

Guyton, A.C.: Textbook of Medical Physiology, W.B. Saunders Company, Philadelphia, 1976.

Hadhazy, C., Benko, K., and Balogh, P.A.: Studies on cartilage formation: XII. Electron microscopic investigation on cartilage neoformation. Acta Biol. Acad. Sci. Hung., 19:323, 1968.

Ham, A.W.: A histological study of the early phases of bone repair. JBJS, 12:827, 1930.

Kase, F., D'Amico, J.C.: A literature search for the methods and materials used to stimulate osteogenesis. JAPA, 66:604, 1976,

Klosterman, E.J.: Hyaline cartilage repair and surgical application. JAPA, 68:178, 1978.

Luben, R.A., Sherman, J.K. and Wadkino, C.L.: Studies of the mechanism of biological calcification. Calcif. Tissue Res., 11:39, 1973.

McClean, F.C. and Urist, M.R.: Bone-Fundamentals of the Physiology of Tissue, University of Chicago Press, Chicago, 1968.

Mercado, O.A.: What Podiatrist Should Know About Bone Healing. Audio Tape Cassette and Slide Program, Teach'Em Inc., Chicago 1977.

Mercado, O.A.: Intramedullary Cortical Graft for Adductory Wedge Osteotomy. Hosp. Podiatry Review Vol. I, Spring Issue 1973.

Mohr, R., Scherer, P.N.: Accelerated fracture healing. JAPA, 66:588, 1976.

Mueller, M.E, Allgower, M. and Willenessen, H.H.: Manual of Internal Fixation of Fractures, Springer Verlag, New York, 1970.

Peacock, E.E., Jr. and VanWinkle, W., Jr.: Wound Repair, 2nd Ed., W.B. Saunders Company, Philadelphia, 1976.

Perren, S.M., Allgower, M. and Condey, S.: Development of compression plate techniques for internal fixation of fractures. Prog. Surg., 12:152, 1973.

Ray, R.D., Holloway, J.A.: Bone implants: preliminary reports of an experimental study. JBJS, 39A:119, 1957.

Scherer, P., Weil, L.S., Mohr, R. and Zlotoff, H.: The osteoclasp: a constant compression device for internal stainless steel fixation of bone. JAPA, 65:774, 1975.

Urist, M.R.: Recent advances in physiology of calcification. JBJS, 46A:889, 1964.

Metatarsal Phalangeal Joint Surgery
Chapter 6

Addante, J.B.: Metatarsal osteotomy as a surgical approach for the elimination of plantar keratosis. J. Foot Surg., 8:36, 1969.

Addante, J.B.: Metatarsal osteotomy as an office procedure to eradicate intractable plantar keratosis. JAPA, 60:397, 1970.

Amuso, S.L., Wissinger, H.A., Margolis, H.M., Eisenbeis, C.H. and Stolzer, B.L.: Metatarsal head resection in the treatment of rheumatoid arthritis. Clin. Orthop., 74:94, 1971.

Anderson, R.: The treatment of intractable plantar warts. Plast. Reconst. Surg., 19: 384, 1957.

Bartel, P.F.: Lesser metatarsal osteotomy. JAPA, 67:358, 1977.

Barton, N.J.: Arthroplasty of the forefoot in rheumatoid arthritis. JBJS, 55:126, 1973.

Billig, H.E.: Condylectomy for metatarsalgia — indications and results. J. Int. College Surg., 25:220, 1956.

Brattstrom, H. and Brattstrom, M.: Resection of the metatarsophalangeal joint in rheumatoid arthritis. Acta Orthop. Scand., 41:213, 1970.

Clayton, M.L.: Surgery of the forefoot in rheumatoid arthritis. Clin. Orthop., 16:136, 1960.

Clayton, M.L.: Surgery of the forefoot in rheumatoid arthritis. Arthritis and Rheumatism, 3:84, 1959.

Crenshaw, A.H.: Campbell's Operative Orthopaedics, Vol. 2, 5th Ed., C.V. Mosby Co., St. Louis, 1971.

Davidson, M.R.: A simple method for correcting second, third, and fourth plantar metatarsal head pathology — especially intractable keratomas. J. Am. coll. Foot Surg., 8:14, 1969.

Davidson, M.R.: Non-stabilization metatarsal head osteotomies — a simple method for correcting second, third, fourth, and fifth metatarsal head pathology. J. foot Surg., 10:4, 1971.

Davidson, M.R.: V-osteotomy for correction of metatarsal head pathology. J. Foot Surg., 13:23, 1974.

Davies, H.: Metatarsus quintus varus. Brit. Med. J., 1:664, 1949.

Downey, M.A. and Dorothy, W.L.: A radiographic technique to demonstrate the plantar aspect of the forefoot in stance. JAPA, 59:   , 1969.

DuVries, H.L.: New approach to treatment of intractable verruca plantaris. JAMA, 152:1202, 1953.

DuVries, H.L.: Surgery of the Foot. C.V. Mosby Co., St. Louis, 1973.

Faithful, D.K. and Savill, D.L.: Review of the results of excision of the metatarsal heads in patients with rheumatoid arthritis. Ann. Rheum. Dis., 30:201, 1971.

Gerbert, J., Sgarlato, T.E. and Subotnick, S.I.: Preliminary study of a closing wedge osteotomy of the Fifth metatarsal for correction of a Tailor's Bunion deformity. JAPA, 62:212, 1972.

Gerbert, J., Melillo, T. etal: The Surgical Treatment of the Intractable Plantar Keratoma. Futura Publishing Co., Mt. Kisco, N.Y., 1974.

Giannestras, N.J.: Shortening of the metatarsal shaft for the correctionof plantar keratosis. Clin. Orthop., 4:225, 1954.

Giannestras, N.J.: Shortening of the metatarsal shaft and the treatment of plantar keratosis and end result studies. JBJS, 40A:64, 1958.

Giannestras, N.J.: Foot Disorders: Medical and Surgical Management. Lea and Febiger, Philadelphia, 1973.

Graver, H.H.: Angular metatarsal osteotomy. JAPA, 63:96, 1973.

Hatcher, R.M., Goller, W.L. and Weil, L.S.: Intractable plantar keratoses — a review of surgical corrections. JAPA, 68:377, 1978.

Helal, B.: Metatarsal osteotomy for metatarsalgia. JBJS, 57B:187, 1975.

Jacoby, R.P.: V-osteoplasty for correction of intractable plantar keratoses. JBJS, 49A:61, 1958.

Jacoby, R.P.: V-osteotomy for correction of intractable plantar keratoses. J. Foot Surg., 12:8, 1973.

Kates, A.: Surgery of the rheumatoid foot. Proc. Roy. Soc. Med., 63:679, 1970.

Kelikian, H.: Hallux Valgus, Allied Deformities of the Forefoot and Metatarsalgia, W.B. Saunders Co., Philadelphia, 1965.

Kestler, O.C.: Resection of metatarsal heads for metatarsalgia. Bull. Hosp. Joint Dis., 30:89, 1969.

Lipscomb, P.R., Benson, G.M. and Jones, D.A.: Resection of proximal phalanges and metatarsal condyles for deformities of the forefoot due to rheumatoid arthritis. Clin. Orthop., 82:24, 1972.

Mann, R.A. and DuVries, H.L.: Intractable Plantar Keratoses. Orthop. Clin. N.A., 4:67, 1973.

Mau, C.: Eine Operation des kontrakten Spreizfusses. Zbl. Chir., 67:667, 1940.

McGlamry, E.D. and Ruch, J.A.: Status of implant arthroplasty of the lesser metatarsophalangeal joints. JAPA, 66:3, 1976.

McKeever, D.C.: Operation for plantar callosities and metatarsalgia. JBJS, 34A:129, 1952.

McKeever, D.C.: Excision of the fifth metatarsal head, Clin. Orthop., 13:321, 1959.

Meisenbach, R.O.: Painful anterior ach of the foot — an operation for its relief by means of raising the arch. Am. J. Ortho. Surg., 14:206, 1916.

Mercado, O.A.: Peg and Hole Technique for Metatarsal Shortening. The Journal of Podiatric Medicine, Vol. 60, Nos. 1-4 Jan-April 1974.

Mercado, O.A.: The McKeever Operation, Hosp. Podiatry Review Vol. 1, Fall Issue 1973.

Mercado, O.A.: New Techniques in the Treatment of Intractable Plantar Keratosis. Audio-Cassette Program, Carolando, Oak Park, Illinois 1976.

Reese, H.W.: Surgical treatment of intractable plantar keratosis, J. Foot Surg., 12:92, 1972.

Rutledge, B.A. and Green, A.L.: Surgical treatment of plantar corns. U.S. Armed Forces Med. J., 8L219, 1957.

Rutherford, R.: Metatarsal shrotening for the relief of symptomatic plantar keratosis. J. Foot Surgery, 9:13, 1970.

Seidner, A.N. and Kaplan, B.R.: Use of the Calcan-Nicolle metacarpophalangeal joint implant in the foot — a case report. JAPA, 67:805, 1977.

Sgarlato, T.E.: Compendium of Podiatric Biomechanics, California College of Podiatric Medicine, San Francisco, 1971.

Stess, R.M.: A surgical approach to advanced rheumatoid arthritis of the forefoot. JAPA, 62:259, 1972.

Sullivan, J.D. and O'Donnel, J.E.: The dorsal displacement "floating" metatarsal subcapital osteotomy. J. Foot Surgery, 14:62, 1975.

Thomas, W.H.: Metatarsal osteotomy. Surg. Clin. N.A., 49:879, 1979.

Weinstock, R.E.: Surgical judgement in metatarsal surgery for elimination of intractable plantar keratoses. JAPA, 65:979, 1975.

Wilner, R.J.: Osteoclasis, a discussion. JAPA, 63:1, 1973.

Wolf, M.D.: Metatarsal osteotomy for the relief of painful metatarsal callosities. JBJS, 55A:1760, 1973.

Hallux Valgus Surgery — Chapter 7

Akin, O.F.: The treatment of hallux valgus — a new operative procedure and its results. Med. Sentinel, 33:678, 1925.

Auerbach, A.M.: Review of distal metatarsal osteotomies For hallux valgus in the young. Clin. Orthop., 70:148, 1970.

Barnett, C.H.: Valgus deviation of the distal phalanx of the great toe. J. Anat., 96:171, 1962.

Barnicot, N.A. and Hardy, R.H.: The position of the hallux in West Africans. J. Anat., 89:355, 1955.

Bingold, A.C. and Collins, D.H.: Hallux Rigidus. JBJS, 32B:214, 1950.

Bonney, G. and Kessel, L.: Hallux rigidus in the adolescent. JBJS, 40B:668, 1958.

Booley, B.J. and Berryman, D.B.: Wilson's osteotomy of the First metatarsal for hallux valgus in the adolescent and the young adult. Aust. N.Z.J. Surg., 43:255, 1973.

Butilin, W.E.: Modifications of the McBride procedure for correction of hallux valgus. JAPA, 64:585, 1974.

Carr, C.R.: Correctional osteotomy for metatarsus primus varus and hallux valgus. JBJS, 50:1353, 1968.

Cleveland, M. and Winant, E.M.: An end result study of the Keller operation. JBJS, 32A:163, 1950.

Colloff, B. and Weitz, E.M.: Proximal phalangeal osteotomy in hallux valgus. Clin. Orthop., 54:105, 1967.

Cralley, J.C., McGonagle, W. and Fitch, K.: The role of adductor hallucis in bunion deformity (Part I), JAPA, 66:910, 1976.

Cralley, J.C., McGonagle, W. and Fitch, K.: The role of adductor hallucis in bunion deformity (Part II). JAPA, 68:473, 1978.

Daw, S.W.: An unusual type of hallux valgus (two cases). Br. Med. J., 2:580, 1935.

Dovey, H.: The treatment of hallux valgus by distal osteotomy of the first metatarsal. Acta Orthop. Scand., 40: 402, 1969.

Durman, D. C.: Metatarsus primus varus and hallux valgus. Arch. Surg., 74: 128, 1957.

DuVries, H. L.: Surgery of the Foot. 3rd Ed., V. T. Inman, editor C. V. Mosby Co. St. Louis, 1973.

Ebisui, J. M.: The first ray axis and the first metarsophalangeal joint- an anatomical and pathomechamical study. JAPA, 58: 160, 1968.

Ely, L. W.: Hallux valgus. Surg.Clin. N. A., 6: 425, 1926.

Frankel, J.: Structural or positional hallux abductus? JAPA, 63: 647, 1973.

Funk, J. F. and Wells, R. E. : Bunionectomy with distal osteotomy. Clin Orthop., 85: 71, 1972.

Galland, W. I. and Jordan, H. : Hallux Valgus. Surg. Gyn. and Obst., 66: 95, 1938.

Gerbert, J. Melillo, T. : A modified Akin procedure for the correction of hallux valgus. JAPA, 61: 132, 1971.

Gerbert, J., Spector E., Clark, J. : Osteotomy procedures on the proximal phalanx for correction of the hallux deformity. JAPA, 64: 617, 1974.

Gerbert, J., Mercado, O. A., Solokoff, T. H. : The Surgical Treatment of Hallux-Abducto-Valgus and Allied Deformities. Futura Publishing Company, Mt. Kisco, N. Y. 1973,

Girdlestone, G. R. and Spooner, H. J. : A new operation for hallux valgus and hallux rigidus. JBJS, 19: 30, 1937.

Graver, H. H. : Cuneiform osteomy in correction of metarsus primus varus. JAPA, 68: 111, 1978.

Groman, A. D., Solomon, M. G., Ketai, N. H. : Repiar of cocked hallux secondary to Keller procedure using silicone® rubber implant. JAPA, 66; 181, 1976.

Gudas, C. J. : An etiology of hallux rigidus. J. Foot Surgery, 10: 113, 1971.

Haines, R. W. and McDougall, A. : The anatomy of hallux valgus. JBJS, 36B: 272, 1954.

Hardy, R.H. and Clapham, J.C.R.: Observations on Hallux Valgus. JBJS, 33B:376, 1951.

Hardy, R.H. and Clapham, J.C.R.: Hallux valgus predisposing anatomical causes. Lancet, 1:1180, 1952.

Hawkins, F.B., Mitchell, C.L. and Hedrick, D.W.: Correction of hallus valgus by metatarsal osteotomy. JBJS, 27:387, 1945.

Helal, R. Gupta, S.K. and Gojaseni, P.: Surgery for adolescent hallux valgus. Acta Orthop. Scand., 45:271, 1974.

Hicks, J.H.: The mechanics of the Foot. I. The joints. J. Anat., 87:345, 1953.

Hiss, J.M.: Hallux valgus—its causes and simplified treatment. Am. J. Surg., 11:50, 1931.

Iida, M. and Basmajian, J.V.: Electromyography of hallux valgus. Clin. Orthop., 101:220, 1974.

Inge, G.A.L. and Ferguson, A.G.: Surgery of the sesamoid bones of the great toe; anatomic and clinical study with report of 41 cases. Arch. Surg. 27:466, 1933.

Joplin, R.J.: Sling procedure for the correction of splayfoot, metatarsus primus varus and hallux valgus. JBJS, 32A:779, 1950.

Joplin, R.J.: Surgery of the forefoot in the rheumatoid arthritic patient. Surg. Clin. N.A., 49:847, 1969.

Joplin, R.J.: The proper digital nerve, vitallium® stem arthroplasty and some thoughts about foot surgery in general. Clin. Orthop. Rel. Research, 76:199, 1971.

Kaplan, E.B.: The tibialis posterior muscle in relation to hallux valgus. Bull. Hos. Joint Dis., 16:88, 1955.

Kelikian, H.: Hallux Valgus, Allied Deformities of the Forefoot and Metatarsalgia. W.B. Saunders Co., Philadelphia, 1965.

Keller, W.L.: The surgical treatment of bunions and hallux valgus. N.Y. Med. J., 80:741, 1904.

Keller, W.L.: Further observations on the surgical treatment of hall valgus and bunions. N.Y. Med. J., 95:696, 1912.

Kessel, L. and Bonney, G.: Hallux rigidus in the adolescent. JBJS, 40B:668, 1958.

Ketai, N.H., Ketai, R.S., Sherman, A.M., Tilles, S.J.: Hallux limitus. JAPA, 66:413, 1976.

Kleinburg, S.: The operative cure of hallux valgus and bunions. Am. J. Surg., 15:75, 1932.

Lapidus, P.W.: Operative correction of metatarsus varus primus in hallux valgus. Surg. Gyn. and Obst., 58:183, 1934.

Lapidus, P.W.: "Dorsal bunion": its mechanics and operative correction. JBJS, 22:627, 1940.

Lapidus, P.W.: The author's bunion operation from 1931 to 1959. Clin. Orthop. 16:119, 1960.

LaPorta, G.A., Mellilo, T., Olinsky, D.: X-ray evaluation of hallux abducto valgus deformity. JAPA, 64:544, 1974.

LaPorta, G.A., Pilla, P. Richter, K.P.: Keller implant procedure. A report of 536 procedures using a silastic® intramedullary stemmed implant. JAPA, 66:126, 1976.

Lawton, J. Evans, R.: Modified McBride bunionectomy. JAPA, 65:670, 1975.

Leach, R.E. and Igou, R.: Metatarsal osteotomy for bunionette deformity. Clin. Orthop., 100:171, 1974.

Margo, M.K.: Surgical treatment of conditions of the forepart of the foot. JBJS, 49A:1665, 1967.

Mayo, C.H.: The surgical treatment of bunions. Ann. Surg., 48:300, 1908.

Mayo, C.H.: The surgical treatment of bunions. Minn. Med. I., 3:326, 1920.

McBride, E.D.: A conservative operation for bunions. JBJS, 10:735, 1928.

McBride, E.D.: The conservative operation for "bunions"—end results and refinement of technique. JAMA, 105:1164, 1935.

McBride, E.D.: Surgical treatment of hallux valgus bunion. Am. J. Surg., 44:320, 1939.

McBride, E.D.: Hallux valgus bunion deformity. Am. Acad. Orthop. Surg., 9:334, 1952.

McBride, E.D.: Hallux valgus, bunion deformity—its treatment in mild, moderate and severe stages. J. Int. Coll. Surg., 21:99, 1954.

McBride, E.D.: The surgical treatment of hallux valgus bunions. Amer. J. Orthop., 5:44, 1963.

McBride, E.D.: The McBride bunion hallux valgus operation. JBJS, 49A:1675, 1967.

McElvenny, R.T. and Thompson, F.R.: A clinical study of one hundred patients subjected to simple exostectomy for the relief of bunion pain. JBJS, 22:942, 1940.

McElvenny, R.T.: A study of hallux valgus; its causes and operative management. Quat. Bull. Northwestern Med. School, 18:286, 1954.

McGlamry, E.D.: Hallucial sesamoids. JAPA, 55:693, 1965.

McGlamry, E.D.: Keller bunionectomy and hallux valgus correction. JAPA, 60:161, 1970.

McGlamry, E.D. and Feldman, M.H.: A treatise on the McBride procedure. JAPA, 60:161, 1970.

Mercado, O.A.: An Atlas of Podiatric Anatomy. American Academy of Hospital Podiatry, Chicago, Ill., 1972.

Mercado, O.A.: Hallux valgus surgery: history, polemics and modern techniques. Current Podiatry, Vol. 12, nos. 6 and 7, 1963.

Mercado, O.A.: A Modern Approach to Hallux Valgus Surgery. Audio Tape Cassettes. Teach 'Em Inc., Chicago, 1973.

Mercado, O.A. and Conway, V.H.: The minibunion operation. Current Podiatry, vol. 19, 1970.

Mercado, O.A.: Podiatric Surgical Dissection—Fundamental Skills. Carolando, Oak Park, Illinois, 1976.

Mercado, O.A.: Surgical Considerations of Hallux Valgus. Audio Tape Cassette, Carolando, Oak Park, Illinois, 1977.

Mercado, O.A.: Hallucial Derotation and the modified silver's. Current Podiatry, Oct. 1966.

Mercado, O.A.: Office Foot Surgery. Monograph Published June, 1966, Chicago.

Mercado, O.A.: Surgical Anatomy of Hallux valgus. Audio Tape cassettes and slide program. Teach 'Em Inc., Chicago, 1977.

Miller, F., Arenson, D., Weil, L.S.: Incongruity of the first metarsophalangeal joint—the effect of cartilage contact surface area. JAPA, 67:328, 1977.

Mitchell, C.L., Fleming, J.L., Allen, R., Glenney, C. and Sanford, G.A.: Osteotomy—bunionectomy for hallux valgus. JBJS, 40A:41, 1958.

Mosher, M.R.: Modified Stone bunionectomy. JAPA, 61:207, 1971.

Peabody, C.W.: The surgical cure of hallux valgus. JBJS, 13:273, 1931.

Peabody, C.W. and Muro F.: Congenital metatarsus varus. JBJS., 15:171, 1933.

Piggott, H.: The natural history of hallux valgus in adolescence and early adult life. JBJS, 42B:749, 1960.

Purvis, C.G., Brown, J.H., Kaplan, E.G., Mann, I.: Conbination Bonney-Kessel and modified Akin procedure for hallux limitus associated with hallux abductus. JAPA, 67:236, 1977.

Rega, R. and Green, D.: The extensor hallucis longus and Flexor hallucis longus tendons in hallux abducto valgus. JAPA., 68:467, 1978.

Reverdin, J.: De la deviation en dehors du gros orteil (Hallux valgus, Vulg. "Oignon," "Bunions," "Ballen") et de son traitement chirurgical. Trans. Int. Med. Congress, 2:405, 1881.

Rix, R.: Modified Mayo operation for hallux valgus and bunion—a comparison with the Keller procedure. JBJS, 50A:1368, 1968.

Robinson, H.A.: Etiology of bunion. Milit. Surg. 62:807, 1928.

Rogers, W.A. and Joplin, R.J.: Hallux valgus, weak foot and the Keller operation: an end result study. Surg. Clin. N.A., 27:1295, 1947.

Root, M.L., Orien, W.P., Weed, J.H.: Normal and Abnormal Function of the Foot. Clinical Biomechanics Corp., Los Angeles, 1977.

Seelenfreund, M. and Fried, A.: Correction of hallux valgus deformity by basal phalanx osteotomy of the big toe. JBJS, 55A:1411, 1973.

Sgarlato, T.E.: A Compendium of Podiatric Biomechanics. California College of Podiatric Medicine, San Francisco, 1971.

Shaw, A.M. and Pack, L.G.: Osteotomies of the first ray for hallux abducto valgus deformity. JAPA, 64:567, 1974.

Shine, I.B.: Incidence of hallux valgus in a partially shoe-wearing community. Brit. Med. J., 1:1648, 1965.

Silberman, F.S.: Proximal phalangeal osteotomy for the correction of hallux valgus. Clin. Orthop., 85:98, 1972.

Silver, D.: The operative treatment of Hallux valgus. JBJS, 5:225, 1923.

Smith, S. and Weil, L.S.: Criteria for removal of the fibular sesamoid, Northlake Seminar Notes, 1971.

Sorto, L.A., Balding, M., Weil, L.S., Smith, S.: Hallux abductus interphalangeious, etiology, x-ray evaluation and treatment. JAPA, 66:384, 1976.

Stein, H.C.: Hallux Valgus. Surg. Gyn. and Obst., 66:889, 1938.

Stamm, T.T.: The surgical treatment of hallux valgus. Guy's Hospital Report. 106:273, 1957.

Swanson, A.B.: Implant arthroplasty for the great toe. Clin. Orthop., 85:75, 1972.

Szaboky, G.J. and Raghaven, V.C.: Modification of Mitchell's lateral desplacement argulation osteotomy. JBJS, 51A:1430, 1969.

Tachdjan, M.O.: Pediatric Orthopedics, Volume One and Two, W.B. Saunders Co., Philadelphia, 1972.

Tate, R., Pachniek, R.L.: The accesory tendon of extensor hallucis longus. JAPA, 66:889, 1976.

Thomas, F.B.: Keller's arthroplasty, modified—a technique to insure postoperative traction of the toe. JBJS, 44B:356, 1962.Thomson, S.A.: Hallux varus and metatarsus varus. Clin. Orthop., 16:109, 1069.

Trethowan, J.: Hallux Valgus, A system of Surgery. New York. P.W. Hoeber, 1923.

Truslow, W.: Metatarsus Primus Varus or Hallux Valgus? JBJS, 7:98, 1925.

Vranes, R.: Hallux sesamoids: a divided issue. JAPA, 66:687, 1976.

Wheeler, P.H.: Os intermetatarseum and hallux valgus. Am. J. Surg., 18:341, 1923.

Wilkinson, J.L.: The terminal phalanx of the great toe. J. Anat., 88:537, 1954.

Wilson, J.N.: Oblique displacement osteotomy for hallux valgus. JBJS, 45B:552, 1963.

Wilson, J.N.: Cone arthrodesis of the first metatarso-phalangeal joint. JBJS, 49B:98, 1967.

Yanklowitz, B.A.D., Jaworek, T.A.: The frequency of the interphalangeal sesamoid of the hallux. JAPA, 65:1058, 1975.

Young, J.K.: The etiology of hallux valgus or os intermetatarseum. Am. J. Orthop. Surg., 7:336, 1909.

Zlotoff, H.: Shortening of the first metatarsal following osteotomy and its clinical significance. JAPA, 67:412, 1977.

INDEX

Adductus, metatarsus, 170-175
Akin, 193, 211-217
Albrecht, 186
Anatomy, metatarsal phalangeal joint, 124-126
Anesthesia, local, 3
hallux, 10
lesser toe, 8-9
peroneal nerve, 12
tibial nerve, 10
toxic reaction, 6
perfusion, 13-14
Arthritis, rheumatoid, 176-179
Atropine, 5
Avascular Necrosis, 180-182

Barbiturate, 4
Barker, 186
Belladonna derivatives, 5
Blocks, hallux, 10
lesser toe, 8-9
peroneal nerve, 12
tibial nerve, 10
Bone, bank, 117
cancellous, 94-97
compact, 97
cortical, 94-97
healing, 97
pegs, 116-118
plates, 116
tumor, 183-184
vascularity, 95
Borgreve, 122
Brachman, 170
Brauneck, 186
Breuner, 181
Bunionette, 165-166
Bunion, tailor, 165-166
Bunion (see hallux valgus)

Callus, 97
Capsular dissection, 199
Carpino, Wm, 133
Cartilage, 96-200
Casting, 170-171
Charnley, John, 98
Circulatory collapse, 7
Clayton panmetatarsectomy, 178-179
Cleavage lines, 37
Closing wedge osteotomy, 103, 240-245
Condylectomy, 123
Contracted toe, 46, 55-58
Convulsions, 7
Crescentic osteotomy
distal, 229-232
proximal, 233-239
Crista, 200

Davis, George, 122
Deviated toe, 46, 74-75
Dickson, 122
Digits
block, 8-9
congenital deformities, 46
contracted, 46
pressure deformities, 46
distal heloma durum, 46, 62-65
Dropped metatarsal head, 109
Drugs, 3-7
DuVries, 123, 126, 138, 186

Einhorn, 3
Endosteum, 95, 96
Exostosis subungual, 33, 34
Extensorhallucis capsularis, 198
Extensor osteoarthrotomy, 129
Extensor osteotomy, 129

Fifth toe heloma durum, 46-51
Fixation, 135
external, 113-119
internal, 113-119
Freiberg infraction, 180-182
Freud, Sigmund, 3

Giannestra, 123

Hallux block, 10
Hallux Valgus
acute, 193
angle, 191
etiology, 187
interphalangeal, 193
moderate, 193
simple, 193
surgery acute, 194
basic bunionectomy, 218
closing wedge, 240-245
criteria, 187
distal cresentic, 229-232
inter phalangeal, 194
mini bunionectomy, 194-197
moderate, 194
proximal crescentic, 233-239
Reverdin, 222-228
simple, 194- 197-211
Halsted Wm, 3
Hammer toe, 46-52-55
Haversian canals, 95-96
Hawkins, 186
Hedrick, 186
Heloma molle, 46-60-62
Heyman, Herdom and Strong, 172-173
Hohmann, 186
Hueter, 186

Implants
hemi, 253-266
total, 268-273
Cutter,
Intermetatarsal angle, 190
Intractable plantar keratosis, 127
Etiology, 127

Joints
shapes, 190
metatarsal cunneiform, 190
metatarsal phalangeal, 188
Jones, 186
Juavara, 186

Kaplan, 3
Keller, 186
Keratosis, 122
plantar, 122-127
sub fifth-metatarsal, 165-166
sub first-metatarsal, 131-132
Kirschner wire, 113, 135
Koller, 3

Lacunae, 95, 97, 98
Lamellae, 96
Langer's Lines, 37
Lapidus, 186, 246-253
Ligaments collateral, 200
Loison-Balacesu, 186

Mallet toe, 58-60
Matrix, nail, 16-18
Mau, 122
McBride, 218-221
McKeever, 122
McKeever peg and hole, 129, 146-159
Medullary canal, 95
Meisenbach, 122, 154
Mercado peg and hole, 129, 151-153
Mercado-Smith osteotomy, 100, 129, 143-145
Metatarsal
anatomical neck, 125
anatomy, 124-126
head shape, 188
fifth, 165-169
first dorsiflectory wedge osteotomy, 134-137
parabola, 128
Surgery:
Clayton panmetatarsectomy, 178, 179
criteria, 129, 130
Extensor osteoarthrotomy (EOA), 129, 162-164
Extensor osteotomy (EO), 129, 160-162
Heyman, Herdon and Strong, 172, 173
McKeever peg and hole, 129, 146-151
Mercado peg and hole, 129, 151-153
Mercado-Smith osteotomy, 129, 143-145
Metatarsectomy, 137
Osteoclasis, 129, 154-157
Crescentic osteotomy, 174, 175
V-osteotomy, 158-159

Partial metatarsal head resection, 138, 139
Sesamoidectomy, 131-134
Suppan cap, 140-142
metatarsus primus varus, 190, 191
metatarsus varus, 170-175
Mitchell, 186
Morton, 2, 186
Muhsam, 186

Nail matrix, 16-18
Narcotic, 5
Neuroma, 41-43
Non-barbiturates, 4
Nutrient vessels, 95

Olivecrona, 186
Onychoplasty
complete:
Kaplan, 23-25
Mini-Kaplan, 26-28
Terminal syme, 29-30
Osteotripsy, 31, 32
Partial:
Frost, 19, 20
Winograd, 21, 22
Ostectomy, 201
Osteoclasis, 129
osteocyte, 95
Osteoma, 183, 184
Osteotomy site, 102, 110
Osteotripsy, 31, 32, 64, 65, 194-197
Overlapping fifth toe, 46, 76-83

Papillary lines, 31
Partial phalangectomy, 47-55
Perfusion anesthesia, 13, 14
Periosteum, 95, 96
Peroneal N. block, 12
Pes adductus, 170-175
Phalangectomy, 74, 75
Pinch callus, 46, 66-70
Plantar interphalangeal joint callus, 46, 71-73
Polydactylism, 46, 88-92
Pre anesthesia drugs, 4-6
Pressure deformities, 46
Prober, Edwin, 64

Respiratory depression, 7
Reverdin osteotomy, 103, 186, 222-228
Rheumatoid arthritis, 176-179
Riordan pin (fixation), 114

Scopolamine, 5
Screws, 115, 116
Sesamoidectomy, 131-134
Severino, Marco, 2
Shede, 186
Silver, 186
Spay foot, 174, 175
Spooner, 186
Stainless steel wire, 114
Staples, 114, 115

Steinberg, 3
Steinman, 113
Student hole, 199
Supernumerary toe, 88-92
Suppan cap, 105, 129, 140-142
Swanson, 253
Syndactylism, 46, 83-87
Syncope, 7

Tailor's bunion, 165-166
Tibial nerve, 10
Toxic reaction, 6

Transfer lesion, 122
Transverse metatarsal ligament, 125

Vasoconstrictor drugs, 3
Verruca
mosaic, 40
plantar, 36
surgery, 38-40
Volkman's canals, 95, 96

Webbed toes, 83-87
Wells, Horace, 2